Early Childhood
Oral Health

11/3/09

Dear Ellie,

I could never thank you enough for all the many wonderful things you do for us each day. Your ever present smile and positive energy is captured by all of us around you.

Wishing you only the best, always,

[signature]

Early Childhood Oral Health

Edited by

Joel H. Berg, DDS, MS

Department of Pediatric Dentistry
University of Washington School of Dentistry
Seattle, WA 98195

Rebecca L. Slayton, DDS, PhD

Department of Pediatric Dentistry
The University of Iowa College of Dentistry
Iowa City, IA 52242

⊛WILEY-BLACKWELL

A John Wiley & Sons, Ltd., Publication

Edition first published 2009
© 2009 Wiley-Blackwell

Blackwell Publishing was acquired by John Wiley & Sons in February 2007. Blackwell's publishing program has been merged with Wiley's global Scientific, Technical, and Medical business to form Wiley-Blackwell.

Editorial Office
2121 State Avenue, Ames, Iowa 50014-8300, USA

For details of our global editorial offices, for customer services, and for information about how to apply for permission to reuse the copyright material in this book, please see our website at www.wiley.com/wiley-blackwell.

Library of Congress Cataloging-in-Publication Data
Early childhood oral health / [edited by] Joel Berg, Rebecca L. Slayton.
     p. ; cm.
  Includes bibliographical references and index.
  ISBN-13: 978-0-8138-2416-1 (alk. paper)
  ISBN-10: 0-8138-2416-8 (alk. paper)
  1. Children—Dental care.   2. Dental caries.   3. Teeth—Care and hygiene.
I. Berg, Joel H.   II. Slayton, Rebecca L.
  [DNLM: 1. Dental Care for Children—methods.   2. Child.   3. Dental Caries—diagnosis.   4. Dental Caries—therapy.   5. Infant.   6. Oral Health.   7. Oral Hygiene—methods. WU 480 E12 2009]
  RK55.C5E27 2009
  617.6′45—dc22

                                                                    2008045795

A catalog record for this book is available from the U.S. Library of Congress.

Set in 9.5/12 pt Palatino by Aptara® Inc., New Delhi, India
Printed and Bound in Singapore by Markono Print Media Pte Ltd.

Disclaimer
The contents of this work are intended to further general scientific research, understanding, and discussion only and are not intended and should not be relied upon as recommending or promoting a specific method, diagnosis, or treatment by practitioners for any particular patient. The publisher and the author make no representations or warranties with respect to the accuracy or completeness of the contents of this work and specifically disclaim all warranties, including without limitation any implied warranties of fitness for a particular purpose. In view of ongoing research, equipment modifications, changes in governmental regulations, and the constant flow of information relating to the use of medicines, equipment, and devices, the reader is urged to review and evaluate the information provided in the package insert or instructions for each medicine, equipment, or device for, among other things, any changes in the instructions or indication of usage and for added warnings and precautions. Readers should consult with a specialist where appropriate. The fact that an organization or Website is referred to in this work as a citation and/or a potential source of further information does not mean that the author or the publisher endorses the information the organization or Website may provide or recommendations it may make. Further, readers should be aware that Internet Websites listed in this work may have changed or disappeared between when this work was written and when it is read. No warranty may be created or extended by any promotional statements for this work. Neither the publisher nor the author shall be liable for any damages arising herefrom.

1   2009

Dedication

We dedicate this book to the babies of today and tomorrow, and to their parents, caregivers, and health care providers on whom they rely. May they all benefit from the advice herein and may those babies suffer less oral pain, thus setting them on the path to overall well-being.

Contents

Acknowledgments

Much of the work behind the scenes that led to the creation of this book was managed by Amanda Jane Ryan. We are grateful for her expertise, her hard work, and her ever-present enthusiasm.

Contributor List

Editors

Joel H. Berg, DDS, MS
Professor
Lloyd and Kay Chapman Chair for Oral Health
Department of Pediatric Dentistry
University of Washington School of Dentistry
Seattle, WA 98195

Rebecca L. Slayton, DDS, PhD
Professor and Chair
Department of Pediatric Dentistry
The University of Iowa College of Dentistry
Iowa City, IA 52242

Contributing authors

Tegwyn H. Brickhouse, DDS, PhD
Associate Professor
Department of Pediatric Dentistry
School of Dentistry
Virginia Commonwealth University
Richmond, VA 23298

Paul S. Casamassimo, DDS, MS
Professor and Division Head
Pediatric Dentistry
The Ohio State University
Columbus, OH 43218

Courtney H. Chinn, DDS, MPH
Assistant Professor of Dental Medicine (Community Health)
Columbia University College of Dental Medicine
New York, NY 10027

James J. Crall, DDS, ScD
Professor and Chair, Section of Pediatric Dentistry
UCLA School of Dentistry
Los Angeles, CA 90095

David K. Curtis, DMD, PA
300 Hospital Drive
Columbus, MS 39705

Kevin J. Donly, DDS, MS
Professor and Chair
Department of Pediatric Dentistry
Dental School
University of Texas Health Science Center at San Antonio
San Antonio, TX 78229

Burton L. Edelstein, DDS, MPH
Professor of Clinical Dental Medicine (Community Health) and Clinical
    Health Policy and Management
Chair of the Section of Social and Behavioral Sciences
Columbia University College of Dental Medicine
New York, NY 10027

Robert J. Laughlin, DDS, MPH
Pediatric Dentistry Resident
National Children's Medical Center
Washington, DC 20010

Jessica Y. Lee, DDS, MPH, PhD
Associate Professor
Department of Pediatric Dentistry
University of North Carolina
Chapel Hill, NC 27599

Russell Maier, MD
Program Director
Central Washington Family Medicine Residency
Yakima, WA 98902
Clinical Professor
Department of Family Medicine
University of Washington School of Medicine
Seattle, WA 98195

Wendy E. Mouradian, MD, MS
Associate Dean for Regional Affairs
Director, Regional Initiatives in Dental Education (RIDE)
Professor of Pediatric Dentistry, Pediatrics, Dental Public Health Sciences
    and Health Services (Public Health)
University of Washington School of Dentistry
Seattle, WA 98195

Arthur J. Nowak, DMD, MA, FAAPD
Professor Emeritus
Departments of Pediatric Dentistry and Pediatrics
University of Iowa
Iowa City, IA 52242

Rocio Quiñonez, DMD, MS, MPH
Clinical Assistant Professor
Department of Pediatric Dentistry
School of Dentistry
University of North Carolina
Chapel Hill, NC 27599

Adriana Segura, DDS, MS
Professor and Interim-Chair
Department of Community Dentistry
Dental School
University of Texas Health Science Center at San Antonio
San Antonio, TX 78229

Norman Tinanoff, DDS, MS
Chair, Department of Health Promotion and Policy
University of Maryland Dental School
Baltimore, MD 21201

Early Childhood Oral Health

Introduction—why this book?

Joel H. Berg

This book represents the first published textbook on the topic of the name it carries—*Early Childhood Oral Health*. This topic has caught the attention of a large host of stakeholders, as evidence of its importance to those who encounter the youngest members of our society. We hope that after reading this book, you will agree there is nothing more important in dentistry than early intervention, with the connected comprehensive prevention and management of the prevalent early childhood caries. We have the tools available to us to prevent most dental caries in children at a very early age, yet we have seen an increase in dental caries in preschoolers in recent years. This book will guide you from the epidemiology of caries in young children through ways in which preventive programs for infants and toddlers can be established in a variety of settings. You will note a prevailing theme of interaction between members of a team of providers—from a variety of health care delivery disciplines—to avert what is essentially a behavioral disease. You will notice that our approach in early intervention is one of managing a disease well before it manifests itself in the form of a cavity, the way in which many children, generally later than at a toddler age, might encounter their first visit to a dentist. You will also perceive a prevailing theme of education—including the family and all related caregivers, to the community of health care providers, all of whom need to be educated in the prevention of early childhood caries.

There is new science related to the prevention and management of early childhood caries that you will read in this book. There is also repetition of science that has been known for decades, indicating what the new science confirms—that early childhood caries is essentially preventable (Carrico, 2007; Sohn et al., 2007; Tiberia et al., 2007). Only now when various societal, academic, and political forces are properly aligned are we ready to recognize the clear value of a much earlier entry into the dental world.

Dr Edelstein in his chapter on the epidemiology of early childhood caries (Chapter 2) talks about why the disease has reached a pandemic stage. He talks about the changing representation of early childhood caries in populations around the world. This awareness, and his description of why the early childhood caries has reached the levels that it has, explains why we have reached a point where we all need to start much earlier in life if we are to make an important difference for so many children.

Many parties are becoming aware of the costs associated with the treatment of the effects of early childhood caries. These costs have historically been apparent only after children present to their dentist or to an emergency room somewhere, at the age of 2 or 3, with a mouthful of cavities. As a society, we have accepted the fact that children present somewhere with many cavities in their primary teeth at a young age, never having had any form of prevention attempted (Ramos-Gomez, 2005; Hallett and O'Rourke, 2006; Kowash et al., 2006; Selwitz et al., 2007). Only recently have we started to ask why we cannot change the way in which the profession views the management of early childhood caries as an opportunity for prevention versus waiting for the devastation to occur. We believe this book provides a guide for making the transition to manage the disease before it devastates the mouth and potentially beyond. We talk about the relationship between oral health and overall health. With so much more being discovered each day connecting the mouth to the rest of the body, early intervention becomes ever more important.

Another important factor that has instilled increased enthusiasm around the early management and prevention of early childhood caries is the realization by many of how rapidly an infant with no clinically evident disease can progress to a toddler with multiple caries-affected teeth (Donaldson and Fenton, 2006; Weber-Gasparoni et al., 2007; Gussy et al.,

2008; Twetman, 2008). Few chronic diseases persist and progress over such a long period, and yet so rapidly as does early childhood caries. Drs Mouradian and Maier describe the important role of physicians in prevention and management of early childhood caries. In the years ahead, health care providers from all perspectives will play a role in the identification of children at the greatest risk of disease. Chapter 11 will guide us through the ways in which existing encounters in conjunction with well-baby checkups in pediatrician and family physician offices can work in concert with referrals to dental homes to avert disease in early childhood.

In spite of greater attention to early childhood oral health, there remains a need for greater awareness which we hope this book will fulfill. The focus needs to be on the youngest children which will require the participation of families, teachers, and health care professionals.

An extra course for students and practicing dentists beyond pediatric dentistry in "general" should include a discreet emphasis on early childhood oral health. Early childhood oral health, as this book elucidates, is primarily an effort to prevent and manage early childhood caries. Although pediatric dentistry in more general terms includes a multitude of other aspects of assessing the health of children, as well as managing their oral care in a variety of ways, the emphasis in early childhood' and within the pages of this book' is essentially on dental caries prevention and treatment. Caries is the disease we speak of and which dominates the oral disease morbidity in early childhood. Problems that occur later in children's lives regarding their oral health will include caries in a significant way and along with many other diseases and problems that are rarely seen in early childhood. The subsequent 12 chapters provide a complete landscape of views regarding dental caries and its prevention, management, and outcomes of treatments in early childhood.

Many organizations tout the dental visit at age of 1 year, or even earlier. The American Academy of Pediatric Dentistry as well as the American Dental Association proclaim that a child's first dental visit should be soon after the first tooth erupts, and no later than age 1 (American Academy of Pediatric Dentistry Liaison with Other Groups Committee, 2005–2006). The American Academy of Pediatrics says that the first oral health screening should take place at or around 6 months of age (Oral Health Risk Assessment Timing and Establishment of the Dental Home, 2003), likely in conjunction with a well-baby checkup already on the docket as part of the normal periodicity of examinations.

It sounds like integration of an oral assessment into an existing examination that occurs for other purposes is the right thing to do, yet historically this has not occurred. Only after the relatively recent emphasis on oral health have physicians begun to think about their own role in the comprehensive management of oral health for the children they have seen many times at a very young age. Physicians are now well integrated into the messages that go out to health care team about oral health in early childhood. Yet, the work is not yet complete. As in any "system" of health care delivery, access to the most appropriate care for all must target those at the greatest risk as early as possible in the course of potential disease, and there must be a mechanism in place to provide continuous, comprehensive, and effective preventive and surgical care where needed most. The system must facilitate not only the best possible access to care for the greatest in need, but must also have the assurances in place that higher-risk patients will be treated more aggressively. This would focus more attention and cost on those infants and toddlers deemed to be at the greatest risk. Dentistry as a whole is new to risk-based management of patients as it relates to dental caries. There is no better opportunity to implement a risk-based approach to caries management than in the preschool population to avert the devastation of early childhood caries. In Chapter 8, by Quiñozez and Crall, an approach to managing the youngest children related to their dental caries-risk level is described.

A decade of discussion has not "tipped" the situation yet. Although many in the business of dealing with preschoolers and their oral health would say that we have reached the point of dealing with caries management effectively in the youngest children, clearly there is a long way to go. Third-party payers, holding an enormous amount of influence over the determination of who gets care when and how often, are also beginning to recognize the value of early intervention—as it should occur in managing caries at the youngest possible age.

Parents are engaged early on, yet we have not talked with them enough and at each possible opportunity about their critical role in preventing and managing early childhood caries in their infant or toddler.

For the dental professional, bringing early childhood oral health into their practice might amount to a change in practice philosophy. Dr Curtis tells us in Chapter 12 how to make an infant and toddler practice work in anyone's office. Dental practices may not yet be accustomed to the notion that patients will be treated at an age and from a perspective that most will not need restorative surgical intervention. The idea that a visit with infants or toddlers and their parent(s) will generally be without any "treatment" to deliver may be a foreign one. Clearly, however, we are moving toward a new kind of dentistry, a kind where our words and actions regarding anticipatory guidance and prevention will be the care we deliver that will be the most impactful for the child's entire life.

Third-party payers, as noted, are recognizing the problem of waiting until children are older before intervention takes place. Because there are fewer teeth in the mouth at a very young age, it is far simpler to engage parents to comply with oral hygiene regimens that can be implemented early for lifelong prevention. Drs Nowak and Casamassimo tell us how anticipatory guidance can be brought to parents early on to engage their enthusiasm toward better health outcomes for their child and to demonstrate their role in preventing disease. Chapter 7 talks about the blend of risk assessment and referral of the most at risk to a dental home—something from which all children will benefit, and from which the highest risk patients will particularly benefit.

STAKEHOLDERS

What is likely to be the primary factor in "tipping" the access to care issue for infants and toddlers in the direction of a dental home for all children by the first birthday is the multitude of stakeholders engaged in making this happen. Whereas a decade ago it was the dental professional community speaking alone toward this end, today and even more in the future, a long list of interested parties is striving to make this happen. In Chapter 10 by Dr Lee, we learn of community programs that connect a long list of stakeholders, all with the common interest of early childhood oral health.

Parents are at the head of this list. Infants and toddlers are dependent on their families to maintain their health. Parents are becoming aware of their role in establishing a dental home early in life and the difference that can make in preserving good oral health. In Chapter 9, Dr Brickhouse shows the essential role of parents and families in protecting their child's oral health early in life. We learn therein specific means of communicating with parents and the responses to the questions they might receive. Early childhood oral health in the office is about communication with the parents and the family. Dr Segura tells us about the complete list of elements in the examination of an infant's or toddler's mouth, and therein one sees the importance of communication with the parents and family as a critical component of achieving success.

Now is a very good time for every stakeholder who cares about early childhood oral health to ask the questions he or she will need to ask. By encouraging parents, families, and all who encounter the youngest children to ask questions about the child's oral health alongside their overall health, we will provide the answers to effective solutions. Stakeholders, by definition, have a vested interest in the well-being of the young children around whom they hold stake. Given that position of caring, and with the multitude of touch points collectively managed by the various stakeholders, we have both the opportunity and the obligation to educate each stakeholder individually about his or her component role in preventing and managing the oral health of children.

As generations of stakeholders have changed, so have the expectations regarding health in general. What was expected in terms of oral health decades ago is not necessarily expected today. Whereas parents placed their own health and the health of their children "solely" into the hands of professionals in the past, today they understand their inextricable role in maintaining the good health of their child. Again, this provides both the opportunity and the obligation to educate all stakeholders so that they possess the tools necessary to maintain good oral health along with the overall health of all children.

Several decades ago, fluoridated toothpaste commercials on television not only raised the awareness about oral health, cavity prevention, and fluoride's great benefit in general, but also perhaps provided another message. When we heard the famous line "look mom, no cavities" after the child in the advertisements returned from the dentist, we were ingrained with the appropriate powerful message that good oral health maintenance including a regimen of fluoridated toothpaste can prevent cavities. We also learned that the outcome measure of success—no cavities—was a conclusion reached by the dentist only after the child's examination. Today, when we talk about early childhood oral health we recognize the role of fluoride in various forms, including toothpaste, in preventing early childhood caries and maintaining good oral health. We also know, however, as we did then, that there is a process of caries progression that leads toward what might become a "cavity." What has changed today, and what might be a good way to describe, in a nutshell, the difference in the way we should talk with our patients/parents today, is in the communication about the caries process. Only in this way can we effectively integrate all the various components of a comprehensive and patient-specific prevention program that includes information about a proper fluoride regimen, as described in Chapter 4 by Dr Tinanoff. This may be the first look at a complete fluoride program with infants and toddlers specifically in mind. And only when we think about the process of dental caries progression as one we want to communicate to our families, can we provide the right information about other aspects of a comprehensive preventive program that includes information about the child's diet and oral hygiene, and the role of the parents/family in changing behavior—behavioral change that increases interaction with their child to achieve the desired healthy outcome (Weinstein et al., 2006).

Although it is not universally true, there is clearly a trend in the practice of dentistry for children for parents to be present in the operatory during a dental visit. This automatically provides an opportunity to communicate with parents of children of all ages. Clearly, a parent must be present in the operatory to allow an effective infant or toddler examination, but importantly to allow the right kind of communication to effect behavioral change that will result in good oral health. Given the expectation that parents will be present in the operatory for a dental visit with an older child, there is an additional opportunity to engage the parent in communication concerning the establishment of a dental home for younger siblings.

There is a culture of interaction with today's parents that will make them feel more comfortable in asking the right questions about the health of all of their children, including, of course, the baby in their arms while they are attending a visit of their older child. Additionally, as we educate more and more parents about the importance of early intervention toward good oral health, peer pressure from other parents about the essential role of a parent in maintaining oral health might further encourage early establishment of dental home.

Our communication to families individually and collectively and the way we talk with consumers in general should make it no longer acceptable to have "rotten" teeth. Many parents of the past may have had the expectation that a child would get cavities, and/or that it was not really a problem. As discoveries are made about the morbidity of dental caries in the youngest children, combined with the host of changing expectations, we might effectively engage more parents to establish a dental home for their child early on.

This book will not provide a repeat discussion of the dental caries process and the biology or microbiology of dental caries. There are many resources available to provide such information. Our intent in writing this book is rather to bring information available from the collective body of science today into programs delivered in different venues that collectively result in improved oral health of children at a very young age.

Bacteria from mom? There is developing body of science related to the familial transmission of the caries-causing oral flora from parent to child during what Caufield calls the "window of infectivity," which takes place during the establishment of the primary dentition in the mouth in the first years of life. One can learn much scientifically and can imagine the discoveries and resultant therapies that will be in place, extending from Caufield's important work (Ercan et al., 2007). And in the context of this book, one might imagine the opportunity to educate families about the implications of transmission of bacterial flora from parent to child as an opportunity for their own engagement in their child's oral health. This opportunity exists not only in the dental home, but also in the many places a young child encounters various stakeholders.

Who is supposed to brush whom? In Chapters 5 and 12 by Drs Segura and Curtis, we learn not only about the various elements of an infant or toddler examination, but also about the education on effective oral hygiene for babies. Parents must be educated on their essential role in brushing their child's teeth. Although we might all assume that this important parental duty is well known, we could certainly spend much more time not only educating about toothbrushing, but also demonstrating how to do it well. Additionally, we should document how well parents can actually brush their child's teeth. Only by witnessed "coaching" on this absolutely essential parental duty—with subsequent documentation and follow-up—can we expect that parents will perform adequately. Because parents are so important in the role of brushing their baby's teeth, one might argue that early childhood oral health is really "parent education for early childhood oral health." Rarely can there be good oral health outcomes for children without parental engagement.

Fluoride is all around us (Riordan, 1993; Ismail, 1994; Levy, 1994; Stookey, 1994; Duperon, 1995; Levy et al., 1995). It exists in water, in toothpaste, in rinses, and in professionally delivered varnishes and gels. Chapter 4 by Dr Tinanoff's gives us an understanding of the importance and interaction of these and other forms of fluoride (Levy, 2003; Douglass et al., 2004; Hallett and O'Rourke, 2006; Zhan et al., 2006). Because fluoride is available from so many places, and is also administered professionally in many instances by health care professionals beyond the dental home, the dental home must be cognizant of the various oral health "touch points" and must assume the role of managing the child's oral health comprehensively (Duperon, 1995; Spencer, 1996; Davies, 1998; Stookey, 1998; Duggal and van Loveren, 2001; Featherstone et al., 2003; Tinanoff and Palmer, 2003). Chapters 4, 6, and 7 by Tinanoff and Casamassimo and Nowak give us effective ways of managing each child's oral health individually, given the existence of a team of providers. Teachers are becoming important stakeholders in maintaining oral health. In school-age children, they might be the first to note problems related to tooth decay that manifests in the classroom, either as a toothache that first becomes known to anyone besides the child or perhaps what might be originally noticed as a deterioration in performance. Pediatric dentists will commonly report anecdotal stories of school-age children whose performance deteriorates, only later to discover that a toothache was the cause. A body of evidence is being developed toward this end, and teachers may be some of the first to report dental problems in their students. For infants and toddlers, many of whom may be in preschool or some type of day care scenario, it may similarly be the teacher who plays an important role. In this latter instance, however, the preschool teacher is also vital in establishing and maintaining behaviors that are effective in improved oral health. It is, therefore, important to note the dental community's obligation to properly educate all teachers about their important role in oral health maintenance, regardless of the child's age. In fact, for the preschooler, the teacher's role in dental caries prevention is more important than ever. Teachers today also have better oral health themselves than their predecessors years and decades ago. Therefore, their expectations regarding oral health will be different for the children they encounter than those of their predecessors. A different set of expectations is in place for the many stakeholders who encounter our children today, and today's stakeholders, therefore, have a new vested interest in children's oral health. Our opportunity to intervene early on in life has never been greater.

PARTNERSHIPS

Partnerships within and among the various stakeholders are key to implementing all of the many measures this book discusses related to improved oral health for infants and toddlers. Pediatricians and family physicians are principal players in the oral health team. They see patients early in life, and on many occasions in the first years of life, during which time historically, dental teams have not been engaged in the process. Because of this, they have been seeing the problem for a long time—the problem being early childhood caries in the primary dentition—often within a year of the time the teeth emerge into the mouth. Although dental offices need to serve as a dental home starting in early childhood for all patients, not enough of dentistry has participated in engaging patients into their practices early in life.

Now that dentistry clearly understands its need not only to participate, but also to lead the team of caregivers, how we communicate and refer interactively becomes a critical component of successful oral care delivery at a young age. We must take advantage of the fact that children are encountered by their pediatrician or family physician many more times in their early years than by their dentist, even when properly managed in the context of a dental home. Drs Mouradian and Maier guide us through a discussion of what the interactive role of the medical and dental teams in maintaining oral health in their patients have in common. Questions raised and answered include the following: Who is responsible for what (Alm et al., 2008)? How much time do I have to do what? What expertise/training do I need/have? The question of being compensated for services provided is important and is an emerging topic prominent on the agenda of third-party payers. Most notably, the role of the medical office in risk assessment is critical. Given the challenges of obtaining a dental home for all children soon after the first tooth erupts and no later than the child's first birthday, it certainly makes good sense to identify the infants at the greatest risk for dental caries and provide them with all the elements of a dental home as early on as possible.

Family physicians see the minority of young children, with pediatricians seeing the majority. Mouradian and Maier talk about their respective and mutual responsibility to assist all patients in maintaining good oral health and the role of their medical teams. As in dentistry, family physicians have the advantage that they can treat parents as well as infants/toddlers in their practice. General dental practices see 70% of the population of children, with pediatric dentists seeing the minority of (older) children, the reverse of the situation in medicine.

Historically, we have poorly trained our general dentistry graduates in predoctoral curricula in dental schools. Now, not only is there an interest, but there also is a desire to learn about early childhood caries prevention in the predoctoral dental curriculum, as well as now in the medical school curriculum. Additionally, pediatrics as well as family medicine residents are exposed to curricula showing them how to provide oral health assessment and referral in their practices. In many parts of the United States and certainly around the world, there is no specialist pediatric dentist or pediatrician. In these areas and others, it is important for generalists in medicine and dentistry to work together to maintain oral health while establishing a referral mechanism for special needs and complex restorative treatment patients.

There is a great need for regular and easy access to continuing education for medical and dental teams in all aspects of early childhood oral health. This book is intended to provide a comprehensive view on the management of patients in early childhood in order to maintain oral health. Communities must establish their own mechanisms to guarantee that teams of providers remain up-to-date with the latest scientific methods in early childhood oral health.

DENTAL INDUSTRY ROLE

Industry cares about oral health, particularly for the youngest of children. Not only is there a profit motive, an essential component for product development and distribution in industry, but also early childhood oral health-related products provide a means to "do well by doing good." Given the relative newness of the world's attention to oral health for the youngest of children, we are only now seeing the possibilities in the creation of what will likely be a plethora of products to help parents and health care professionals maintain the oral health of the babies they treat. Although we are well aware of the benefits of fluoride delivery (Garrison et al., 2007; Oliveira et al., 2007; Sledd, 2007; Azarpazhooh and Main, 2008; Peres et al., 2008) to infants and toddlers as discussed in this book by Tinanoff, there are other agents in various developmental stages that may also be of benefit. The effectiveness of other agents may be dependent not only on their actual clinically measured efficacy as demonstrated via clinical trials, but also by their ease of use in the context of the environment in which they are to be delivered. Additionally, as the U.S. Food and Drug Administration further allows additional methods of assessing the outcomes for newly developed products in terms of clinical endpoints, we will likely see many new products that will benefit the youngest of children, and especially those with the greatest risk. Dr Donly talks about various pharmaceuticals that either are available for use in young children or are under development. More attention to the oral health of infants and toddlers will ultimately result in the demand by dental professionals for new and better products. If one sees a child at the greatest risk, there will be a need for products, in addition to behavioral change, to provide the desired results.

Likely one of the most valuable roles of the dental industry in improving oral health for infants and toddlers is in its ability to reach consumers/ parents with important oral health messages. Just as the toothpaste advertisements of decades ago shaped the behavior of millions of (older) children and their parents, there will be a need to reach all of the above-referenced stakeholders with newly emerging oral health messages. Perhaps the most important message is simply the need for early engagement and intervention. The dental industry, particularly the consumer products/

over-the-counter (OTC) component therein, has the means and the need to reach families with oral health messages as they relate to product marketing. By working together as partners with the dental industry, we can, therefore, help shape the important messages that will ultimately improve access to care for all children at ever younger ages.

For example, teaching parents about the caries process, not just the results of caries in the form of cavities, can be promulgated in a significant way by the dental industry. As new products are created that manage caries in a variety of venues, the need to educate consumers about the process of dental caries progression, and hopefully regression, will be in the hands of the dental industry.

The attention given to cosmetic dentistry products in the OTC dental business is demonstrative of how effective the industry can be in reaching consumers quickly. By partnering with the OTC dental industry as new products for infant and toddler oral health become available, we can collectively reach the targeted audience with important oral health messages.

MEDIA

The media collectively have a role similar to that of industry.

A good story will reach a lot of people very quickly. One could then imagine how future oral care product introductions that are intended for infants and toddlers might be promoted by media as well. Similarly, as we discover more about the morbidity related to dental caries in young children, it likely would not be the scientific literature that ultimately affects change in consumer behavior in the direction of improved oral health for infants and toddlers. It will most likely be the media that reports on discoveries that will create the necessary information access. "Wouldn't you rather have a rinse than a drill?" might be a message that can be promulgated by the media to engage in change. As the consumers, including all of the stakeholders mentioned in this book, learn of the caries process and their own role in managing that process, they will be more likely to engage their youngest patients to achieve oral health as early as possible.

TODAY'S CHILDREN AS ADULTS

In Chapter 13 of this book. Dr Slayton takes us into the future. As adults, today's children will ask more questions of their caregivers. They will likely be even more diligent than their parents about health; such health achievement will include oral health. Beauty and health are often connected in the eyes of the consumer, and the current generation of parents will continue to strive for improved health in their own children not only for health's sake alone, but also for esthetics. Whereas dental professionals today encounter many parents who do not seem as concerned as we would like them to be about a decayed, and therefore unhealthy, primary dentition, we hope that as we move forward into the future it will be an increased desire for health, also as measured by improved esthetics, that will drive a change in behavior.

ADVOCATES

The fact that oral health is no longer an option is being recognized by a variety of stakeholders. Oral health is medically necessary, and all who have an interest in health should therefore have an interest in oral health.

Legislators are learning about the importance of oral health, and it is likely that as funding priorities are adjusted in the future, an increased awareness about the importance of early childhood intervention to achieve oral health in all children will direct more financial investment in the various aspects of managing the elements of dental caries prevention in all the ways we discuss in this book.

Organized dentistry is also refocusing its attention on the youngest of our children. In part, this is happening because of the recent reported increases in caries rates in preschool children. It is also a result of the fact that dental school curricula, as noted by Dr Lee in Chapter 10, includes more information and hands-on training on how to manage dental caries in infants and toddlers. As many specialties of dentistry consolidate around restorative management, particularly related to implantology and esthetic dentistry, prevention will consolidate as well, and the attention therein will focus on the youngest of all children.

THE INTERNET

We have seen many examples recently of how so-called viral marketing on the Internet can achieve mass awareness change on a variety of product or health care ideas. If one looks at what happened with tooth whitening, it is easy to see how communication between many different age groups has effected behavioral change. Similarly, if we want to reach consumers who are the stakeholders for our infants and toddlers, the Internet and all of its reach will be an important tool in spreading the word about early childhood oral health.

WHAT WE HOPE THIS BOOK WILL ACCOMPLISH

More engagement related to early childhood oral health by a variety of important stakeholders is our main objective.

Parental engagement is the most important of all, and it is only through education of all the other stakeholders and their own engagement that we can change parental behavior so as to allow better oral health for their children, and early in life. We need to continue to discover more ways to bring greater time and attention to this most important aspect of dentistry. It is also the intent of this book to bring an isolated focus on prevention at an early age, which is different in its form and frequency of encounter than other aspects of oral disease prevention. Clearly, one will see the need for more research in risk assessment and how to manage costs accordingly to reduce dental caries in children that often occurs at a very young age.

THIS BOOK'S AUDIENCE

Many will benefit from this book. The primary audience is intended to be students in various places. Of course, it is our intent that this book will be used as a textbook for dental and dental hygiene students, and be considered as an integral part of their training to be an effective general dentist. Additionally, trainees in medicine, including residency trainees in pediatrics and/or family medicine, will benefit from the contents of this book. Many others, including nurses, social workers, teachers, dental auxiliaries, and also parents will benefit from certain specific chapters herein that may be specific to their needs.

REFERENCES

Alm A, Wendt LK, Koch G, and Birkhed D. 2008. Oral hygiene and parent-related factors during early childhood in relation to approximal caries at 15 years of age. *Caries Res* 42(1):28–36.

American Academy of Pediatric Dentistry Liaison with Other Groups Committee; American Academy of Pediatric Dentistry Council on Clinical Affairs. 2005–2006. Guideline on fluoride therapy. *Pediatric Dent* 27(7, Suppl): 90–91.

Azarpazhooh A and Main PA. 2008. Fluoride varnish in the prevention of dental caries in children and adolescents: A systematic review [review]. *J Can Dent Assoc* 74(1):73–9.

Carrico S. 2007. Fluoride: A review of therapeutic actions and use in infant oral health programs. *JMich Dent Assoc* 89(1):38, 40.

Casamassimo P. 2007. Floundering in fluoride fog. *Pediatr Dent* 29(1):5–6.

Chussid S. 2003. Optimizing infant and toddler oral health. The importance of early intervention [review]. *Dent Today* 22(7):122–5.

Davies GN. 1998. Early childhood caries—a synopsis [review]. *Community Dent Oral Epidemiol* 26(1, Suppl):106–16.

Donaldson ME and Fenton SJ. 2006. When should children have their first dental visit? *J Tenn Dent Assoc* 86(2):32–5.

Douglass JM, Douglass AB, and Silk HJ. 2004. A practical guide to infant oral health [review]. *Am Fam Physician.* 2004 Dec 1; 70(11):2113–20. Summary for patients in *Am Fam Physician* 70(11):2121–2.

Duggal MS and van Loveren C. 2001. Dental considerations for dietary counselling [review]. *Int Dent J* 51(6, Suppl 1):408–12.

Duperon DF. 1995. Early childhood caries: A continuing dilemma [review]. *J Calif Dent Assoc* 23(2):15–16, 18, 20–22 passim.

Ercan E, Dülgergil CT, Yildirim I, and Dalli M. 2007. Prevention of maternal bacterial transmission on children's dental-caries-development: 4-year results of a pilot study in a rural-child population. *Arch Oral Biol* 52(8):748–52.

Featherstone JD, Adair SM, Anderson MH, Berkowitz RJ, Bird WF, Crall JJ, Den Besten PK, Donly KJ, Glassman P, Milgrom P, Roth JR, Snow R, and Stewart RE. 2003. Caries management by risk assessment: Consensus statement, April 2002 [review]. *J Calif Dent Assoc* 31(3):257–69.

Garrison GM, Loven B, and Kittinger-Aisenberg LG. 2007. Clinical inquiries. Can infants/toddlers get enough fluoride through brushing? [review] *J Fam Pract* 56(9):752, 754.

Gussy MG, Waters EB, Riggs EM, Lo SK, and Kilpatrick NM. 2008. Parental knowledge, beliefs and behaviours for oral health of toddlers residing in rural Victoria. *Aust Dent J* 53(1):52–60.

Hallett KB and O'Rourke PK. 2006. Caries experience in preschool children referred for specialist dental care in hospital. *Aust Dent J* 51(2):124–9.

Ismail AI. 1994. Fluoride supplements: Current effectiveness, side effects, and recommendations [review]. *Community Dent Oral Epidemiol* 22(3): 164–72.

Kowash MB, Toumba KJ, and Curzon ME. 2006. Cost-effectiveness of a long-term dental health education program for the prevention of early childhood caries. *Eur Arch Paediatr Dent* 7(3):130–35.

Lee JY, Bouwens TJ, Savage MF, and Vann WF, Jr. 2006. Examining the cost-effectiveness of early dental visits [review]. *Pediatr Dent* 28(2):102–5; discussion 192–8.

Levy SM. 1994. Review of fluoride exposures and ingestion [review]. *Community Dent Oral Epidemiol* 22(3):173–80.

Levy SM. 2003. An update on fluorides and fluorosis [review]. *J Can Dent Assoc* 69(5):286–91.

Levy SM, Kiritsy MC, and Warren JJ. 1995. Sources of fluoride intake in children [review]. *J Public Health Dent* 55(1):39–52.

Oliveira MJ, Paiva SM, Martins LH, Ramos-Jorge ML, Lima YB, and Cury JA. 2007. Fluoride intake by children at risk for the development of dental fluorosis: Comparison of regular dentifrices and flavoured dentifrices for children. *Caries Res* 41(6):460–66.

Oral Health Risk Assessment Timing and Establishment of the Dental Home (Policy Statement). 2003. *Pediatrics* 111(5):1113–6.

Peres RC, Coppi LC, Volpato MC, Groppo FC, Cury JA, and Rosalen PL. 2008. Cariogenic potential of cows', human and infant formula milks and effect of fluoride supplementation. *Br JNutr* 25:1–7.

Ramos-Gomez FJ. 2005. Clinical considerations for an infant oral health care program. *Compend Contin Educ Dent* 26(5, Suppl 1):17–23.

Riordan PJ. 1993. Fluoride supplements in caries prevention: A literature review and proposal for a new dosage schedule [review]. *J Public Health Dent* 53(3):174–89.

Selwitz RH, Ismail AI, and Pitts NB. 2007. Dental Caries [review]. *Lancet* 369(9555):51–9.

Sledd JL. 2007. Applying fluoride varnish to pediatric patients to prevent caries. *Northwest Dent* 86(1):4, 66.

Sohn W, Ismail AI, and Taichman LS. 2007. Caries risk-based fluoride supplementation for children. *Pediatr Dent* 29(1):23–31.

Spencer JP. 1996. Practical nutrition for the healthy term infant [review]. *Am Fam Physician* 54(1):138–44.

Stookey GK. 1994. Review of fluorosis risk of self-applied topical fluorides: Dentifrices, mouthrinses and gels [review]. *Community Dent Oral Epidemiol* 22(3):181–6.

Stookey GK. 1998. Caries prevention. *J Dent Educ* 62(10):803–11.

Tiberia MJ, Milnes AR, Feigal RJ, Morley KR, Richardson DS, Croft WG, and Cheung WS. 2007. Risk factors for early childhood caries in Canadian preschool children seeking care. *Pediatr Dent* 29(3):201–8.

Tinanoff N and Palmer CA. 2003. Dietary determinants of dental caries and dietary recommendations for preschool children [review]. *Refuat Hapeh Vehashinayim* 20(2):8–23, 78.

Twetman S. 2008. Prevention of early childhood caries (ECC)—Review of literature published 1998–2007. *Eur Arch Paediatr Dent* 9(1):12–18.

Weber-Gasparoni K, Kanellis MJ, Levy SM, and Stock J. 2007. Caries prior to age 3 and breastfeeding: A survey of La Leche League members. *J Dent Child* 74(1):52–61.

Weinstein P, Harrison R, and Benton T. 2006. Motivating mothers to prevent caries: Confirming the beneficial effect of counseling. *J Am Dent Assoc* 137(6):789–93.

Zhan L, Featherstone JD, Gansky SA, Hoover CI, Fujino T, Berkowitz RJ, and Den Besten PK. 2006. Antibacterial treatment needed for severe early childhood caries. *J Public Health Dent* 66(3):174–9.

Early childhood caries: Definition and epidemiology

Burton L. Edelstein, Courtney H. Chinn, and Robert J. Laughlin

INTRODUCTION

Tooth decay experience among toddlers and preschoolers—regardless of what it is called, how it is measured, and which children are most impacted by it—is of epidemic proportions in the United States and worldwide. All of the various interventions needed to address this disease require an understanding of its characteristics, correlates, occurrence, and distribution. This is true across the spectrum from prevention to rehabilitation, whether addressing the needs of an individual child or an entire population of children. This chapter explores the various terms used for this condition, describes distinct patterns of disease within early childhood caries (ECC), summarizes information on ECC prevalence and distribution among U.S. children, and elucidates the social, behavioral, and biologic correlates of this condition.

"ECC": WHERE THE NAME CAME FROM AND WHY

Since the first published descriptions of cavities in the primary teeth of young children, the terminology for this condition has ranged from the florid "bottle rot" to the generic "early childhood caries." Names for this disease have combined various words to suggest (1) causality, for example, "baby bottle," "nursing bottle," "nursing," and "night bottle"; (2) disease activity and outcome, for example, "caries," "cavities," and "tooth decay"; (3) lesion location, for example, "labial," and "maxillary anterior"; (4) aggressiveness, for example, "rampant," and "severe"; and (5) complexity, for example, "syndrome." Mixing and matching these terms has resulted in a variety of names that have been employed at various times and for various purposes. Examples include nursing or baby bottle mouth, nursing bottle or milk bottle syndrome, early infant decay, and labial caries. Some names have been criticized as being inappropriately narrow because they indicate a specific causal behavior while others have been indicted for being overly broad and "vague" (Wyne, 1999).

To address the problem of naming this disease, three federal health agencies convened an expert workshop in 1999 charged to establish diagnostic and reporting criteria that would be useful in research (Drury et al., 1999). The workshop built on prior work including findings of a national *Conference on Early Childhood Caries* (Community Dentistry and Oral Epidemiology, 1998) and a systematic review of 95 studies of this condition by Ismail and Sohn (Ismail and Sohn, 1999). Twenty-six participants concluded that the term "Early Childhood Caries" (ECC) should be adopted as standard nomenclature and should be used to indicate "the presence of one or more decayed noncavitated or cavitated, missing due to caries, or filled tooth surfaces in any primary tooth" in children under 6 years of age. In short, ECC was defined as any cavity in any tooth of any child younger than age 6.

The group recognized that this very broad definition failed to distinguish a clinically significant and extensive form of this disease. Calling this extreme presentation "atypical," the group coined the term "severe early childhood caries" or "S-ECC" to identify those children whose clinical presentation was primarily cavities on smooth surfaces or whose disease experience was more extensive than that of 50% of same-aged children. The resulting taxonomy considers a child to have S-ECC if (1) the child is younger than age 3 and demonstrates any evidence of disease experience on any smooth surface of any tooth; (2) the child is 3, 4, or 5 years of age and demonstrates any evidence of disease experience on a maxillary incisor smooth surface; or (3) the total number of affected surfaces is equal to or greater than four surfaces at age 3, five surfaces at age 4, or six surfaces at age 5.

Despite this effort to codify terminology based on a single set of diagnostic criteria and case definitions, there remains a profusion and confusion of terms for this disease (Cleaton-Jones, 2002). Dental epidemiologists continue to exclude noncavitated lesions in national prevalence studies (Dye et al., 2007) despite the definition's inclusion of such lesions. The lay press, child advocates, and child health professionals often seek more descriptive and causally related terms than ECC when communicating to the public and policy makers. For example, the American Dental Association (http://www.ada.org/public/topics/decay_childhood_faq.asp), American Academy of Pediatrics (http://www.medem.com/MedLB/article_detaillb.cfm?article_ID=ZZZKBW52R7C&sub_cat=11), and American Academy of Family Physicians (http://www.aafp.org/afp/20000101/20000101b.html)—all employ "baby bottle tooth decay" rather than ECC on their consumer web sites; the American Academy of Pediatric Dentistry offers "baby bottle caries" as a synonym for ECC (AAPD, 2007b); and the Children's Dental Health Project describes the condition explicitly as "dental cavities in the teeth of preschoolers" when communicating with federal and state policy makers (Children's Dental Health Project, 2007). There is no single term that fully satisfies the competing needs to express the etiology, risk, extent, seriousness, varieties, and levels of aggressiveness of this disease that can be utilized when communicating with both health professionals and the general public (Wyne, 1999).

The term ECC itself is intended to be clear on its face in describing dental disease in young children. Yet both the words "early childhood" and "caries" require some elucidation as they themselves are subject to variant usages. The term ECC is inclusive of children from birth through age 5 years, while the pediatric medical literature excludes infants (children younger than age 1) and sometimes 5-year-olds from its use of the term "early childhood" (Pierce et al., 2002). The term "caries" is defined by Dorland's Medical Dictionary for Health Consumers (2007) as "a destructive *process* . . . leading to . . . cavitation of the tooth." By emphasizing that caries is the underlying oral pathogenic process that later manifests as damaged teeth, this definition closely parallels the nineteenth century terminology employed before caries was fully understood as an infectious disease. Modern dentistry's founder G.V. Black employed the term "cavities of decay" (Ring, 1985) to distinguish a pathological process (decay) that must exist before lesions (cavities) occur. He predicted 150 years ago that at some future time the decay process would be treated independently of treating the resultant cavities—a prescient prediction that has yet to be fully realized. Yet common twentieth century usage has corrupted the term "caries" so that it has lost its clarity as a disease *process* and has become synonymous for cavities. There is today no unique terminology in common usage by either the health professions or the public that captures solely the notion of a disease process that causes cavities. Without such a term, clinical efforts to identify the disease process prior to cavity formation, anticipate its development, and prevent or treat it independently of treating cavities are hampered in both clinical and public health settings. This failure to separately treat the disease process that causes cavities before repairing cavities explains the high incidence of postrepair recurrence experienced by children who have been treated in the operating room for extensive damage from this disease (Berkowitz, 2003). It is doubtful that such high recurrence rates would be as widely accepted for other surgical procedures that are provided under general anesthesia to young children.

ECC terminology is further complicated by the need to determine the earliest point in disease progression at which it can be said to definitely exist. The Ismail and Sohn systematic literature review concluded that the "measurement of dental caries has not kept up with the evolving understanding of the disease process" (Ismail and Sohn, 1999). This is evident in the Workshop experts' determination that ECC identification should extend to the earliest possible stages and therefore include noncavitated lesions that appear as demineralized white spots. As earlier and earlier caries diagnostic modalities are developed and validated, criteria used for case identification will need to be updated and moved even further "downstream" than white spots to include indicators of disease initiation that occur even before white spots are evident. The case definition could already be extended to include the presence of visible plaque at the gingival margin of maxillary incisors in very young children. In a study of 92 children with an average age of 19 months at baseline, the presence or absence of plaque correctly classified children who would or would not subsequently develop cavities over 18 months in 91% of cases (Alaluusua and Malmivirta, 1994). Based on an understanding of caries pathogenesis, it may be possible to identify children who will develop cavities even earlier than the timing of plaque accumulation. While there is not yet a fully valid and reliable risk test for ECC, multiple efforts are underway to diagnose the caries process prior to the development of any clinical signs or symptoms. This potential is suggested by a cross-sectional study that employed salivary mutans testing and a history of bottle usage to correctly identify 88% of children with cavities and 91% of children without cavities in a population with high cavity experience (prevalence of 60%) (O'Sullivan and Tinanoff, 1993; Tinanoff and O'Sullivan, 1997). Similarly, a longitudinal study that measured salivary mutans levels among 1,206

18-month-old Japanese children successfully predicted caries incidence over a 2-year period (Nishimura et al., 2008). When coupled with information on breast-feeding, bottle usage, frequency of sugar intake, and oral hygiene, salivary mutans levels further identified children with existing and developing cavities. These findings suggest that very early risk prediction models can be developed to identify disease activity prior to plaque accumulation, white spots, or loss of tooth integrity. Such a test could help the clinician monitor and manage disease activity without awaiting the need for dental repair and be used in public health settings to identify those groups of children who should be targeted with the most intense interventions.

ECC CLINICAL PRESENTATIONS—DISEASE PATTERNS WITHIN ECC

The currently accepted case definition of ECC—evidence of one or more incipient or cavitated lesion in children under age 6—subsumes a variety of different clinical presentations that appear as different disease patterns. Patterns are important because each pattern may relate to differences in likelihood of progression (O'Sullivan and Tinanoff, 1996; Warren et al., 2006), social determinants (Psoter et al., 2006), biologic and behavioral etiologic risk factors (Thibodeau and O'Sullivan, 1996; Psoter et al., 2003), morbidities, and possible preventive or management interventions at both individual and community levels (Psoter et al., 2004).

The historical evolution of naming this condition is revealing as it evidences a progression from specificity coupled with descriptiveness to generality and inclusiveness. Prior to 1962 when the term "nursing bottle mouth" was introduced by Fass (Fass, 1962) to denote causality, a more generic term, "rampant caries," was used to describe the rapidity and progressiveness of one clinical pattern (Fass, 1962). Fass' decision to use the word "mouth" suggests that the locus of the caries process is the entire mouth, while the disease is manifest as lesions on specific tooth surfaces. This observation is supported by the observation of bilateral symmetry (Vanobbergen et al., 2007) and by the clinically recognizable tooth-to-tooth progression of cavity sequence within the primary dentition of various patterns. Clinically, the locations of lesions in the primary dentition relate to varying susceptibilities of different tooth surfaces that are determined by the sequence of eruption (Veerkamp and Weerheijm, 1995), the microenvironmental niche occupied by each tooth type (vanHoute, 1994), the integrity of tooth surfaces (Johnsen, 1984), and dental anatomy.

Fass' framing of ECC as an oral disease associated with both a specific feeding practice and a specific pattern of expression led to reports of the sweetened pacifier (Winter et al., 1966), the nursing bottle (Goose, 1967), and breast-feeding as etiologic correlates (Kotlow, 1977) and the suggestion that the condition be defined by a positive history of nursing habits (Powell, 1976). During three decades of employing terms suggestive of causality, attempts were made to add further specificity by requiring that a minimum number of lesions on specific anterior tooth surfaces be affected (Cleaton-Jones et al., 1978; Richardson et al., 1981; Holt et al., 1982). Even greater causal linkage and pattern specificity next emerged with the widespread use of the term "baby bottle tooth decay" or "night bottle cavities" and the recurrent requirement of a minimum number of affected maxillary incisor surfaces (Kelly and Bruerd, 1987). The term "syndrome," linked to the terms "baby bottle" or "nursing," later appeared (Cone, 1981) suggesting that the condition presents clinically as a common constellation of signs and symptoms. As a result of these different case definitions, diagnostic criteria, and populations surveyed, reports of prevalence varied remarkably—from less than 1% to 81% (Ismail and Sohn, 1999).

It was this problem of variability in reporting the occurrence of disease that instigated the 1999 Workshop's decision to move away from terms that are specific and descriptive and to adopt a term that is more general and inclusive. As a result, everything from an incipient and isolated carious lesion associated with focal hypoplasia to a fully manifest case of bottle-associated devastation of the entire primary dentition is now included within the broad catchment of ECC. By taking this action, the Workshop experts established a single operational definition that advanced the needs of research "to investigate epidemiologic, etiologic, and clinical aspects of dental caries in primary teeth of preschool-age children." But they did so at the cost of masking specific patterns that have strong clinical and public health significance. This trade-off was mitigated somewhat when the experts also distinguished S-ECC to recognize a more rampant variant that relates to either the specific locations or the numbers of teeth affected.

Whether manifest as a clinically insignificant lesion or a rampant case with acute pain and infection, the underlying caries process that causes the various presentations is the same in nature if not in intensity. The caries process is a dynamic, progressive, diet-dependent, fluoride-mediated infectious disease that results in dental lesions that are reversible at early stages. While this is true of all carious lesions, regardless of their presentation, the clinical value of recognizing specific patterns of lesions within the primary dentition may be greater than knowing the total number of lesions for purposes of making clinical decisions about disease management, dental repair, and prognosticating future disease. Patterns, which constitute subsets of ECC, are clinically associated with differences in lesion location, speed of progression, sequence of manifestation, timing of signs and symptoms, consequence on quality of life, and impact on the integrity of the developing dentition. Patterns have been associated with severity of disease (Rule, 1982), incidence of additional lesions on specific tooth surfaces (Johnsen et al., 1986a; O'Sullivan and Tinanoff, 1996), and variations in eruption patterns (Douglass et al., 2001).

IDENTIFYING PATTERNS OF ECC

Two approaches to identifying caries patterns in young children have yielded very similar results. The first starts with presumed patterns that are based on knowledge of caries etiology and then fits the clinically observed distributions of cavities into those patterns. The second presumes no patterns a priori but simply asks the computer to cluster cavity occurrence into patterns based on how frequently lesions tend to occur together.

Early work employing the first approach categorized children's presentations by type of tooth surface as "pit and fissure, hypoplasia, faciolingual (intended to show bottle caries), molar approximal, and faciolingual plus molar approximal" (Johnsen et al., 1986b). The last pattern was also named "habit-associated lesions" referring to the nursing or bottle habit (Johnsen et al., 1984). A subsequent analysis revealed that the majority (126) of 155 children demonstrated caries patterns that did fit into one of these presumed patterns (Johnsen et al., 1993). The relative frequency of pattern types by age suggests that during the years of early childhood, the faciolingual and hypoplastic patterns predominate first, becoming overwhelmed later by pit and fissure lesions, and then subsequently by molar approximal lesions (Johnsen et al., 1987).

The alternative approach to determining patterns developed them by using a computerized classification technique called multidimensional scaling. This approach identified a similar set of patterns, which were more tooth-type specific and were termed "maxillary incisor, first molar occlusal, second molar pit and fissure, and smooth surfaces other than the maxillary incisors" (Psoter et al., 2003). This study partially explained ECC variants as being influenced by the sequence of primary tooth eruption and noted a specific progression by tooth type and age (Figure 2.1).

An entirely different approach to classifying the range of conditions encompassed by the term ECC offers a three-level hierarchical typology based on lesion location, relative contribution of diet and hygiene, and age. In this rubric, "Type I ECC" captures the isolated carious lesion(s) involving molars and/or incisors caused by solid food and lack of hygiene and typically found in children ages 2–5. "Type II ECC" captures faciolingual lesions of the maxillary incisors, with or without molar caries depending on the child's age and stage of disease typically associated with inappropriate bottle-feeding or at-will breast-feeding occurring as early as the first teeth erupt. "Type III ECC" captures rampant presentations affecting all or almost all teeth in association with a cariogenic diet and poor oral hygiene, typically among 3- to 5-year-olds (Wyne, 1999).

No single taxonomy has succeeded in capturing all young children's clinical presentations. However, distinguishing at least the following three overall patterns holds strong utility for diagnosis and disease management:

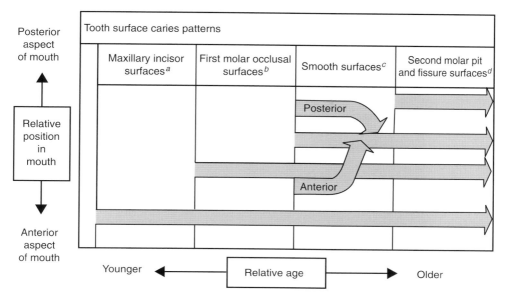

Figure 2.1 Conceptional map of caries patterns in the primary dentition derived from multidimensional scaling in children 5–59 months of age. [a] Proximal, facial, lingual; [b] maxillary and mandibular; [c] smooth, other than maxillary incisor; [d] occlusal, maxillary lingual, mandibular facial (Psoter et al., 2003).

1. Nursing habit–associated pattern, also called maxillary anterior pattern/faciolingual pattern, and faciolingual/molar pattern (Figure 2.2)

   The nursing habit–associated pattern is the earliest (Grindefjord et al., 1995), most aggressive, most destructive, and most consequential pattern within ECC. It can be identified clinically first as soft glutinous plaque accumulation at the gingival margin of maxillary incisors, then as decalcified bands underlying that plaque, and soon thereafter as facial and lingual cavitations of the maxillary incisors. The sequence of teeth affected by this subset of ECC typically follows the sequence of primary tooth eruption with the exception of the relative immunity of the mandibular incisors. These lower incisors are physically protected by the lip and tongue and kept awash in protective saliva from the sublingual and labial mucosal salivary glands. Thus, a common progression begins on the smooth surfaces of maxillary central incisors and extends sequentially to the maxillary lateral incisors, maxillary first primary molars, mandibular first primary molars, maxillary canines, and then second primary molars. The feeding habits associated with this pattern are frequent use of the nursing bottle, sippy cup, or ad libitum breast-feeding.

2. Molar occlusal/pit and fissure patterns and hypoplasia pattern (Figure 2.3)

(a)   (b)   (c)

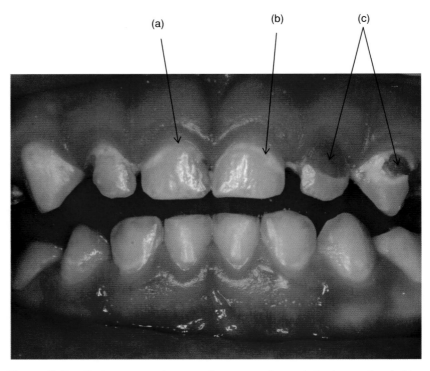

Figure 2.2   Caries progression on primary anterior teeth in the nursing habit–associated pattern. (a) Plaque accumulation at the gingival margin of maxillary incisors in a young child; (b) gingival margin white spots/decalcification; (c) cavitation of maxillary incisors, followed by maxillary first molars, mandibular first molars, maxillary canines, and then second molars. (Photo courtesy of Dr Simon Lin, University of Washington, Seattle, WA.)

This cluster of presentations relates to irregularities in the surfaces of primary teeth either from normal presence of pits and fissures or from defective development associated with hypoplasia. The molar occlusal and pit and fissure patterns describe the occurrence of lesions on the occlusal surface of the first primary molars and in the various pits and fissures of the second primary molars. It may occur independently of the nursing habit–associated pattern in association with frequent consumption of cariogenic solid foods, which become mechanically retained in these defects. It is also likely to occur subsequent to the nursing habit–associated pattern (O'Sullivan and Tinanoff, 1993) as the child transitions to solid foods. Nearly a third of noncavitated pit and fissure lesions progress to cavitation or repair over 4 years—a rate 6 times higher than for noncavitated smooth surface lesions. Hypoplastic enamel, commonly observed on the facial aspects of mandibular primary canines but also the second primary molars (Slayton et al.,

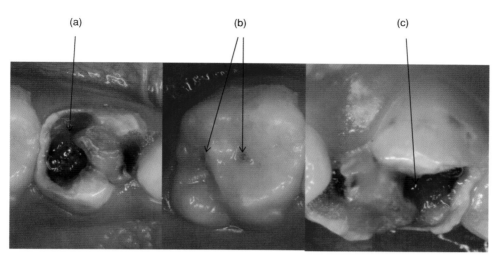

Figure 2.3   Caries progression on the occlusal surface of primary molars in the molar occlusal/pit and fissure patterns. (a) Cavitation on the occlusal surface of first molars; (b) pits and fissures of second molars with progression to cavitation (c). (Photos courtesy of Dr Simon Lin, University of Washington, Seattle, WA.)

2001), has been noted to be more susceptible to dental caries and has been considered as a specific ECC caries type (Johnsen et al., 1987).

3. Molar proximal pattern (Figure 2.4)

Cavities located between the primary molars typically present late in the primary dentition and are classically associated with lack of interdental spacing. They may also occur as smooth surface lesions in the presence of intermolar spacing when the nursing habit–associated pattern is extensive. In a group of children under 3 years of age, this pattern was seen only among children who had first developed the nursing habit–associated pattern on anterior teeth (Douglass et al., 2001). The intermolar space, if present early in the primary dentition, typically closes as the first permanent molars move into place when children reach the end of the early childhood period. Therefore, children who erupt their first permanent molars prior to their sixth birthday are more susceptible to this ECC pattern. Among a diverse group of first grade, 6- to 7-year-old children in Iowa, more than half (57%) had erupted their first molars sufficiently to be sealed and therefore had likely closed their intermolar spaces while still within the ECC age range. Girls were more likely to have erupted their first molars than were boys, but no differences in the Iowa children were noted by race or ethnicity (Warren et al., 2003) although differences in first permanent molar eruption timing by race have also been reported (Maki et al., 1999).

(a)

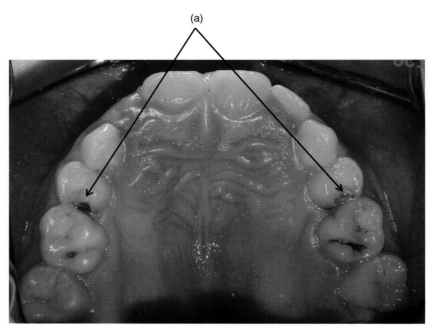

Figure 2.4   Caries progression on the proximal surface of primary molars in the molar proximal pattern. Proximal molar caries (a) frequently occurs following the eruption of permanent molars and the subsequent closing of space between primary molars. This pattern may follow the nursing habit–associated pattern in some children. (Photo courtesy of Dr. Rebecca Slayton, University of Iowa, Iowa City, IA.)

CHARTING ECC PATTERNS WITHIN CHILDREN'S DENTITIONS

No two children with ECC are exactly alike. Children differ by which pattern or patterns they manifest, by how many teeth are affected within each pattern, by how extensively each tooth is affected, and by how impacted their lives are by symptoms that result from their cavities. Various efforts have been attempted to capture this complexity in charting a child's clinical presentation.

Medicine typically uses the concept of "disease staging" to capture such variations and to aid in treatment selection and prognosticating outcomes. Using this approach, one clinically useful substratification of the nursing habit–associated pattern classifies this condition into four stages based on the number of teeth involved and the severity of the lesions. The four stages are described as "initial," typically occurring at ages 10–20 months; "damaged" at 16–24 months; "deep" at 20–36 months; and "traumatic" at 30–48 months (Veerkamp and Weerheijm, 1995).

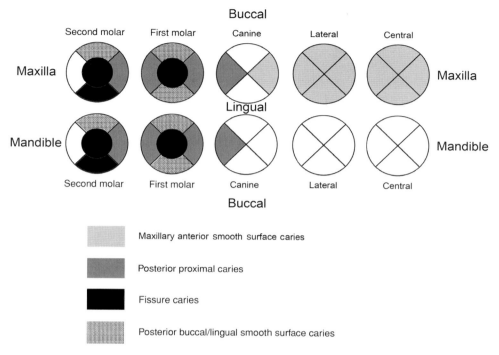

Buccal

Second molar   First molar   Canine   Lateral   Central

Maxilla   Maxilla

Lingual

Mandible   Mandible

Second molar   First molar   Canine   Lateral   Central

Buccal

Maxillary anterior smooth surface caries

Posterior proximal caries

Fissure caries

Posterior buccal/lingual smooth surface caries

Figure 2.5   The caries analysis system (Douglass et al., 1994). Source: Douglass et al. (1994).

Another approach, the "caries analysis system," has been proposed to distinguish ECC patterns within the dentitions of individual children (Douglass et al., 1994). This system (Figure 2.5) utilizes the traditional, circular tooth surface charting form and differentiates each ECC subtype by using different shading schemes for each pattern.

An alternative clinical approach to assessing the occurrence (presence or absence of various patterns), extent (degree to which surfaces associated with each pattern are affected), and impact (symptoms at presentation) of ECC could distribute tooth surfaces from each of the three patterns as concentric rings. The nursing habit–associated maxillary anterior pattern, which would be located at the center of the chart, typically happens first. Cavitation may then sequentially "spread" outward through the dentition next to the occlusal pattern, which would form the second ring and then to the molar proximal pattern, located in a third ring. By charting cavities, white spots, and areas of plaque accumulation on each ring and indicating presence of symptoms associated with specific teeth, a visual representation of the child's status would be readily apparent. Such a chart could also indicate the next teeth that are most likely to be affected if the underlying caries process is not arrested.

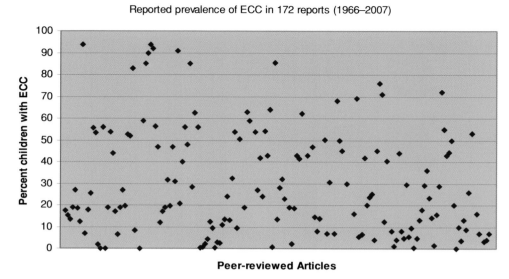

Figure 2.6   Scatterplot of 172 studies conducted between 1982 and 2007 that report prevalence of ECC.

ECC OCCURRENCE AND DISTRIBUTION IN U.S. CHILDREN

How many children are affected?

By any standard, the burden of tooth decay in young U.S. children is simply too high. Any occurrence of this disease can be considered excessive since all forms of ECC are preventable or treatable well before irreversible damage is done.

The overall reported prevalence of ECC varies dramatically depending on case definition, population studied, and research methods employed. Figure 2.6 shows the reported prevalence from 172 studies including the 95 reviewed by the federal expert workgroup in 1999 (Figure 2.6). The tremendous variation evident in the scatterplot suggests that these studies are reporting on very different criteria. In fact, a closer look at these studies show that they capture different age groups, include both convenience and representative samples of both entire child populations and specific subpopulations, consider the entire dentition or only specific teeth or tooth surfaces, report on different ages and age groups, employ single or multiple examiners who may or may not have been calibrated, do or do not count noncavitated lesions, and span the full range of research methodologies from case-control studies to cohort studies and controlled trials. The only conclusion regarding prevalence is that it depends on exactly what is meant by this condition.

For its studies of decay experience in young children, the U.S. federal government employs a conservative standard that holds greatest promise

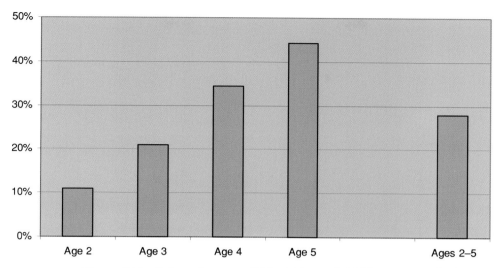

Figure 2.7   Estimated percent of U.S. children with ECC by age. Note that because of the NHANES methodology, age-specific rates are considered only rough estimates of ECC prevalence, while the aggregate rate for 2- to 5-year-olds is a more reliable estimate across the entire age group. Source: NHANES III as analyzed by Iida et al. (2007).

of valid and reliable findings across sequential surveys. It employs a representative sample of all 2- to 6-year-olds in the United States and counts children as having decay experience only if they have one or more visible cavities (without radiographs), have one or more visible fillings, or have one or more teeth missing because of decay. White spots, even if readily evident, are not counted. Young children are examined in the knee-to-knee position. The Center for Disease Control and Prevention (CDC), which conducts this National Health and Nutrition Examination Survey (NHANES), notes that examining such young children is often challenging and that findings may be less reliable for this very young age group than for older, more cooperative children.

Using these stringent criteria for identifying the prevalence of decay experience, the CDC reported in 2007 that during its 1999–2004 NHANES survey, more than one-quarter of all 2- to 6-year-old U.S. children (27.9%) have experienced cavities and nearly three-quarters of these affected children (73.4%) have unrepaired teeth (Figure 2.7) (Dye et al., 2007). These percentages represent 4.5 million affected U.S. toddlers and preschoolers of whom well over 3 million are in need of dental repair before the age of kindergarten. Among 1-year-olds alone, earlier federal findings (1988–1994) suggested that between 36,000 and 62,000 toddlers have experienced tooth decay (Kaste et al., 1999). Of great concern, the situation is worsening and the disease is heavily concentrated in socially disadvantaged children who are least likely to have access to dental services. Dental caries remains the single most common disease of early childhood that is not self-limiting or amenable to a course of antibiotics (Edelstein and Douglass, 1995). It appears from findings of another federal study, the National Survey of Children's Health, that many parents are unaware of their children's poor dental health as only 6.7% of parents of children ages 1–5 years report that their children's dental condition is fair or poor (U.S. Department of Health and Human Services, 2005).

NHANES is used as the official governmental yardstick for measuring progress toward reaching federal Healthy People 2010 objectives. The Healthy People 2010 objective for dental caries experience in children is to see a reduction in prevalence from 24% to 9%. Rather than moving toward this target, the prevalence of cavities in children 2–6 years of age increased by 15.2% from the 1988–1994 baseline to 27.9%.

Children ages 2–5 were recruited into this federal study as a single age group and not as separate cohorts for each of ages 2, 3, 4, and 5 years. As a result, the federal data are neither sufficiently representative nor sufficiently robust to confidently stratify findings by age. Nonetheless, because caries is well understood to progress with age, it would be expected that prevalence is higher among 5-year-olds than 2-year-olds. Consistent with this expectation in the finding that cavity experience increases by roughly 10% Iida et al. reports age stratified the 1999–2004 NHANES data, finding that with each age group, from approximately 10% at age 2 to over 40% at age 5 (Iida et al., 2007).

Looking again at the full set of international studies, they can be sorted by age to determine whether the expected increase with age is found

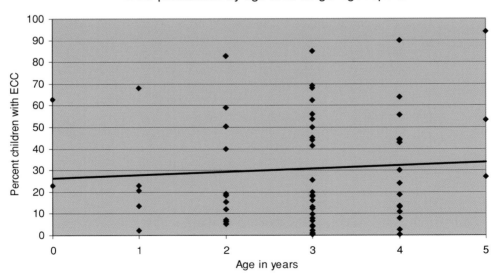

Figure 2.8   Scatterplot of 67 studies that report ECC prevalence for specific ages. The trend line shows that across these studies ECC rates increase by child age.

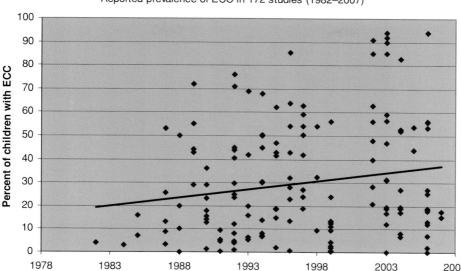

Figure 2.9   Scatterplot of 172 studies that report ECC prevalence by year of publication. The trend line may suggest that caries ECC rates are increasing over time.

across such a diverse collection of reports. Figure 2.8 shows a scatterplot of data from 67 studies of the 172 studies that report for specific age cohorts (Figure 2.8). It reveals a modest trend line suggesting increasing disease with age. These same data can be sorted by year of study report to determine whether ECC may be increasing over time. The trend line best fit to Figure 2.9 may suggest temporal increases in ECC or may be specious as it may be explained by differences among the reported studies (Figure 2.9).

Which children are most affected?

Looking closely at the 172 studies represented in the scatterplots, a number of observations can be made about which children are most affected:

1. Caries experience increases dramatically with age.
2. Very high rates are reported globally for native and aboriginal populations that have become exposed to western diets.
3. Populations of low-income children like those in Head Start have higher disease experience than high-income children.
4. Populations exposed to water fluoridation have lower rates than those without access to community water fluoridation.
5. Prevalence rates are highest in populations that most often engage in inappropriate use of the baby bottle.

Many of these findings are well illustrated in a study of ECC experience among young children in Arizona (Tang et al., 1997). Figure 2.10 illustrates

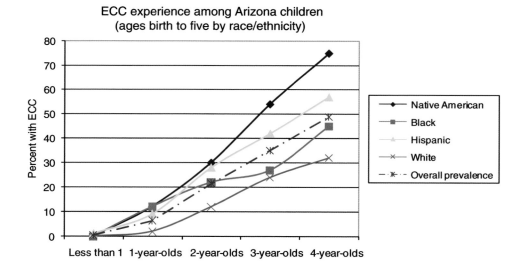

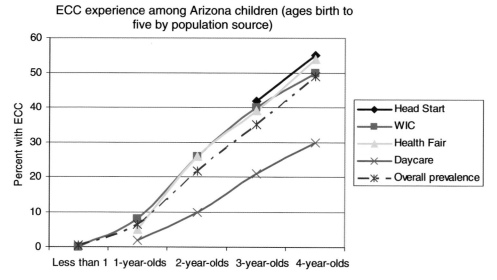

Figure 2.10   Variations in ECC experienced by subpopulations of children in Arizona from Tang et al. (1997). While ECC prevalence increases with age for all subgroups, the prevalence of ECC varies considerably between subgroups, whether those subgroups are defined by program (Head Start, WIC, Child Care, Health Fair) or race and ethnicity (Native American, Black, White, Hispanic).

variations in ECC experience by age, population source, and race/ethnicity among subpopulations in that state (Figure 2.10). These plots demonstrate both the wide variation in disease experience by population subgroups and the "tyranny of the mean,"—that averages mask differences between subgroups. Like the NHANES' nationally representative data, this Arizona study also found that three-quarters (74%) of children with ECC are in need of treatment. It also reported that almost none under the age of 3 had evidence of partial or complete repair. By age of 5 years, approximately 53% of children with cavities had experienced no dental repair, 27% had experienced partial repair, and 20% had experienced complete repair.

Using national NHANES III data from 1,302 U.S. children ages 2–6 years in 1999–2002, a multivariate logistic regression model for ECC reported significant differences in disease occurrence by age, race/ethnicity, family income, maternal smoking, and time since last dental visit (Iida et al., 2007). From age 2, the odds of having cavities doubled at age 3, tripled at age 4, and quintupled at age 5. The odds of having cavities if the child was Mexican American (the only Hispanic group represented in NHANES) was double that of non-Hispanic White children, while Black children were no more likely than White children to be affected. Children living in poor families were 3.5 times more likely, and children in working-poor families were twice as likely to have ECC as children from more affluent families. The finding that children whose mother's smoke are 1.7 times more likely to have ECC may suggest a causal link between environmental smoke and cavities or may reflect confounding because of possible independent relationships between smoking and poverty or smoking and ethnicity. Discovering that children with ECC are twice as likely to have had a dental visit in the past year is reflective of parents seeking care for their affected children. When this descriptive modeling approach was repeated for 1,298 children with S-ECC, the relationship between cavities and Mexican American status and between cavities and poverty remained strong. An analysis of earlier NHANES data (1988–1994) that were limited to children ages 12–23 months also reported that a higher percentage of affected children was Mexican-American than other race/ethnicities by a factor of 4.6 times, but at this young age there was not significant difference noted by income (Kaste et al., 1999).

Higher rates of disease among poor children and among Mexican American children are evident across the years of the primary dentition. For children ages 2–11, the percentage of affected children is 54.3% for children in poverty, 48.8% for children of working-poor families, and 32.3% for more affluent children. Similarly, 55.4% of Mexican American children are affected, while 43.3% of Black children and 38.6% of White children have experienced cavities. While all of these prevalence findings are very high relative to other diseases that children suffer, the disproportionate burden among poor and Hispanic children suggests both the need to better understand etiology and to target aggressive interventions to children at greatest risk and needs (http://drc.hhs.gov/report/17_1.htm) (Figure 2.11).

Low-income and minority children also have more *untreated* decay experience than do their more socially advantaged peers. Among 2- to 11-year-olds, approximately 60% of poor and working-poor children have

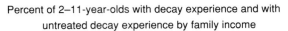

Percent of 2–11-year-olds with decay experience and with untreated decay experience by family income

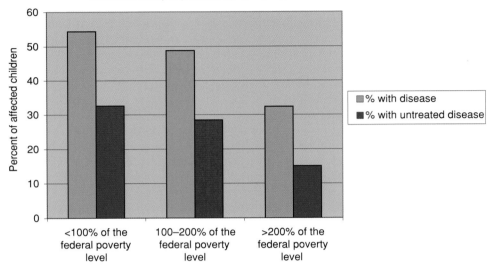

Percent of 2–11-year-olds with decay experience and with untreated decay experiences by race/ethnicity

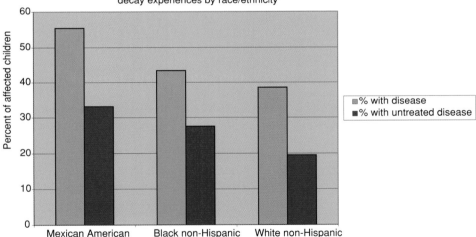

Figure 2.11   Variation in decay experience and untreated decay in 2- to 11-year-olds at different levels of family income and different racial/ethnic backgrounds.

untreated cavities in their primary teeth compared to 47% of children from more affluent families. Similarly, 60% of Mexican American children and 64% of Black children have untreated cavities compared to 51% of White children. These findings are consistent with a 2007 federal report that only

25.1% of young children received one or more dental visit in 2004 (Manski and Brown, 2007).

The U.S. populations with the greatest ECC experience are Native American and Alaskan Native children (Indian Health Service, 1999) with rates that are 5 times the U.S. average. ECC is virtually universal among these children (97% prevalence) with two-thirds experiencing S-ECC. Because of the intensity of dental services provided by the Indian Health Service, a somewhat smaller proportion of these children, 68%, have untreated disease.

While there are lesser available data on Asian and Pacific Islander (API) children in the United States, these groups also experience very high rates of ECC. A California study of preschool-age children reported that API children had ECC rates 3 times the level of White children (Shiboski et al., 2003) and a Hawaii study of school-age children reported both higher experience of ECC and lower treatment rates than non-API children (Greer et al., 2003).

How extensive is the disease occurrence?

The average numbers of affected teeth and tooth surfaces among 2- to 6-year-olds reported by CDC are 1.17 teeth and 2.58 tooth surfaces. A clinical perspective on these findings is that among young children who have decay experience, the average number of decayed teeth is 4.2 out of 20 teeth. This represents more than one-fifth of all primary teeth and more than one-quarter of all susceptible teeth if the mandibular incisors are excluded because they rarely decay. Among young children with decay experience, 9.2 surfaces are affected.

These national reports of average decay experience hint at ECC's overall destructiveness but mask differences in extent by ECC pattern. The extent of tooth destruction within patterns varies significantly. Nursing habit–associated lesions tend to extend to the most numbers of susceptible tooth surfaces, while occlusal molar or proximal molar cavities tend to be less extensive. For example, among 4-year-old Connecticut children, the percent of available surfaces that were found to be carious within the range of all surfaces that are susceptible to each pattern was 42.2% for the maxillary anterior pattern, 37.5% for the posterior proximal pattern, and 33.3% for the fissure pattern. This saturation of lesions within each pattern was found to vary somewhat by age and race/ethnicity, suggesting that there are specific differences in disease extent, as there are in disease prevalence, within each subpopulation (Douglass et al., 1994). These differences are of clinical importance for dentists who care for young children because they need to be aware of the common patterns of disease presentation and progression within the population of children they treat in order to best anticipate, prevent, and manage this disease.

Earlier nationally representative data from 1980 to 1987 detailed the specific primary tooth surfaces of 5-year-olds affected by decay (Li et al.,

1993). These findings clearly reflect how caries moves through the dentition within each of the recognized patterns and will be familiar to clinicians experienced in diagnosing and repairing primary teeth. The nursing habit–associated pattern revealed highest caries rates for the lingual surface of maxillary central incisors followed by the facial aspect of that tooth, then the lingual and facial aspect of the maxillary lateral incisor, then canine facial surfaces, and finally first molar facial surfaces. The pit and fissure patterns revealed that the occlusal surfaces of the mandibular second molars were most affected followed by the maxillary second molars, mandibular first molars, maxillary first molars and then the buccal groove of the mandibular second molar, and finally the lingual groove of the maxillary first molar. The proximal caries pattern revealed highest attack on the distal aspects of the first molars, then mesial aspects of the second molars followed by lesser attack rates on the mesials of the first molars, distals of the second molars that typically have no adjacent tooth at this age. Among proximal lesions of the anterior teeth, the mandibular teeth were virtually unaffected while the mesial aspect of the maxillary central incisors were most affected, followed by the distal of the maxillary centrals, mesial of the maxillary laterals, distal of the maxillary laterals, and mesial aspects of the maxillary canines.

What are some of the key biologic correlates of ECC?

Breast-feeding and bottle-feeding

Clinical observation of a relationship between ad libitum nocturnal breast-feeding and ECC beginning with case reports in 1977 (Kotlow, 1977) has led to American Dental Association and American Academy of Pediatric Dentistry policies warning parents that unrestricted at-will nocturnal breast-feeding after eruption of the child's first tooth should be avoided as it puts children at risk for ECC. Yet epidemiological studies of the U.S. (Dye et al., 2004; Iida et al., 2007) and European (Kramer et al., 2007) populations show no relationship between breast-feeding and ECC. These seemingly contradictory findings are reconcilable when considering the limitations and values of both case reports and epidemiological studies. Case reports are of necessity limited to small numbers of individuals but are able to carefully investigate nuances that are missed by epidemiological studies. Epidemiological studies have the advantage of large numbers but a more limited set of variables to analyze. Reconciling these findings is further complicated by the multifactorial nature of caries pathogenesis. What is clear from the literature is that some children nurse in ways that either correlate with or lead directly to ECC, while the majority of breast-fed children do not experience ECC. Similarly, the majority of children who present with the nursing habit–associated pattern have a positive history of inappropriate bottle or sippy cup usage while the converse (that the majority of children who have a positive history of inappropriate bottle or sippy cup usage have ECC) is not true.

Diet

The relationship between fermentable carbohydrates and caries is well established, but less well understood is the relationship between diet and caries in young children. A valuable approach to investigating dietary correlates of ECC is the case-control method in which children with cavities are compared with children with no decay experience. One such study conducted in Iowa with 39 children who have severe ECC and 39 caries-free children identified caries relationships among 4- to 7-year-olds with regular ingestion of soda and other sugared beverage intake, greater frequency of starch foods, and greater frequency of eating occasions (Mariri et al., 2003). The relationship between the quality of fluid intake and primary tooth caries was also found in a population-level survey in which children in a "high-carbohydrate soft drink" group had higher caries experience than children in a high-juice group, high-water group, and high-milk group, with the last having the least caries experience (Sohn et al., 2006). As suggested by the social determinants of health approach to understanding risk for ECC, other indicators of poor diet and nutrition have also been correlated with cavities in young children. For example, not eating breakfast on a daily basis and not consuming the recommended five fruits and vegetables daily are associated with overall ECC experience (Dye et al., 2004).

Salivary mutans streptococci levels and visible plaque

As with high-sugar diets, the associations between *mutans streptococci*, plaque, and caries are very well established (Berkowitz, 2003). Multiple studies since the mid-1970s relate mutans levels in children to mutans levels in the mouths of their primary caregivers (Douglass et al., 2008), suggesting that managing adult reservoirs and interfering with transmission may hold strong promise to reduce disease onset and experience.

Social determinants of ECC

Successful prevention and management of ECC will require effective strategies that consider not only the biologic but also the underlying social, sociopsychological, socioeconomic, and socioenvironmental causes of illness known as social determinants of health (SDH). SDH describe the conditions in which people live and work and may include a range of nonbiologic factors in the contexts of the child's family, community, and society. Disease risk and protective factors include inherent characteristics such as age, gender, race, and ethnicity as well as acquired characteristics such as education, occupation, employment, income, religion, and housing. Psychosocial risk factors consist of low self-esteem, low self-efficacy, depression, anxiety, insecurity, loss of sense of control, high physical demand, chronic stress, isolation, anger/hostility, coping, and perceptions/expectations. Moving from the individual to societal characteristics, community risk factors include poor social networks, limited support structures, inadequate social participation and civic involvement, a sense of political disempowerment, intolerance of diversity, poverty, crime, domestic violence, and unemployment (Ansari et al., 2003). Such factors have been validated as etiologic determinants in pathogenesis of a variety of conditions independent of biologic factors (Marmot and Wilkinson, 1999).

These determinants go beyond the individual child, yet have a direct impact on children's health behaviors, environment, and access to care—ultimately defining their general health, as well as their oral health outcomes (Urban Child Institute, 2006). For example, preschoolers in poverty are 2 times more likely to have tooth decay and half as likely to visit a dentist than their more affluent counterparts (Edelstein, 2002). In addition, children of low socioeconomic status have 12 times the number of days when dental disease, such as tooth decay, is consequential to their daily activities of learning, eating, speaking, and sleeping (CDC, http://www.cdc.gov/oralhealth/publications/pdf/dental_caries.pdf).

Early-life influences of social class, family income, and parental education greatly impact childhood dental caries (Peres et al., 2005). Thus, socially disadvantaged children of lower-income families, who are least able to afford dental services or access dental care, are those same children experiencing the greatest burden of dental disease and experiencing the largest impact on daily living.

Throughout the course of life, each individual accumulates exposures from positive and negative social determinants that cumulatively impact health outcomes. The study of social influences over time relies on a technique called "life course analysis." A dental example is a study of oral health status at age 26 years as a reflection of oral health at age 5 years, adjusted for changes in socioeconomic status. In this study, Thomson and colleagues found the following:

- Childhood socioeconomic status (SES) impacts childhood dental caries. Low-SES 5-year-olds have higher caries prevalence and more extensive untreated disease than high-SES children (62.6% vs 52.6% prevalence).
- Childhood socioeconomic status impacts adult dental caries. Mean Decayed or Filled Surfaces (DFS) and Decayed Surfaces (DS) were significantly greater at age 26 years for those who were of low SES as children compared to high SES (11.54 vs 10.52 and 1.88 vs 1.60, respectively).
- Changes in socioeconomic status throughout the life course results in differing levels of adult dental caries. Considering childhood "SES origin" and adult "SES destination," those children with improvements in SES (low to high) had lower mean dental caries rates (DFS 10.09) compared to those whose SES worsened (high to low) (DFS 10.62). The

worst caries rates were seen for those children in the low-SES group who remained in the low SES into adulthood (DFS 12.38). However, those advantaged children who continued to be in the high-SES group into adulthood had higher DFS rates compared to the upwardly mobile group (DFS 10.41 vs 10.09). These findings validate the claim that the social origin of children, such as their socioeconomic status, greatly impacts the caries outcomes in their permanent dentition (Thomson et al., 2004).

The trajectory of tooth decay from early childhood through at least the fourth decade of life tends to follow a linear course suggesting that caries is a steady state phenomenon once established in early childhood (Broadbent et al., 2008). Individuals tend to cluster into one of three such trajectories, which have been labeled low, medium, and high and which reflect different levels of underlying caries activity that is established before the eruption of the first permanent tooth.

The pathway between SES and oral health status is explained in part by differences in the availability of dental care for populations of different economic means. SES relates to barriers to dental access that, in turn, relate to utilization of dental care and ultimately to the numbers of sound teeth (Donaldson et al., 2008). These findings suggest that addressing social determinants of oral health during critical early developmental periods in a child's life can result in a life course of greater advantage well into adulthood.

A second method of understanding the overall impact of SDH is the "common risk factor approach." Risk factors for early childhood caries development, such as social conditions and unhealthy behaviors, are well documented and are similar to those that impact general health outcomes. For example, the dietary consumption of high amounts of non-milk extrinsic sugars increases not only the likelihood of dental decay, but also obesity and diabetes (Sheiham and Watt, 2000). According to the CDC, the prevalence of overweight children has doubled in the last 20 years, and approximately 1 in 400–500 children suffers from diabetes. Equally alarming, overweight children are more likely to experience obesity, heart disease, cancer, strokes, diabetes, and osteoarthritis as adults (CDC, http://www.cdc.gov/diabetes/pubs/estimates.htm). A common risk factor approach focusing on the elimination of SDH disparities and reversing unhealthy behaviors, therefore, holds promise to improve a number of unique health outcomes. If addressed, these common risk factors may decrease disease burden within the oral cavity, such as ECC, along with comorbidities of the whole child, while reducing the risk of associated health problems later in life.

A shift in focus from the long-established, lone surgical treatment model to the broader social determinants of oral health, including the life course and common risk factor approaches, has significant implications in the prevention of early childhood caries and promotion of oral health.

Prevention of ECC requires the establishment of the dental home and proper timing for the first and follow-up visits. The American Academy of Pediatric Dentistry states that every child should see a dentist at 1 year of age, or at the time of the first tooth eruption, whichever occurs earlier. This first dental visit establishes the "dental home," defined as a source of care that "provides regular, ongoing, comprehensive oral health care throughout the child's growing years" (AAPD, 2007a). During the first 2 years of life, the child is especially at risk for establishing a virulent caries process through establishment of cariogenic flora associated with introduction of high-sugar diets involving frequent feedings, including inappropriate use of the baby bottle or breast as pacifiers. By establishing the dental home during this critical time, the pediatric dentist can assess the social context of the whole child, perform a caries-risk assessment, determine the current oral health behaviors of the child and family, and develop a tailored plan to anticipate, prevent, or suppress caries activity even before cavitations are evident. Ultimately, the dental home will lay the groundwork for the practitioner to prevent unhealthy practices, thereby limiting early childhood caries, improving function, and altering the life course of potential disadvantage and disease. Oral health promotion necessitates a focus on SDH and consideration of common risk factors as well as biologic factors. For example, early childhood interventions that address dietary and nutritional concerns rather than caries alone hold promise to simultaneously address risks for obesity and diabetes. Envisioned, therefore, are models of care that address risk rather than specific diseases. Through coordination with other health disciplines, program objectives can be more effective in addressing the whole child while also addressing ECC. Efficiency of services can be improved by avoiding duplication across programs, thereby improving the health benefit for each dollar spent on health promotion. Sheiham and Watt propose a health promotion framework based on these strategies that include (1) focusing on common determinants of disease and avoiding blaming the patient; (2) organizing interventions at the community rather than professional office level; (3) targeting populations at greatest risk and disease experience; (4) working in partnerships across sectors and disciplines; and (5) adopting a range of complementary public health policies rather than individually focused health education.

CONSEQUENCES OF ECC

The consequences of ECC are numerous and significant on children's growth, function, and quality of life. It has been typical in the past to describe the consequences of pediatric dental caries from a temporal perspective, examining the both short- and long-term effects dental caries has on the individual child. However, an even more telling perspective is to portray the consequences of ECC in a more contextual and holistic manner, describing its impact within a series of levels beginning with the tooth, mouth, and child and then progressing to its impact on families, community, and society in general.

Consequences to the dentition

ECC results in progressive destruction of tooth structure leading to dental abscesses, facial cellulitis, pain, tooth loss, and development of malocclusion (Acs et al., 1999). Because the pathogenic process underlying ECC continues unabated even with dental repair, tooth decay in the primary dentition is the single strongest predictor of cavities in the permanent dentition (Hollister and Weintraub, 1993).

Consequences to the child

ECC is associated with a child's overall quality of life (Reisine, 1988; Low et al., 1999; McGrath et al., 2004) including the ability to eat, speak, and socialize without discomfort or embarrassment. Chronic dental pain associated with ECC may also cause irritability and disruption of normal sleep patterns. In a convenience study of children presenting to pediatric dentistry residency programs in pain, 86% of families reported that cavities interfered with their child's ability to eat; 50% reported that it affected their child's ability to sleep; and 32% reported that it affected their child's ability to participate in school activities (Edelstein et al., 2006). The relationship between ECC and diet is complex as poor diets may both result in and result from having cavities. Dental pain from untreated dental caries may impact the growth as well as the cognitive development of young children (Sheiham, 2006) although studies of the association between ECC with failure to thrive are inconclusive. One research group found that young children with advanced dental caries weigh significantly less than controls (Acs et al., 1992) but are able to "catch up" following comprehensive dental treatment (Acs et al., 1999), while others reported that 75% of children with S-ECC were of normal size based on body mass indexes (Clarke et al., 2006). In the latter study, children with S-ECC were also found to demonstrate various physiological signs of malnutrition including iron deficiency anemia, which has permanent negative effects on childhood growth and development. ECC is also associated with an increase in the number of days with restricted activity or being absent from school (Low et al., 1999). Parents report that dental repair results in positive social outcomes for their children including more smiling, improved school performance, and increased social interaction (White et al., 2003). Extension of infection from ECC that compromises the airway, creates sepsis, or results in a brain abscess is rare but nonetheless life threatening. Complications of ECC treatment, particularly deep sedation and general anesthesia mishaps, also occasionally result in disability and death.

Consequences beyond the child

Children are by nature vulnerable and dependent. Their health and well-being, therefore, have direct impacts on family members and their communities. As future adults, children's oral health will impact their social functioning and economic productivity. ECC may add to family stress, particularly when it affects a child's behavior, sleeplessness, or pickiness at meals, and it has been associated with increased risk of domestic violence. Caring for dental emergencies resulting from ECC can add further stress as parents need to adjust work and other obligations to care for or comfort their child suffering from dental pain. ECC has both a direct and an indirect economic impact related to both the cost of care and missed income opportunities related to loss of parental work time. There has been little research done on the indirect costs of oral health as measured by productivity; however, the total time lost from work due to oral health care is associated with having poorer oral health and having greater treatment need (Reisine, 1989). While the time lost in work productivity may seem trivial on an individual basis, as an aggregate, the impact of indirect costs nationally are significant (Gift et al., 1992). In the larger societal picture, such costs speak to the extent that ECC has contributed to the overall rising oral health costs in the United States. For example, dental Medicaid expenditures in California are disproportionately consumed by children requiring dental repair for ECC as 35% of dental expenditures are attributable to just 5% of children who receive dental care (Reforming States Group, 1999).

REFERENCES

Acs G, Lodolini G, Kaminski, and Cisneros GJ. 1992. Effect of nursing caries on body weight in a pediatric population. *Pediatr Dent* 14:302–5.

Acs G, Shulman R, Ng MW, and Chussid S. 1999. The effect of dental rehabilitation on the body weight of children with early childhood caries. *Pediatr Dent* 21:109–13.

Alaluusua S and Malmivirta R. 1994. Early plaque accumulation-a sign of caries risk in young children. *Community Dent Oral Epidemiol* 22(5):273–6.

American Academy of Pediatric Dentistry (AAPD). 2007a. *Policy on the Dental Home. Pediatr Dent 29 (7) Reference Manual 2007–2008*. Available at http://www.aapd.org/media/Policies_Guidelines/P_DentalHome (accessed December 24, 2007).

American Academy of Pediatric Dentistry (AAPD). 2007b. *Oral Health Policies—Early Childhood Caries. Pediatr Dent 29 (7) Reference Manual 2007–2008*. Available at http://www.aapd.org/media/Policies_Guidelines/P_ECCClassifications.pdf (accessed October 22, 2008).

Ansari Z, Carson NJ, Ackland MJ, Vaughan L, and Serraglio A. 2003. A public health model of the social determinants of health. *Soz.-Praventivmed* 48: 242–51.

Berkowitz RJ. 2003. Causes, treatment and prevention of early childhood caries: A microbiologic perspective. *J Can Dent Assoc* 69(5):304–7.

Broadbent JM, Thomson WM, and Poulton R. 2008. Trajectory patterns of dental caries experience in the permanent dentition to the fourth decade of life. *J Dent Res* 87:69–72.

Children's Dental Health Project. 2007. *CDC Study Finds Dental Health Among Young Children Worsening*. Available at www.cdhp.org (accessed December 24, 2007).

Clarke M, Locker D, Berall G, Pencharz P, Kenny DJ, and Judd P. 2006. Malnourishment in a population of young children with severe early childhood caries. *Pediatr Dent* 28:254–9.

Cleaton-Jones P. 2002. No Consensus on definition of early childhood caries. *Evidence-Based Dent* 3:75.

Cleaton-Jones P, Richardson BD, McInnes PM, and Fatti LP. March 1978. Dental caries in South African white children aged 1–5 years. *Community Dent Oral Epidemiol* 6(2):78–81.

Cone TE. 1981. The nursing bottle caries syndrome. *JAMA* 245(22):2334.

Community Dentistry and Oral Epidemiology. 1998. *Conference on Early Childhood Caries, Bethesda, MD*. October 1997. Community Dentistry and Oral Epidemiology 1998;16(Suppl 1).

Donaldson AN, Everitt B, Newton T, Steele J, Sherriff M, and Bower E. 2008. The effects of social class and dental attendance on oral health. *J Dent Res* 87(1):60–64.

Dorland's Medical Dictionary for Health Care Consumers. 2007. Saunders: Elsevier Press.

Douglass JM, Li Y, and Tinanoff N. 2008. Association of mutans streptococci between caregivers and their children. *Pediatr Dent* 30(5):375–87.

Douglass JM, Tinanoff N, Tang JMW, and Altman DS. 2001. Dental caries patterns and oral health behaviors in Arizona infants and toddlers. *Community Dent Oral Epidemiol* 29:14–22.

Douglass JM, Wei Y, Zhang JM, and Tinanoff N. 1994. Dental caries in preschool Beijing and Connecticut children as described by a new caries analysis system. *Community Dent Oral Epidemiol* 22:94–9.

Drury TF, Horowitz AM, Ismail AI, Maertens MP, Rozier RG, and Selwitz RH. 1999. Diagnosing and reporting early childhood caries for research purposes. *J Pub Health Dent* 59(3):192–7.

Dye BA, Shenkin JD, Ogden CL, Marshall TA, Levy SM, and Kanellis MJ. 2004. The relationship between healthful eating practices and dental caries in children aged 2–5 years in the United States, 1988–1994. *J Am Dent Assoc* 135:55–66.

Dye BA, Tan S, Smith V, Lewis BG, Barker LK, Thornton-Evans G, Eke PI, Beltrán-Aguilar ED, Horowitz AM, and Li CH. 2007. Trends in oral health status: United States, 1988–1994 and 1999–2004. National Center for Health Statistics. *Vital Health Stat* 11(248).

Edelstein BL. 2002. Dental care considerations for young children. *Spec Care Dent* 22(3, Suppl):11S–25.

Edelstein BL and Douglass CW. 1995. Dispelling the myth that 50 percent of US schoolchildren have never had a cavity. *Public Health Rep* 110(5):522–30.

Edelstein BE, Vargas CM, Candelaria D, and Vemuri M. 2006. Experience and policy implications of children presenting with dental emergencies to US pediatric dentistry training programs. *Pediatr Dent* 28(5):431–7.

Fass EN. 1962. Is bottle feeding of milk a factor in dental caries? *J Dent Child* 29:245–51.

Gift HC, Reisine ST, and Larach DC. 1992. The social impact of dental problems and visits. *Am J Public Health* 82(12):1663–8.

Goose DH. 1967. Infant feeding and caries of the incisors: An epidemiological approach. *Caries Res* 1:166–73.

Greer MH, Tegan SL, Hu K, and Takata JT. 2003. Early childhood caries among Hawaii public school children, 1989 versus 1999. *Pac Health Dialog* 10:17–22.

Grindefjord M, Dahllof G, and Modeer T. 1995. Caries development in children from 2.5 to 3.5 years of age: A longitudinal study. *Caries Res* 29:449–54.

Hollister MC and Weintraub JA. 1993. The association of oral status with systemic health, quality of life, and economic productivity. *J Dent Educ* 57:901–9.

Holt RD, Joels D, and Winter GB. 1982. Caries in pre-school children. The Camden study. *Br Dent J* 153(3):107–9.

Iida H, Auinger P, Billings R, and Weitzman M. 2007. Association between infant breastfeeding and early childhood caries in the United States. *Pediatrics* 120(4):e944–52.

Indian Health Service. 1999. *Oral Health Survey of American Indian and Alaskan Native Dental Patients.* 2002 Division of Dental Services. Rockville, MD: Indian Health Service.

Ismail AI and Sohn W. 1999. A systematic review of clinical diagnostic criteria of early childhood caries. *J Pub Health Dent* 59(3):171–91.

Johnsen D. 1984. Dental caries patterns in preschool children. *Dent Clin North Am* 28:3–20.

Johnsen D, Schultz D, Schubot D, and Easley M. 1984. Caries patterns in Head Start children in a fluoridated community. *J Public Health Dent* 44:61–6.

Johnsen DC, Bhat M, Kim MT, Hagman FT, Alice LM, Credong RL, and Easley MW. 1986a. Caries levels and patterns in Head Start children in fluoridated and non-fluoridated, urban and nonurban sites in Ohio, USA. *Community Dent Oral Epidemiol* 14:206–9.

Johnsen DC, Gerstenmaier JH, DiSantis TA, and Berkowitz RJ. 1986b. Susceptibility of nursing-caries children to future approximal molar decay. *Pediatr Dent* 8:168–71.

Johnsen DC, Schechner TG, and Gerstenmaier JH. 1987. Proportional changes in caries patterns from early to late primary dentition. *J Public Health Dent* 47(1):5–9.

Johnsen DC, Schubot D, Bhat M, and Jones PK. 1993. Caries pattern identification in primary dentition: A comparison of clinician assignment and clinical analysis groupings. *Pediatr Dent* 15(2):113–5.

Kaste LM, Drury TF, Horowitz AM, and Beltran E. 1999. An evaluation of NHANES III estimates of early childhood caries. *J Public Health Dent* 59(3):198–200.

Kelly M, and Bruerd B. 1987. The prevalence of baby bottle tooth decay among two Native American populations. *J Public Health Dent* 47(2): 94–7.

Kotlow LA. 1977. Breastfeeding: A cause of dental caries in children. *ASDC J Dent Child* 44(3):192–3.

Kramer MS, Vanilovich I, Matush L, Bogdanovich N, Zhang X, Shishko G, Muller-Bolla M, and Platt RW. 2007. The effect of prolonged and exclusive breast-feeding on dental caries in early school-age children: New evidence from a large randomized trial. *Caries Res* 41:484–8.

Li S-H, Kingman A, Forthofer R, and Swango P. 1993. Comparison of tooth surface-specific dental caries attack patterns in US schoolchildren from two national surveys. *J Dent Res* 72(10):1398–405.

Low W, Tan S, and Schwartz S. 1999. The effect of severe caries on the quality of life of young children. *Pediatr Dent* 21:325–6.

Maki K, Morimoto A, Nishioka T, Kimura M, and Braham RL. 1999. The impact of race on tooth formation. *ASDC J Dent Child* 66(5):353–6.

Manski RJ and Brown E. 2007. *Dental Use, Expenses, Private Dental Coverage, and Changes, 1996 and 2004.* Rockville, MD: Agency for Healthcare Research and Quality. MEPS Chartbook No. 17. Available at http://www.meps.ahrq.gov/mepsweb/data_files/publications/cb17/cb17.pdf (accessed December 29, 2007).

Mariri BP, Levy SM, Warren JJ, Bergus GR, Marshall TA, and Broffitt B. 2003. Medically administered antibiotics, dietary habits, fluoride intake, and dental caries experience in the primary dentition. *Community Dent Oral Epidemiol* 31:40–51.

Marmot M and Wilkinson R (eds). 1999. *Social Determinants of Health.* New York, NY: Oxford University Press.

McGrath C, Broder H, and Wilson-Genderson M. 2004. Assessing the impact of oral health on the life quality of children: Implications for research and practice. *Community Dent Oral Epidemiol* 32:81–5.

Nishimura M, Oda T, Kariya N, Matsumura S, and Shimono T. 2008. Using a caries activity test to predict caries risk in early childhood. *J Am Dent Assoc* 139:63–71.

O'Sullivan DM and Tinanoff N. 1993. Maxillary anterior caries associated with increased caries risk in other primary teeth. *J Dent Res* 72(12):1577–80.

O'Sullivan DM and Tinanoff N. 1996. The association of early dental caries patterns with caries incidence in preschool children. *J Public Health Dent* 56(2):81–3.

Peres MA, do Rosario M, de Oliveira Latorre D, Sheiham A, Peres KG, Barros FC, Hernandez PG, Nunes Maas AM, Romano AR, and Victora CG. 2005. Social and biological early life influences on severity of dental caries in children aged 6 years. *Community Dent Oral Epidemiol* 33:53–63.

Pierce KM, Rozier GR, and William FV. 2002. Accuracy of pediatric primary care providers' screening and referral for early childhood caries. *Pediatrics* 109(5):e82.

Powell D. January 1976. Milk: Is it related to rampant caries of the early primary dentition? *J Calif Dent Assoc* 4(1):58–63.

Psoter WJ, Morse DE, Pendrys DG, Zhang H, and Mayne ST. 2004. Historical evolution of primary dentition caries pattern definitions. *Pediatr Dent* 26(5):508–11.

Psoter WJ, Pendrys DG, Morse DE, Zhang H, and Mayne ST. 2006. Associations of ethnicity/race and socioeconomic status with early childhood caries patterns. *J Public Health Dent* 66(1):23–9.

Psoter WJ, Zhang H, Pendrys DG, Morse DE, and Mayne ST. 2003. Classification of dental caries patterns in the primary dentition: A multidimensional scaling analysis. *Community Dent Oral Epidemiol* 31:231–8.

Reforming States Group. 1999. *Pediatric Dental Care in CHIP and Medicaid: Paying for What Kids Need, Getting Value for State Payments*. New York, NY: Milbank Memorial Fund.

Reisine ST. 1988. The impact of dental conditions on social functioning and quality of life. *Annu Rev Public Health* 9:1–19.

Reisine ST. 1989. The impact of dental conditions on patients' quality of life. *Comm Dent Health* 17(1):7–10.

Richardson BD, Cleaton-Jones PE, McInnes PM, and Rantsho JM. 1981. Infant feeding practices and nursing bottle caries. *ASDC J Dent Child* 48(6):423–9.

Ring ME. 1985. *Dentistry: An Illustrated History*. New York, NY: Abrams.

Rule J. 1982. Recognition of dental caries. *Pediatr Clin North Am* 29:439–56.

Sheiham A. 2006. Dental caries affects body weight, growth and quality of life in pre-school children. *Br Dent J* 201:625–6.

Sheiham A and Watt RG. 2000. The common risk factor approach: A rational basis for promoting oral health. *Community Dent Oral Epidemiol* 28:399–406.

Shiboski CH, Gansky SA, Ramos-Gomez F, Ngo L, Isman R, and Pollick HF. 2003. The association of early childhood caries and race/ethnicity among California preschool children. *J Public Health Dent* 63:38–46.

Slayton RL, Warren JJ, Kanellis MJ, Levy SM, and Islam M. 2001. Prevalence of enamel hypopolasia and isolated opacities in the primary dentition. *Pediatr Dent* 23(1):32–6.

Sohn W, Burt BA, and Sowers MR. 2006. Carbonated soft drinks and dental caries in the primary dentition. *J Dent Res* 85:262–6.

Tang JM, Altman DS, Robertson DC, O'Sullivan DM, Douglass JM, and Tinanoff N. 1997. Dental caries prevalence and treatment levels in Arizona preschool children. *Pub Health Rep* 112:319–29.

Thibodeau EA and O'Sullivan DM. 1996. Salivary mutans streptococci and dental caries patterns in pre-school children. *Community Dent Oral Epidemiol* 24(3):164–8.

Thomson WM, Poulton R, Milne BJ, Caspi A, Broughton JR, and Ayers KMS. 2004. Socioeconomic inequalities in oral health in childhood and adulthood in a birth cohort. *Community Dent Oral Epidemiol* 32:345–53.

Tinanoff N and O'Sullivan DM. 1997. Early childhood caries: Overview and recent findings. *Pediatr Dent* 19(1):12–6.

Urban Child Institute. 2006. *A Closer Look at the Social Determinants of Health*. Issue Brief. September 13, 2006.

U.S. Department of Health and Human Services, Health Resources and Services Administration, Maternal and Child Health Bureau. 2005. *The National Survey of Children's Health 2003*. Rockville, MD: U.S. Department of Health and Human Services.

vanHoute H. 1994. Role of microorganisms in caries. *J Dent Res* 67:2–81.

Vanobbergen J, Lesaffre E, Garcia-Zattera MJ, Martens JA, and Declerck D. 2007. Caries patterns in primary dentition in 3-, 5- and 7-year-old children: Spatial correlation and preventive consequences. *Caries Res* 41(1):16–25.

Veerkamp JSJ and Weerheijm KL. 1995. Nursing-bottle caries: The importance of a developmental perspective. *J Dent Child* 62:381–6.

Warren JJ, Levy SM, Broffitt B, and Kanellis MJ. 2006. Longitudinal study of non-cavitated carious lesion progression in the primary dentition. *J Public Health Dent* 66(2):83–7.

Warren JJ, Slayton RL, Yonezu T, Kanellis MJ, and Levy SM. 2003. Interdental spacing and caries in the primary dentition. *Pediatr Dent* 25(2):109–13.

White H, Lee JY, and Vann WF, Jr. 2003. Parental evaluation of quality of life measures following pediatric dental treatment using general anesthesia. *Anesth Prog* 50:105–10.

Winter GB, Hamilton MC, and James PMC. 1966. Role of the comforter as an aetiological factor in rampant caries of the deciduous dentition. *Arch Dis Child* 41:207–12.

Wyne AH. 1999. Early childhood caries: Nomenclature and case definition. *Community Dent Oral Epidemiol* 27:313–5.

Managing caries: Obtaining arrest

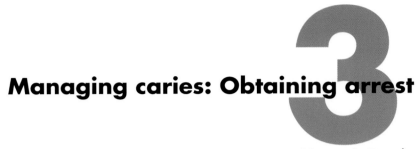

Kevin J. Donly

DIAGNOSTIC TECHNIQUES

To aid in the reduction of dental caries, the disease must be viewed as an infectious disease. As with all infectious diseases, prevention is paramount in controlling disease initiation and progression. When disease is established, early diagnosis and reversal of lesion progression is critical to maintaining a sound oral balance. The diagnosis of children to be at high risk for the development of caries is important. The American Academy of Pediatric Dentistry (2007a) developed a caries-risk assessment tool referred to as the CAT, which can be very helpful in identifying children that may be at a higher risk for the development of caries. Clinical diagnostic techniques are of absolute importance so that early lesions can be identified prior to cavitation and an attempt for repair can be initiated.

Visual examination

Visual examination has been the primary method for diagnosing primary and secondary caries. The specificity of visual examination shows great variance through clinical trials (Wenzel et al., 1991; Verdonschot et al., 1992; Lussi, 1993, 1996; Le and Verdonschot, 1994). A reason for the significant differences in the visual examination is the differences in the status of occlusal surfaces. Dentinal caries under an apparent intact occlusal surface is difficult to detect. Low diagnostic sensitivity is associated with these types of carious lesions (Creanor et al., 1990; Kidd et al., 1992a; Weerheijm et al., 1992a, b).

The combination of visual examination and probing the enamel surface with a dental explorer, although traditionally the standard of care, is not recommended today because the dental explorer can transfer cariogenic microorganisms from one site to another and damage the integrity of the enamel surface, which can promote caries development (Loesche et al., 1979; Ekstrand et al., 1987; van Dorp et al., 1988).

Secondary caries is very difficult to detect at early stages. Secondary caries along the margins of restorations, referred to as wall lesions, cannot be easily detected until it has progressed to an advanced stage (Kidd et al., 1992b). Probing with dental explorers has been demonstrated to be not an accurate method for diagnosing secondary caries (Merrett and Elderton, 1984).

Discoloration has been an integral component to clinical visual examination. White spot lesions are the earliest signs of enamel demineralization. Although these white spot lesions indicate early enamel demineralization visually, the typical white spot lesion is approximately 500 μm in depth before it becomes visually apparent. Discoloration is also an integral component to the diagnosis of secondary caries (Kidd et al., 1995). Stained restoration margins and ditched restoration margins are not necessarily signs of dental caries, although they are indicators of greater risk for caries development (Kidd and Beighton, 1996).

Transillumination

Bitewing radiographs have been the standard of care for evaluating proximal surfaces of teeth. Fiber-optic transillumination (FOTI) has also been recommended for use in the evaluation of proximal tooth surfaces (Peers et al., 1993; Pine and ten Bosch, 1996). Likewise, FOTI has been recommended for the evaluation of occlusal tooth surfaces (Verdonschot et al., 1992). The FOTI method has been found to be a good adjunctive diagnostic technique to visual examination, particularly when lesions are restricted to enamel (Wenzel et al., 1992; Côrtes et al., 2000).

Digital imaging fiber-optic transillumination (DIFOTI) has also been recommended for use in the diagnosis of proximal tooth surfaces, as well as occlusal surfaces. This diagnostic method has been found to be superior to bitewing radiographs (Schneiderman et al., 1997).

Laser fluorescence

Infrared laser fluorescence has become an increasingly popular method utilized for caries diagnosis. The specific device is DIAGNOdent (KaVo, Biberach, Germany). DIAGNOdent is a noninvasive technique for detection and quantification of demineralization, which utilizes the illumination of a tooth with a laser light (655 nm) that is absorbed by both inorganic and organic tooth substance, as well as metabolites from oral bacteria (Hibst and Gall, 1998; Longbottom et al., 1998; Lussi et al., 1998; Hibst and Paulus, 2000). Different tips can be placed on the DIAGNOdent handpiece that emits a near-infrared fluorescent light. As tooth demineralization progresses, an increase in emitted fluorescent light occurs. The DIAGNOdent instrument detects this light and presents a digital readout number—the higher the number the greater the emitted fluorescent light, which is interpreted as the extent of demineralization.

Studies report that laser fluorescence can be useful for the diagnosis of caries in both the permanent dentition and the primary dentition, particularly when lesions have progressed into dentin (Heinrich-Weltzien et al., 2002; Rocha et al., 2003). Lesions that have progressed into dentin have been shown to be detected significantly better with laser fluorescence compared to visual inspection (Lussi and Francescut, 2003). However, other studies report that laser fluorescence presents similar accuracy when compared to visual inspection (Sheehy et al., 2001; Anttonen et al., 2003; Rocha et al., 2003; Burin et al., 2005). At this point, we can accept the recommendation that laser fluorescence is a good adjunctive diagnostic method to confirm the presence of dental caries that has progressed to dentin.

Laser fluorescence has also been evaluated as a means of detecting secondary caries adjacent to restorations (Ando et al., 2004). Laser fluorescence showed values higher or similar to visible inspection, resulting in the recommendation that laser fluorescence may improve the ability to detect early secondary caries.

Laser fluorescence has been evaluated for monitoring the remineralization of incipient carious lesions in primary teeth (Mendes et al., 2003). This is important so that the clinician can ascertain whether the lesion is progressing and needs aggressive intervention or if remineralization is occurring. The study found that laser fluorescence was not able to detect remineralization of natural incipient caries lesions. This would appear to agree with the concept that DIAGNOdent is much more accurate in detecting lesions extending to dentin. Lesions with DIAGNOdent readings of less than 20, which have been shown to be related to dentin lesions less than 50% of the time, are less accurate than readings above 20 (Lussi et al., 2001; Heinrich-Weltzien et al., 2002).

Quantitative light fluorescence

Quantitative light-induced fluorescence (QLF) is another noninvasive technique for detection and quantification of demineralization, which utilizes the illumination of a tooth with filtered visible light (van der Veen and de Josselin de Jong, 2000). Teeth are illuminated with an arc lamp using a light guide with peak intensity of 370 nm. A filter (520 nm) is placed in front of a charge-coupled device microcamera that captures the tooth image and displays the image on a computer screen (Figure 3.1). Images can be saved on the hard drive of the computer.

Demineralized enamel will fluoresce less than sound intact enamel, and the loss of fluorescence can be detected, quantified, and longitudinally monitored (Pretty et al., 2002). The analysis program detects less fluorescent areas of the image and simulates the fluorescence radiance of sound enamel at the lesion site with a reconstruction algorithm. This is accomplished by a two-dimensional linear interpolation of sound enamel values adjacent to the lesion. Decrease in fluorescence is calculated from the percentage loss between actual and reconstructed fluorescence, being expressed as change in fluorescence (ΔF). Area of the lesion is also calculated; this value being defined as the fluorescence radiance loss integrated over the lesion area, representing the total mineral loss from the lesions as measured by transverse microradiography (TMR). TMR is considered the current gold standard from demineralization analysis. QLF has been validated against TMR in enamel evaluation and has demonstrated excellent agreement, the analysis method being proved as reliable and reproducible (van der Veen and de Josselin de Jong, 2000; Pretty et al., 2001).

QLF has also been evaluated for the detection of secondary caries (Ando et al., 2004). This study suggests that QLF can improve the ability to detect early secondary caries.

Overall, studies have demonstrated that QLF is excellent for detecting very early mineral loss (less than 100 μm), as well as more aggressive loss of enamel, and offers the opportunity to monitor lesions longitudinally.

Radiographs

Radiographs can be very difficult to obtain on children of age 3 years and less. When spacing is seen between teeth, and direct visual evaluation can be made, radiographs are not necessary. However, when teeth are in

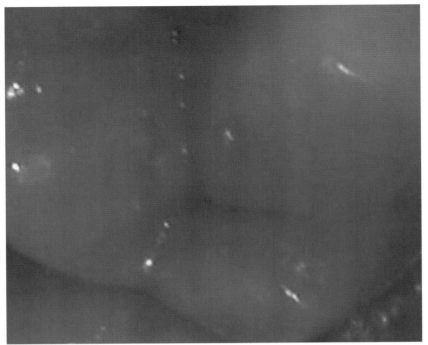

(a)

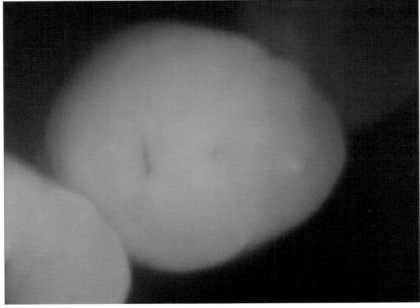

(b)

Figure 3.1   (a) A close-up view (×10 magnification) of the distal pit and fissure of a maxillary first molar. (b) The same tooth viewed with quantitative light fluorescence. Note the demineralized area of the distal pit and fissure that was not apparent by visual examination (a).

TYPE OF ENCOUNTER	PATIENT AGE AND DENTAL DEVELOPMENTAL STAGE				
	Child with Primary Dentition (prior to eruption of first permanent tooth)	Child with Transitional Dentition (after eruption of first permanent tooth)	Adolescent with Permanent Dentition (prior to eruption of third molars)	Adult Dentate or Partially Edentulous	Adult Edentulous
New patient* being evaluated for dental diseases and dental development	Individualized radiographic exam consisting of selected periapical/occlusal views and/or posterior bitewings if proximal surfaces cannot be visualized or probed. Patients without evidence of disease and with open proximal contacts may not require a radiographic exam at this time.	Individualized radiographic exam consisting of posterior bitewings with panoramic exam or posterior bitewings and selected periapical images.	Individualized radiographic exam consisting of posterior bitewings with panoramic exam or posterior bitewings and selected periapical images. A full mouth intraoral radiographic exam is preferred when the patient has clinical evidence of generalized dental disease or a history of extensive dental treatment.		Individualized radiographic exam, based on clinical signs and symptoms.
Recall patient* with clinical caries or increased risk for caries**	Posterior bitewing exam at 6-12 month intervals if proximal surfaces cannot be examined visually or with a probe			Posterior bitewing exam at 6-18 month intervals	Not applicable
Recall patient* with no clinical caries and no increased risk for caries**	Posterior bitewing exam at 12-24 month intervals if proximal surfaces cannot be examined visually or with a probe		Posterior bitewing exam at 18-36 month intervals	Posterior bitewing exam at 24-36 month intervals	Not applicable
Recall patient* with periodontal disease	Clinical judgment as to the need for and type of radiographic images for the evaluation of periodontal disease. Imaging may consist of, but is not limited to, selected bitewing and/or periapical images of areas where periodontal disease (other than nonspecific gingivitis) can be identified clinically.				Not applicable
Patient for monitoring of growth and development	Clinical judgment as to need for and type of radiographic images for evaluation and/or monitoring of dentofacial growth and development		Clinical judgment as to need for and type of radiographic images for evaluation and/or monitoring of dento-facial growth and development. Panoramic or periapical exam to assess developing third molars	Usually not indicated	
Patient with other circumstances including, but not limited to, proposed or existing implants, pathology, restorative/endodontic needs, treated periodontal disease and caries remineralization	Clinical judgment as to need for and type of radiographic images for evaluation and/or monitoring in these conditions				

*Clinical situations for which radiographs may be indicated include but are not limited to:

A. Positive Historical Findings
1. Previous periodontal or endodontic treatment
2. History of pain or trauma
3. Familial history of dental anomalies
4. Postoperative evaluation of healing
5. Remineralization monitoring
6. Presence of implants or evaluation for implant placement

B. Positive Clinical Signs/Symptoms
1. Clinical evidence of periodontal disease
2. Large or deep restorations
3. Deep carious lesions
4. Malposed or clinically impacted teeth
5. Swelling
6. Evidence of dental/facial trauma
7. Mobility of teeth
8. Sinus tract ("fistula")

9. Clinically suspected sinus pathology
10. Growth abnormalities
11. Oral involvement in known or suspected systemic disease
12. Positive neurologic findings in the head and neck
13. Evidence of foreign objects
14. Pain and/or dysfunction of the temporomandibular joint
15. Facial asymmetry
16. Abutment teeth for fixed or removable partial prosthesis
17. Unexplained bleeding
18. Unexplained sensitivity of teeth
19. Unusual eruption, spacing or migration of teeth
20. Unusual tooth morphology, calcification or color
21. Unexplained absence of teeth
22. Clinical erosion

**Factors increasing risk for caries may include but are not limited to:
1. High level of caries experience or demineralization
2. History of recurrent caries
3. High titers of cariogenic bacteria
4. Existing restoration(s) of poor quality
5. Poor oral hygiene
6. Inadequate fluoride exposure
7. Prolonged nursing (bottle or breast)
8. Frequent high sucrose content in diet
9. Poor family dental health
10. Developmental or acquired enamel defects
11. Developmental or acquired disability
12. Xerostomia
13. Genetic abnormality of teeth
14. Many multisurface restorations
15. Chemo/radiation therapy
16. Eating disorders
17. Drug/alcohol abuse
18. Irregular dental care

Figure 3.2 Guidelines on prescribing dental radiographs for infants, children, adolescents, and persons with special health care needs. Reprinted from *Pediatric Dentistry* with permission from the American Academy of Pediatric Dentistry (American Academy of Pediatric Dentistry, 2007b).

contact, making visual evaluation impossible, radiographs are recommended according to American Academy of Pediatric Dentistry Guidelines (2007b) (Figure 3.2). Risk assessment and behavior of the child become important factors. Every attempt should be made to obtain radiographs on children at high risk with closed contacts between the teeth. Parents holding the child may comfort the patient and improve the possibility of obtaining radiographs. Likewise, using Snap-O-Ray (Dentsply Rinn, Elgin, IL) radiographic film holders offer a thick "biting surface," which decreases gagging and allows for obtaining radiographs easier.

When caries is clinically diagnosed, radiographs are important. When carious lesions appear to extend to the tooth pulp, a periapical radiograph is indicated. A periapical radiograph is also indicated when trauma occurs. This allows the clinician the opportunity to evaluate the root of the tooth and surrounding structures, as well as the extent of trauma to the tooth and pulp. Children experiencing active caries should have radiographs exposed more frequently, such as 6-month intervals, than children not experiencing caries activity. Caries-free children may have radiographic evaluation extended up to 2 years, should they remain at low risk during caries-risk assessment.

Children treated in the operating room follow the same radiographic evaluation recommended guidelines. Teeth with caries should have radiographs. Bitewing radiographs are recommended for posterior teeth in proximal contact and periapical radiographs are recommended for teeth that have carious lesions encroaching on or involving the pulp.

EARLY INTERVENTION

Early diagnosis of enamel demineralization allows for early intervention to remineralize enamel and to evaluate the reason for demineralization. The oral balance of demineralization/remineralization must be controlled to prevent progression of early lesions and the initiation of new lesions.

Rebalancing the oral cavity

The oral cavity exists in a state of perpetual change. The biofilm is a community of bacteria that is constantly changing. As dental disease occurs, there has been a shift in the oral cavity that needs to be rebalanced to create a healthy oral environment. This would include adjusting pH, affected by diet and aciduric/acidogenic bacteria. Remineralization minerals can be adjusted by increasing salivary flow or adding remineralizing ions such as calcium, phosphate, and fluoride to the oral environment. Risk assessments, including the presence of white spot lesions, are early identifiers that the patient needs to be further assessed for causative factors and appropriately treated to rebalance the system.

Bacterial testing

Research has indicated that patients with high levels of *mutans streptococci* are at higher risk to develop caries (Berkowitz, 1996). Children that acquire *mutans streptococci* by 2 years of age are at higher risk to develop caries by age 4 than those that had not acquired the bacteria by age 2 (Kohler et al., 1988). Likewise, children of mothers that have high levels of intraoral bacteria are more susceptible to dental caries, the transmission of the bacteria from mother to child being associated with the increased risk for caries (Berkowitz et al., 1981; Berkowitz and Jones, 1985; Caufield et al., 1988). There are bacterial testing systems available that can indicate bacteria levels in the oral cavity and can be helpful in completing a risk assessment. These diagnostic systems are specific to actual bacteria presence and to bacterial acid production.

Antimicrobials

Chlorhexidine

Chlorhexidine has demonstrated antimicrobial effectiveness through numerous well-controlled clinical trials (Lang and Brecx, 1986; Anderson, 2003). Chlorhexidine is 1,6-bis-4-chloro-phenyldiguanidohexane, a synthetic cationic detergent. It has great bacteriostatic and bacteriocidal features and was originally used to treat dermatologic infections, wound surfaces, and eye and throat infections.

When chlorhexidine was originally tested for efficacy in plaque control, 10 mL of a 0.2% chlorhexidine digluconate rinse demonstrated successful plaque control with subsequent inhibition of gingivitis (Davies et al., 1970; Löe and Schiött, 1970). Other studies have demonstrated the effectiveness of 0.12% chlorhexidine digluconate solution, the formulation available in the United States, to effectively reduce plaque and gingivitis (Lang and Briner, 1984; Siegrist et al., 1986).

The cationic chlorhexidine molecule binds to anionic compounds, such as free sulfates, carboxyl and phosphate groups, and salivary glycoproteins (Rölla and Melsen, 1975). This action will reduce the adsorption of proteins to the tooth surface, delaying the formation of the dental pellicle. Chlorhexidine molecules also coat salivary bacteria, which alter the mechanisms of adsorption of bacteria to the tooth.

Chlorhexidine is active against gram-positive and gram-negative microorganisms, as well as yeast cells. Due to the high cationic nature of chlorhexidine, it has an affinity for the cell wall of bacteria and changes the surface structures, whereby osmotic equilibrium is lost. This consequently extrudes the cytoplasmic membrane and the cytoplasm precipitates, which inhibits the repair of the cell wall (Davies, 1973).

The main side effects of chlorhexidine are staining of the teeth and, taste and the content of ethyl alcohol. The stain on the teeth can be easily removed with a pumice prophylaxis. Since chlorhexidine can temporarily affect taste sensations, use around mealtimes is not recommended. The high-alcohol content of chlorhexidine becomes a factor when using it with children. Children must be of the age where they can expectorate the rinse and not swallow it. Since this is a problem with very young children, the chlorhexidine can be carefully applied to the teeth with cotton-tipped swabs, limiting the amount of agent exposure.

It has been recommended that high-risk patients with high intraoral bacterial levels rinse 10 mL of 0.12% chlorhexidine digluconate solution once per day for 1 week every 6 months (Featherstone, 2006). Since children less than 3 years of age would not be appropriate for rinsing, this would be more pertinent to mothers at high risk for caries development with high intraoral bacterial levels.

Chlorhexidine is also available in gels and varnish; however, these are not currently available in the United States marketplace. The gels containing chlorhexidine have contained 1 or 2% chlorhexidine digluconate. The 2% gel has been shown to be effective when used as a dermatologic wound healing agent (Asboe-Jörgensen et al., 1974). Gels with 1% chlorhexidine digluconate incorporated into the gel have shown efficacy in reducing caries when applied for 5 min per day over a period of 2 weeks (Zickert et al., 1982). The chlorhexidine does not diffuse as rapidly from a gel as a rinse; therefore, it needs a longer contact time, as well as direct application to the tooth surface, to be effective.

In a longitudinal study using 0.2% chlorhexidine gel weekly in 10-month-old infants, it was found that no differences were observed when compared to a placebo group and to a treatment group at follow-up evaluations after 3 months (Wan et al., 2003).

A clinical trial evaluating the use of a 40%, by weight, chlorhexidine varnish in Chinese preschool children indicated a positive anticaries effect. The preschool children received 6-monthly applications of the 40% chlorhexidine varnish and a control group received a placebo varnish at the same application intervals. At 2 years, the chlorhexidine group demonstrated a 37% reduction in caries compared to the control. This chlorhexidine varnish anticariogenic effect was also seen in children evaluated in other studies (Achong et al., 1999; Forgie et al., 2000).

Iodine

Studies have indicated that topical iodine agents can significantly suppress levels of *mutans streptococci* (Lopez et al., 1999, 2002). Therefore, studies have examined the effectiveness of iodine agents to inhibit the development of early childhood caries. The application of 10% povidone iodine, to the tooth surfaces of 83 high-caries-risk children (12–19 months), was performed every 2 months in a study for duration of 12 months. The children that received this treatment developed significantly fewer white spot lesions than a control group that received treatment with a placebo agent. Further research will indicate the long-term effects of iodine treatment, when it is being applied and when it has been removed as an antibacterial agent.

Xylitol

Xylitol is a sugar substitute that has 40% fewer calories than sucrose (Lindley et al., 1976). Xylitol is a sugar alcohol that is produced from birch trees, or other trees containing xylan, corncobs, fruits, and sugarcane bagasse. The U.S. Food and Drug Administration (FDA) has approved xylitol for human consumption and it is safe, with no known side effects when used at the doses appropriate for sweetening effects (Ly et al., 2006). Diarrhea can occur when xylitol is consumed in large quantities.

Sugar alcohols, such as xylitol, sorbitol, mannitol, and maltitol, have been shown to be noncariogenic (Hayes, 2001; Roberts et al., 2002). The literature indicates that xylitol also reduces the level of *mutans streptococci* in plaque and reduces the level of lactic acid produced by bacteria (Trahan, 1995).

Xylitol consumption in the range of 6–10 g per day, divided into at least three time periods, is effective in reducing bacteria levels and subsequent drop in acid production (Ly et al., 2006). The delivery of xylitol for caries protection is usually gum. Although xylitol-containing gums have demonstrated great success in reducing caries, very young children may have difficulty chewing gum and may have a tendency to swallow the gum. Further evaluation of xylitol-sweetened snacks and drinks may prove beneficial for younger children.

The influence of maternal xylitol consumption on the mother's transmission of bacteria to their child has also been evaluated (Söderling et al., 2000, 2001). Xylitol has been shown to reduce bacteria in the oral cavity; therefore, the potential for this to reduce the transmission from mother to child would be a means to reduce early childhood caries. Mothers that regularly chewed xylitol-sweetened gum for 21 months, starting 3 months after birth of their infant, had reduced mother–child transmission of *mutans streptococci*. Further investigation revealed that this significant reduction in bacterial transmission continued with the children of mothers who had chewed xylitol gum, with 27% being colonized by 3 years of age and 51% being colonized by 6 years of age.

Xylitol is also available in wipes to clean the teeth of infants. This can be an effective means of providing oral hygiene maintenance and xylitol at the same time. There are many other products that contain xylitol that is noted in Figures 3.3 and 3.4 (Ly et al., 2006).

Saliva

Saliva is very important in providing remineralization effects for tooth structure. Since saliva is supersaturated with calcium and phosphate, which bathes the teeth, remineralization can occur with the deposition of minerals into subsurface enamel lesions.

Saliva is also important as a buffering agent. This is critical to control the pH of the oral environment. Buffering can be attributed, in part, to bicarbonate in stimulated salivary secretions and peptides, as well as amino acids in unstimulated saliva (Van Wuyckhuyse et al., 1995). Furthermore, salivary proteins aid in antimicrobial activity by inhibiting bacterial growth (Tabak, 2006). Examples of these proteins would include histatins, lactoferrin, peroxidase, and lysozyme.

Products[†]	Xylitol per piece (g) [total polyols (g)]	Pieces for 6 (10) g/d	Preventive Potential[‡]	Approximate Cost/10 pieces
Gums				
Epic–xylitol gum (various flavors)	1.05	6 (10)	Yes	$0.70–$1.00 online
Clen-Dent/Xponent gum (various flavors)	0.67	10 (15)	Yes	$1.60–$1.70 retail
Fennobon Oy "XyliMax Gum"	0.86	7 (12)	Yes	$0.80–$1.00 online
Hershey "Carefree Koolerz Gum" (various flavors)	1.50	4 (7)	Yes	$0.95–$1.50 retail
Lotte–xylitol gum (various flavors)	0.65	9 (15)	Yes	$0.70–$0.80 online
Omnii "Theragum"	0.70	9 (14)	Yes	$1.25–$1.50 online
Spry Xylitol gum (various flavors)	0.72	8 (14)	Yes	$0.70–$0.90 online
Tundra Trading "XyliChew Gum"	0.80	8 (13)	Yes	$1.50–$1.65 retail
Vitamin Research "Unique Sweet Gum"	0.72	9 (14)	Yes	$1.00 online
WellDent "Xylitol Gum"	0.70	9 (14)	Yes	$0.90–$1.00 online
Altoids Sugar-Free Chewing Gum	First of 3 polyols (1.0)	NC[§]	Maybe	$0.90–$1.00 retail
B-FRESH Gums (various flavors)	First of 2 polyols (1.0)	NC	Maybe	$0.70 online
Starbucks "After Coffee Gum" Peppermint	First of 2 polyols (1.0)	NC	Maybe	$1.00 retail
Arm & Hammer "Dental Care Baking Soda Gum"	Second of 3 polyols (1.0)	NC	No	$0.80–$1.00 retail
Arm & Hammer "Advance White Icy Mint Gum"	Second of 3 polyols (1.0)	NC	No	$1.00–$1.30 retail
Biotene "Dental Gum" and "Dry Mouth Gum"	Second of 2 polyols (1.0)	NC	No	$1.00–$1.40 retail
Eco-Dent "Between Dental Gum" (various flavors)	0.35	17 (29)	No	$1.05–$1.40 online
Warner-Lambert "Trident Gum with Xylitol"	Second of 3 polyols (1.0)	NC	No	$0.60–$0.70 retail
Warner-Lambert "Trident for Kids Gum"	Third of 3 polyols (1.0)	NC	No	$1.20–$1.40 retail
Wrigley "Orbit Sugar-Free Gum"	Third of 3 polyols (1.0)	NC	No	$0.45 REI online
Ford Gum "Xtreme Xylitol Gums"	NC	NC	NC	$0.65–$0.85 online
Wrigley "Everest Mint Gum"	NC	NC	NC	$0.45 REI online
Mints				
Clen-Dent/Xponent "Mints"	0.67	9 (15)	Yes	$0.62–$0.70 online
Epic "Xylitol Mints" 0.50	0.50	12 (20)	Maybe	$0.35–$0.50 online
Omnii "Theramints"	0.50	12 (20)	Maybe	$0.45 online
Spry "Mints"	0.50	12 (20)	Maybe	$0.38–$0.49 online
Tundra Trading "XyliChew Mints"	0.55	11 (18)	Maybe	$0.35–$0.50 retail
VitaDent "Mints"/"Unique Sweet Mints"	0.50	12 (20)	Maybe	$0.62–$0.65 online
WellDent "Xylitol Mints"	0.55	11 (18)	Maybe	$0.38 online
Smint "Mints"	<0.20	30 (50)	No	$0.35–$0.40 retail
Brown & Haley "Zingos Caffeinated Peppermints"	Second of 2 polyols	NC	No	$0.40–$0.50 retail
Oxyfresh "Breath Mints"	Second of 2 polyols	NC	No	$0.35–$0.40 online
Starbucks "After Coffee Mints"	Second of 2 polyols	NC	No	$0.20 Starbucks
Tic Tac "Silvers"	NC	NC	No	$0.35–$0.40 online
Xleardent "Mints"	NC	NC	No	$0.20 Starbucks

*Cost varies based on retail, convenience stores, and Internet vendors. Stated cost based on a few Seattle retailers or Internet vendors.
†Product list is not exhaustive. Xylitol market is rapidly changing and new xylitol containing products appear frequently.
‡"Yes," "no," or "maybe" are based on the potential a person is willing to consume 2 to 3 pieces, 3 to 5 times per day to meet the effective dose range of 6 to 10 g per day. Products with a potential for effectiveness, but for which xylitol dose is either unknown or required consumption, is >10 pieces/day to provide 6 g of xylitol are assigned "maybe."
§NC=not certain. Information cannot be derived from Internet vendor or market packaging, or authors unsuccessful in obtaining information from vendors' information representatives.

Figure 3.3   Xylitol-containing gums and mints available in U.S. markets, their xylitol content, preventive potential, and approximate cost. Reprinted from *Pediatric Dentistry* with permission from the American Academy of Pediatric Dentistry (Ly et al., 2006).

Products*	Xylitol content	Cost/unit†	Availability
Energy bars and food			
Buddha Bars	4-5 g/bar	$3.00/bar	Online
E Enterprises–"E Bar"	14 g/bar	$2.00/bar	Online
Fran Gare's "Decadent Desserts" Mix (various types)	15-25 g/30 g serving	$7.00/canister	Online
Jay Robb Enterprise "Jaybar"	13 g/bar	$3.00/bar	Online
Kraft Jell-O Pudding Sugar Free Chocolate	7 g/serving	$0.65/serving unit	Retail
Nature's Hollow–Sugar Free Jam (various flavors)	4.5 g/20 g serving	$6.00/10 oz	Online
Nature's Hollow–Sugar Free Syrup (various flavors)	2.5 g/40 ml serving (7%)	$5.40/8.5 oz	Online
Nature's Hollow–Sugar Free Ketchup	.8 g/20 g serving (4%)	$5.50/10 oz	Online
Nature's Hollow–Sugar Free Honey	1.2 g/20 g serving (8%)	$5.50/10 oz	Online
Biochem "Ultimate LoCarb 2" bars	Second of 2 polyols	$2.00/bar	Retail and online
Richardson Labs "Carb Solutions" Creamy Chocolate	Third of 3 polyols (13 g)	$1.50/bar	Retail and online
Oral hygiene			
Biotene "Dry Mouth Toothpaste" (±Calcium)	10%	$6.00-$7.00/4.5oz	Retail and online
Crest "Multicare Cool Mint Toothpaste"	10%	$3.50-$4.50/8 oz	Retail and online
Epic Toothpaste (fluoride free)	25% (no fluoride)	$4.50-$5.00/4.9 oz	Online
Epic Toothpaste with fluoride	35%	$7.00-$8.00/4.9 oz	Online
Squigle "Enamel Saver Toothpaste"	36% (.24% sodium fluoride)	$7.25-$8.00/4 oz	Online
Topex Toothpaste "Take Home Care," "White Care"	10% (1.1% sodium fluoride)	$4.50-$5.50/2 oz	Dental office and online
Rembrandt Toothpaste "For Canker Sore"	Only sweetener (fourth ingredient)	$6.50-$7.50/3 oz	Retail and online
Spry Toothpaste "MaxXylitol and Aloe"	NC‡ only polyol (no fluoride)	$4.50-$5.00/4 oz	Online
Tom's of Maine "Baking Soda" Toothpaste line	NC (varies in ingredient list)	$3.50-$4.50/6 oz	Retail and online
Tom's of Maine "Natural Toothpaste" line	NC (varies in ingredient list)	$3.50-$4.50/6 oz	Retail and online
Tom's of Maine "Sensitive Toothpaste" line	NC (varies in ingredient list)	$3.50-$4.50/6 oz	Retail and online
XyliWhite Toothpaste (fluoride free)	25% (no fluoride)	$3.50/6.4 oz	Online
Biotene "First Teeth" Infant Toothpaste	First of 2 polyols	$5.00-$6.00/1.4 oz	Retail and online
Gerber "Tooth and Gum Cleanser"	Second of 2 polyols (sixth ingredient)	$5.00-$5.50/1.4 oz	Retail and online
Spry Infant "Tooth Gel"	NC only polyol (no fluoride)	$4.50-$5.50/2 oz	Online
Biotene "Oral Balance" Dry mouth gel	Second of 2 polyols	$5.00-$6.00/1.5 oz	Retail and online
Biotene "Mouthwash"	First of 2 polyols	$6.00-$7.00/16 oz	Retail and online
Epic "Oral Rinse"	25%	$7.50-$8.50/16 oz	Online
Oxyfresh "Mouthrinse"	Only sugar (second ingredient)	$9.00-$10.00/16 oz	Online
Rembrandt "Dazzling Breathdrops"	Only sugar (second ingredient)	$1.00-$1.50/.22 oz	Retail and online
Spry "Oral Rinse"	First of 2 polyols (no fluoride)	$5.00-$5.50/16 oz	Online
Tom's of Maine "Natural Mouthwash" line	NC (varies in ingredient list)	$4.00-$6.00/16 oz	Retail and online

Figure 3.4 Xylitol-containing diet, oral hygiene, and health care products available in U.S. markets and their xylitol content. Reprinted from *Pediatric Dentistry* with permission from the American Academy of Pediatric Dentistry (Ly et al., 2006).

Some medications can cause xerostomia; therefore, it is important to note all medications taken when completing a medical history and ascertain whether salivary flow has been compromised due to medication side effects.

An adequate salivary flow rate is considered to be approximately 1 mL/min. If salivary flow is reduced to less than 0.5 mL/min, interventions should be considered. Artificial saliva can be utilized, greater consumption of water can be recommended, and chewing gum has been shown to stimulate salivary flow (Donly and Brown, 2005). Reduced salivary flow, which increases the risk of caries, would indicate the appropriateness of increased fluoride exposure and increased exposure to calcium and phosphate-containing agents.

Diet evaluation

Dietary intake plays a role in the status of the oral cavity. Intake of sugar (sucrose) is known to decrease the pH level to the point of causing tooth demineralization. In fact, any fermentable carbohydrate can initiate and progress carious lesions. As a part of risk assessment, intake of fermentable carbohydrates is important to know. Of particular importance is the frequency of intake. Each exposure can drop the pH; therefore, the greater number of times fermentable carbohydrates enter the oral cavity (snacking, juice, and soda drinking), the greater amount of times the pH within the oral cavity is prone to caries initiation/progression.

Practitioners can recommend that frequency of exposure to fermentable carbohydrates be reduced (Featherstone, 2006). Xylitol-sweetened mints or candies, as well as healthy snacks, can replace frequently ingested cariogenic snacks.

REMINERALIZATION OF DEMINERALIZED ENAMEL

Fluorides have been the principal means of remineralizing demineralized enamel and continue in this respect today. Topical fluoride is effective in three basic ways: (1) inhibition of demineralization, (2) enhancement of remineralization, and (3) bacteriostatic/bacteriocidal effects on bacteria. Fluroide exerts antibacterial actions by impairing glycolysis and other metabolic processes within bacteria, forming HF that lowers bacterial intracellular pH, interfering with bacterial membrane permeability to ionic transfer, and inhibiting enzyme systems (Donly and Stookey, 2004). The fluoride ion is uptaken at hydroxyl groups at the enamel surface creating fluoridated hydroxyapatite and fluorapatite, which is more difficult to demineralize than nonfluoridated enamel. Fluoride also enhances the precipitation of calcium and phosphate ions into subsurface enamel lesions. Recommendations have been made for appropriate topical fluoride use in children (Figure 3.5).

Fluoridated dentifrices

Fluoridated dentifrices have proved their effectiveness as an effective anticarious agent. Recent reviews indicate that fluoridated dentifrices reduce

Fluoride regimen	Recommendations
Dietary supplements	• Assay patient's primary source of drinking water; consider other sources of fluoride intake • Consider delaying supplementation until after eruption of permanent first molars • Ensure that parents understand risks/benefits of supplementation • Instruct patient to chew/swish supplement prior to swallowing • Prescribe no more than 120 mg F • No benefit to prenatal administration
Dentifrices	• Use in children <2 ys old should be based on caries risk assessment • Tooth-brushing for young child should be done by adult; brushing by older child should be supervised by adult • Use pea-sized dab of dentifrice in children with immature swallowing reflexes; older children can use larger amounts • Brush with fluoride toothpaste twice daily
Mouthrinses	• Reserve for use in children with moderate/high caries risk • Reserve for use in children who have mastered swallowing reflex • Recommend alcohol-free preparations
Self-applied gels/pastes (5000 ppm F)	• Reserve for patients in fluoride-deficient communities who are at increased risk for caries • Application should be done by adult for young child, and supervised by adult for older child • Application period should be 4 minutes • Allow patient to expectorate freely after application; postpone eating/drinking for 30 minutes • Use with caution in children who have not mastered swallowing reflex • Monitor effectiveness; terminate regimen when feasible
Professionally applied gel/foam (12,300 ppm F)	• Application frequency based on caries risk assessment • Follow a pumice prophylaxis with fluoride application • Use minimum amount of gel/foam necessary to cover teeth • Seat patient upright, use suction to reduce swallowing of product • Apply for 4 minutes • Allow patient to expectorate freely after application; postpone eating/drinking for 30 minutes
Fluoride varnish (22,600 ppm F)	• Use after pumice prophylaxis as noted for gel/foam application • Use in alternative restorative technique to arrest lesions in young, precooperative patients • Have patient refrain from eating/drinking for 30 minutes after application • Have patient postpone brushing teeth until following morning

Table assumes that the baseline recommendation for all patients is twice daily use of a fluoridated dentifrice coupled with once- or twice-yearly professional application of fluoride gel/foam/varnish. Use of all regimens except fluoride dentifrice should be based on a caries risk assessment.

Figure 3.5 Summary of the author's recommendations for the use of fluoride regimens in contemporary pediatric dental practice. Reprinted from *Pediatric Dentistry* with permission from the American Academy of Pediatric Dentistry (Adair, 2006).

caries by approximately 25% (Twetman et al., 2003; Marinho et al., 2005). Fluoridated dentifrices have fluoride available as sodium fluoride, stannous fluoride, and monofluorophosphate. All three of these fluoride compounds are recognized for effectiveness in the reduction of caries by the FDA, and they all exhibit similar cariostatic effects. Most dentifrices have a fluoride level of 1,000 or 1,100 ppm, but 1,500 ppm is also available. There is a 5,000 ppm fluoride dentifrice, but it must be professionally prescribed.

The risk of swallowing fluoridated dentifrices is higher among younger children, and children who tend to use "child-flavored" dentifrices in greater amounts and for longer time of brushing (Levy et al., 1992; Naccache et al., 1992; Adair et al., 1997). For this reason, it is recommended that a pea-sized amount of dentifrice be applied to the toothbrush by the child's caregiver to prevent ingestion of undesirable amounts of toothpaste (American Academy of Pediatric Dentistry, 2007c). Toothbrushing should be performed by an adult caregiver for children until at least age 5, when coordination improves with the child's toothbrushing. When the children begin to brush their own teeth, the dentifrice should still be dispensed by the caregiver, as well as having the brushing evaluated by the caregiver. Toothbrushing should be performed twice per day (Chestnut et al., 1998). When a child is old enough to effectively expectorate, more than a pea-sized amount of dentifrice can be used to increase the level of fluoride exposure.

Professionally applied topical fluoride

Fluoride varnish

Fluoride varnishes, although available in Europe for years as an anticaries agent, is recognized by the U.S. FDA as a device to be used as a desensitizing agent and a cavity-lining varnish (Beltran-Aguilar et al., 2000). Fluoride varnish is available as 5% sodium fluoride (22,600 ppm fluoride) and 1% difluorosilane (1,000 ppm fluoride). There is minimal information regarding the effectiveness of fluoridated varnishes to enhance remineralization; however, early data indicate that fluoride varnish has the potential to aid in the remineralization of incipient caries (Seppä, 1988; Attin et al., 1995).

The slow release of fluoride from fluoride varnish provides a sustained fluoride release over a couple of days and offers excellent safety, since the amount of fluoride released is so slow. Although 50,000 ppm sodium fluoride is a relatively high dose, a minimal amount is applied (0.3–0.6 mL; Figure 3.6) (Roberts and Longhurst, 1987). This can be converted to a range of 5–12 mg of fluoride. Ekstrand and colleagues reported a low plasma fluoride level following placement of a 5% fluoride varnish, which was comparable to plasma fluoride levels experienced after toothbrushing with a fluoridated dentifrice (Ekstrand et al., 1980). This level is significantly lower than plasma fluoride levels seen after a professionally applied 1.23% acidulated phosphate fluoride (Ekstrand et al., 1983).

Since the placement of fluoride trays in young children is difficult, cooperation is difficult with young children to use slow-speed suction to remove excess fluoride from the mouth as it dissipates from the delivery tray and the inability to ensure young children will not swallow fluoride in a tray delivery system—young children can benefit from fluoridated varnish. The ease of varnish application, safety, and efficacy, comparable to 1.23% acidulated phosphate fluoride gel, makes the use of fluoride varnish appropriate for young children.

Professionally applied fluoride gels and foams

There are three professionally applied topical fluorides recognized by the American Dental Association (ADA): 1.23% acidulated phosphate fluoride,

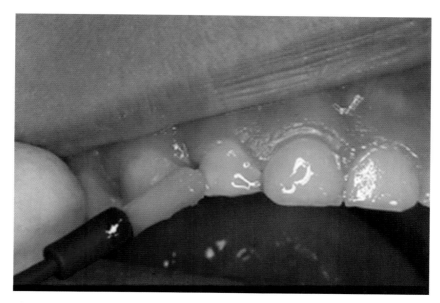

Figure 3.6   A sodium fluoride varnish being applied to the primary dentition.

2% sodium fluoride, and 8% stannous fluoride. All three of these professionally applied topical fluorides have demonstrated success in reducing caries; however, they are difficult to use with small children (Ripa, 1989). As previously discussed, tray-delivered fluoride is difficult in young children; therefore fluoride varnish is preferable as a professionally applied topical fluoride.

Casein phosphopeptide-amorphous calcium phosphate

Casein phosphopeptide-amorphous calcium phosphate (CPP-ACP) has received significant attention over the past decade to aid in the control of caries. Casein phosphopeptide (CPP) stabilizes amorphous calcium phosphate (ACP) in metastable solution (Reynolds, 1998). Through multiple phosphoseryl residues, CPP binds to forming nanoclusters of ACP, preventing their growth to the critical size required for nucleation and phase transformation. The CPP-ACP attaches to plaque, the ACP being released onto the tooth surface. Not only does this provide calcium and phosphate for tooth remineralization, but also acts as a buffering agent when the intraoral pH becomes more acidic.

CPP-ACP rinse

There has been evidence that enamel subsurface lesions can be remineralized with casein phosphopeptide-stabilized calcium phosphate solutions

(Reynolds, 1997). Although these remineralizing solutions can be effective at remineralizing enamel, children at age 3 and less would have a difficult time with a rinse and other delivery systems of CPP-ACP would be more appropriate.

CPP-ACP gum

Studies have also shown the effectiveness of CPP-ACP contained in sugar-free gum to remineralize subsurface enamel lesions (Shen et al., 2001; Lijima et al., 2004). The trademark name for CPP-ACP is Recaldent™. Gums containing CPP-ACP offer benefits from the delivery of bioavailable calcium and phosphate, as well as improving salivary flow, which is supersaturated with calcium and phosphate. An additional benefit can occur if xylitol is used as the sweetener in the gum, xylitol exhibiting anticariogenic effects on bacteria. A clinical trial evaluating a sugar-free gum containing CPP-ACP chewed for 10 min 3 times daily by 2,720 adolescents demonstrated a significant reduction in lesion progression, as well as enhancement of lesion reversal when compared to a sugar-free control gum (Morgan et al., 2006).

Although these gums containing CPP-ACP enhance remineralization of subsurface enamel lesions, children at age 3 and less may not have the ability/coordination to chew gum. If children are unable to chew gum, application of CPP-ACP in another form would be appropriate.

CPP-ACP paste

CPP-ACP is available in a paste form, which is referred to as MI Paste (GC America Inc, Alsip, IL). This CPP-ACP containing MI Paste is not only available in North America, but is also available in Australia and New Zealand with the product name Tooth Mousse. The paste can be applied to the teeth gently with a rubber cup or gloved finger by the dental professional, and can be applied at home by the patient, or parent of the patient, using a finger or toothbrush. The paste is recommended to be placed on the labial surfaces of the teeth, in a pea-sized amount, every day before bedtime (Walsh, 2007). Ingestion of this agent has been classified as safe for patients of all ages. Since saliva flow decreases when sleeping, the CPP-ACP paste would be expected to have a greater contact time and subsequent benefit if applied prior to bedtime.

CPP-ACP paste with fluoride

A new paste was recently introduced to the marketplace that contains CPP-ACP with 900 ppm fluoride (MI Paste Plus, GC America Inc, Alsip, IL). This fluoridated paste has bioavailable calcium and phosphate, yet also has approximately the same amount of fluoride available as that provided in dentifrices. CPP has been shown to stabilize amorphous calcium fluoride phosphate. MI Paste Plus compared to MI Paste remineralizes subsurface enamel lesions better (Walsh, 2007). This is attributed to the fluoride availability that enhances the precipitation of calcium and phosphate. Although this fluoridated CPP-ACP paste is effective in enamel remineralization, it is not indicated in young children. The entire fluoride content of the paste is expected to be swallowed; therefore, the concern for increased potential for fluorosis limits the recommendation for use of fluoridated CPP-ACP in young children.

Other CPP-ACP carriers

CPP-ACP has also been incorporated into dental sealants and dental varnishes. A slow release of the calcium and phosphate would seem to be beneficial; however, little research is presently available for these carriers of CPP-ACP and further information should become available in the near future.

Fluoridated materials

Glass ionomer cement surface protectant

Glass ionomer cements can be used as tooth surface protectants, particularly on the occlusal surfaces (Abadeer et al., 2005). A glass ionomer cement specifically designed for this purpose is marketed in the United States as Triage™ (GC America Inc, Alsip, IL). Glass ionomer cements release fluoride, which can be uptaken by adjacent enamel, which inhibits further demineralization and enhances remineralization (Hicks et al., 2003). The fluoride provided by the glass ionomer cement elevates plaque and salivary fluoride levels that further facilitates remineralization. Glass ionomer cements can be "recharged" with fluoride at the surface of the material with fluoridated dentifrice or other topical fluorides. This allows the fluoride-releasing dental material to act as an intraoral fluoride reservoir.

The placement of glass ionomer surface protectants is particularly valuable when molars are erupting, but cannot be adequately isolated for the placement of a resin-based sealant (Feigal and Donly, 2006). Teeth exhibiting enamel hypoplasia, visible enamel demineralization, or considered at high risk when caries-risk assessment is performed, can benefit from these surface protectants. After full eruption of the tooth, when perfect tooth isolation can be achieved, a resin-based sealant can be placed.

Resin-based sealants

Resin-based sealants are recommended to be placed over "at risk" tooth occlusal surfaces, including surfaces that exhibit noncavitated enamel demineralization (Feigal and Donly, 2006).

RESTORING CAVITATED LESIONS

Utilizing the concept of minimally invasive dentistry, restoration is a last resort when tooth surface cavitation appears. Teeth are restored with a minimally invasive restorative protocol and biomimetic materials. By minimizing the amount of tooth structure removed during cavity preparation, natural tooth structure can be preserved. The selection of the appropriate restorative material should be made in conjunction with the caries-risk assessment.

Secondary caries is responsible for greater than 50% of all restorations that are replaced (Mjor, 1997). Considerable fluoride release occurs during the glass ionomer cement setting reaction and continues at very low levels for years (Arends et al., 1995). The released fluoride is readily up-taken by the cavosurface tooth margins of the restorative material, as well as tooth structure proximally adjacent to a Class II restoration (Hicks et al., 2003). Resistance to secondary caries at the cavosurface margins and adjacent smooth surfaces to the glass ionomer cement restorative material has been demonstrated (Donly et al., 1999a, b). As previously discussed, these materials also uptake fluoride at the restoration surface and rerelease the fluoride, the restorative material acting as a fluoride reservoir. Therefore, there is an advantage of using glass ionomer cement restorations in children who are of moderate caries risk for the prevention of secondary caries.

Glass ionomer cement/resin-modified glass ionomer cement

Glass ionomer cement and resin-modified glass ionomer cement restorative materials offer the advantage of self-adhesive bonding to tooth, as well as the inhibition of adjacent proximal caries and secondary caries. The bond strength of glass ionomer cement to enamel and dentin is not as strong as that of resin-based composite; however, there is less technique sensitivity associated with glass ionomer cements.

Clinicians are advised to use a Centrix (Shelton, CT) syringe to place hand-mixed glass ionomer cements to reduce the concern of creating air voids when placing the relatively "sticky" glass ionomer cement material. After the glass ionomer cement is set or the resin-modified glass ionomer cement is polymerized and set, finishing can be completed with carbide finishing burs and polishing with abrasives. An unfilled resin is then applied to the polished surface to keep the aluminum particles at the restoration surface so that complete set of the acid–base reaction can occur over the next 24 h, improving the compressive strength of the restoration.

Atraumatic restorative technique

The atraumatic restorative technique was initially introduced as a means to restore teeth of individuals in remote locations where access to contemporary comprehensive preventive and restorative dentistry treatment was not readily available (Frencken et al., 1994). Hand instruments were used to remove caries; then chemically cured glass ionomer cement was placed as the restorative material. This restorative technique originated for use in third world countries, where access to dental treatment was very difficult (Frencken et al., 1996; Phantumvanit et al., 1996). The procedure did not require power for air or electrical operated handpieces to remove caries and to light cure the restorative material. There have been clinical outcomes reported with varying results; however, tooth extraction may have been the only alternative treatment in many of these cases (Frencken et al., 1998; Mallow et al., 1998; Holmgren et al., 2000).

In developed countries, where access to comprehensive dental care is more readily available, glass ionomer cement or resin-modified glass ionomer cement restorations can be effectively placed.

Class V restorations

Class V glass ionomer cement restorations can be very effective in the primary dentition (Croll et al., 2001; Berg, 2002). These restorations are not in stress-bearing areas; therefore, the compressive strength of the glass ionomer cement restorative material is not a critical factor. Resin-modified glass ionomer cement Class V restorations would be indicated to be more preferable than resin-based composite restorations where good isolation of the tooth is difficult or impossible (Figures 3.7 and 3.8). This is particularly prevalent when treating young children where behavior can

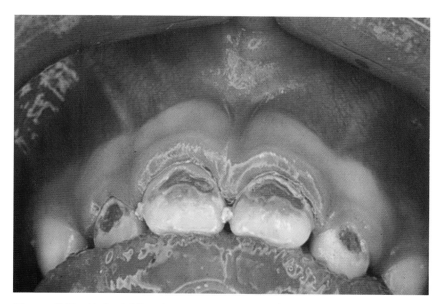

Figure 3.7   Early childhood caries is apparent on the primary maxillary incisors.

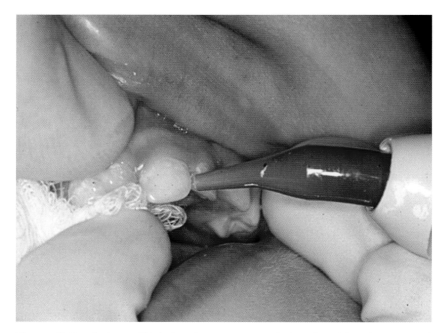

Figure 3.8   Resin-modified glass ionomer cement being placed into the prepared teeth utilizing a Centrix™ syringe.

make it difficult to keep a dry field of operation. Glass ionomer cements and resin-modified glass ionomer cements can set in the presence of water; therefore, minimal saliva contamination will not necessarily lead to restoration failure.

The preparation design for a Class V glass ionomer cement restoration includes butt cavosurface margins and pulpal extension of approximately 1.25 mm or more if caries extends further pulpally. Use of a # 330 carbide or diamond bur provides an undercut that offers additional retention. No bevels are placed at the cavosurface margin of the preparation due to the brittle nature of glass ionomer cements and the potential for fracture at the beveled cavosurface margin.

Class III restorations

Class III glass ionomer cement restorations can also be very effective (Croll et al., 2001; Berg, 2002). Again, these restorations would be appropriate where tooth isolation is not possible for placement of a resin-based composite restoration. Lingual preparation access is recommended for maxillary anterior teeth and labial preparation access is recommended for mandibular anterior teeth. The box of the preparation should only extend as far as caries progresses.

Occlusal restorations

Occlusal glass ionomer cement restorations have demonstrated clinical success (Croll et al., 2001; Berg, 2002). Contemporary heavily filled glass ionomer cements and resin-modified glass ionomer cements have compressive strengths to withstand occlusal load and provide adequate wear properties for the posterior primary dentition. Occlusal glass ionomer cement restorations would be indicated when a tooth cannot be adequately isolated to place a resin-based composite restoration. These are particularly useful in children less than the age of 4, when cooperative behavior is not anticipated.

Class II restorations

The clinical evaluation of Class II glass ionomer cement restorations in the primary dentition has been promising (Vilkinis et al., 2000; Welbury et al., 2000; Berg, 2002). Resin-modified glass ionomer cements have demonstrated clinical success, some studies showing that it is as effective as amalgam Class II restorations after 3 years (Donly et al., 1999b; Croll et al., 2001). The advantages of not needing to acid-etched tooth structure before restoration placement and knowing that the chemical setting reaction will occur, even in the absence of light, makes the glass ionomers favorable for the pediatric patient, where speed is critical and tooth isolation difficult. Glass ionomer cements have varying degrees of radiopacity, which is important when radiographically evaluating the proximal surfaces of Class II restorations.

Class II glass ionomer cement preparation design is very similar to an amalgam preparation design in the primary dentition (Figure 3.9). The proximal box should be deep enough to break contact and the axial wall should ideally extend 1.25 mm, unless caries removal creates the need to extend further. The lateral walls should slightly converge toward the occlusal, offering mechanical retention. The proximal box should be deep

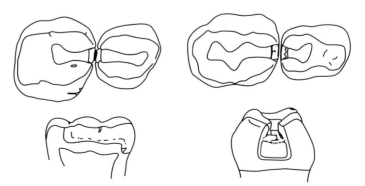

Figure 3.9   Schematic diagram of a Class II glass ionomer cement preparation.

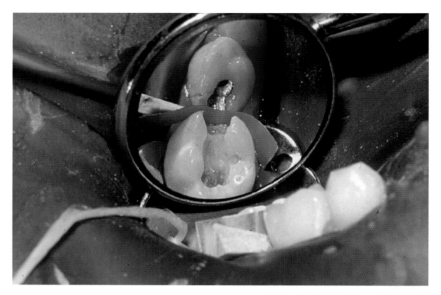

Figure 3.10   A Class II glass ionomer cement preparation in a primary molar.

enough to break contact and the axial wall should ideally extend 1.25 mm, unless caries removal creates the need to extend further. The lateral walls should slightly converge toward the occlusal, offering mechanical retention. The proximal box buccal and lingual extension should remain within the line angles and breaking buccal and lingual contact is not necessary (Figure 3.10). Since glass ionomer cement is brittle, an occlusal extension of the proximal box provides more "bulk" of restorative material to lessen the chance of restoration breakage. Slot preparations, where only the proximal box is prepared with no occlusal extension, is not recommended for glass ionomer cement preparations Likewise, no bevels should be placed on cavosurface margins of glass ionomer cement preparations. A matrix band or T-band can be adapted interproximally and secured firmly with a wedge to create a good postoperative contact with the adjacent tooth (Figure 3.11).

Resin-based composite

Class V restorations

Resin-based composite has been recommended for Class V restorations in the primary dentition (Burgess et al., 2002; Donly and Garcia-Godoy, 2002). Adequate isolation is critical in obtaining a satisfactory restoration. Saliva and/or blood contamination can have negative effects on bonding to acid-etched enamel. The cavity preparation should extend as far as caries has progressed in the enamel and dentin. Ideally, the axial wall would extend

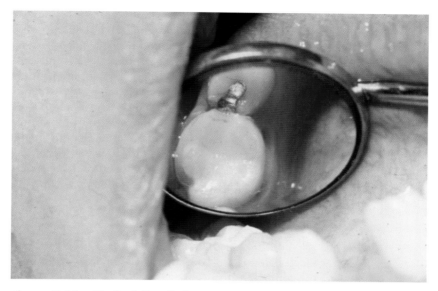

Figure 3.11   The final Class II glass ionomer cement restoration.

1.25 mm and all internal walls should be rounded. Preparation with a size # 330 bur will create natural mechanical retention. All enamel cavosurface margins should have a 45° 0.5–1.0 mm bevel (Donly and Garcia-Godoy, 2002). A glass ionomer liner/base can be placed over all prepared dentin or a dentin adhesive can be placed over all prepared dentin, being careful to follow manufacturers' specific instructions (Garcia-Godoy and Donly, 2002; Swift, 2002). All enamel should be acid etched with 35–40% phosphoric acid for 15–30 s. This etch time is adequate for both primary and permanent enamel (Redford et al., 1986). Following a thorough 10 s water rinse, with subsequent compressed air drying, adhesive may be placed and polymerized. Filled resin-based composite is then placed and polymerized, being sure that no increment is greater than 2 mm in depth. Halogen lights can typically polymerize filled resin up to 2 mm in depth. Finishing of resin restorations can be completed with fluted carbide finishing burs and then abrasives can achieve an optimal polish. After finishing and polishing, a final acid etch of the restoration surface and cavosurface margins is recommended, with the subsequent placement and polymerization of an unfilled resin. This allows for any imperfections, created during finishing and polishing, to have resin incorporated in the restorative surface and for the surface of the resin to reach maximum polymerization.

Class III restorations

Resin-based composites have also been recommended for Class III restorations in the primary dentition (Burgess et al., 2002; Donly and

Garcia-Godoy, 2002). These restorations are appropriate for teeth that can be adequately isolated, to prevent contamination during restoration placement, for teeth that have a sound incisal edge following tooth cavity preparation, and in situations where the patient is not considered to be at high risk for caries. Children at high risk, experiencing multiple caries and other risk factors, may need more aggressive treatment, such as full tooth coverage restorations (Tinanoff and Douglass, 2002). Lingual preparation access is recommended for maxillary anterior teeth and labial preparation access is recommended for mandibular anterior teeth. The box of the preparation should extend as far as caries has progressed and a cavosurface 45°, 0.5–1.0 mm bevel should be placed (Donly and Garcia-Godoy, 2002). Resin-based composite placement can be completed in the same manner noted for Class V restorations.

Occlusal restorations

Resin-based composite is the material of choice for occlusal restorations when the tooth can be adequately isolated (Burgess et al., 2002; Donly and Garcia-Godoy, 2002). Composites have good strength and wear characteristics and have demonstrated success as both occlusal and Class II restorations.

Preparations only need to extend as far as caries has progressed. Simonsen describes the restoration of occlusal surfaces in a minimally invasive method as the preventive resin restoration (Simonsen, 1980). A Group A preventive resin restoration merely opens pits and fissures where caries is present. This can be completed with as small of a bur necessary to remove the carious tooth structure, such as a one-fourth round bur. Group A preventive resin restorations have the surface acid etched with phosphoric acid; then a sealant is flowed into the pits and fissures to restore the prepared area and to prevent caries in susceptible pits and fissures that were not prepared.

Group B preventive resin restorations restore caries that are more extensive in the pits and fissures than the caries associated with Group A preventive resin restorations. Again, only carious tooth structure is removed. Resin-based composite is placed in areas where significant tooth structure was removed; then a sealant is placed over the entire occlusal surface to prevent caries in caries susceptible pits and fissures. The resin-based composite should contain a filler percentage that is appropriate for the restored area. Stress-bearing areas, where significant wear might be expected, should receive a higher filled resin (greater than 70% by weight). Group C preventive resin restorations extend well into dentin and involve a number of pits and fissures. All caries are removed. A glass ionomer cement liner/base can be placed over all prepared dentin, or a dentin adhesive may be applied, as recommended by the manufacturer. The occlusal enamel is then etched for 15–30 s with 35–40% phosphoric acid and the bonding adhesive is applied. Filled resin-based composite is then placed in increments of no more than 2 mm depth and polymerized. The restoration is finished and polished, as previously explained, and sealant is placed into pits and fissure not included in the preparation to prevent future decay.

Class II restorations

Resin-based composite has been shown to be effective as a Class II restorative material in the primary dentition (Nelson et al., 1980; Oldenburg et al., 1987; Tonn and Ryge, 1988; Barnes et al., 1991; Barr-Agholme et al., 1991; Attin et al., 2001). The ADA statement on posterior resin-based composites clearly states that recommendations for Class II restorations were associated with preparations that did not include restoration margins exhibiting heavy occlusal wear (ADA Council on Scientific Affairs and ADA Council on Dental Benefit Programs Statement on Posterior Resin-Based Composites, 1998). This can be interpreted as Class II restorations that do not extend beyond the line angles, or approximately one-half the intercuspal distance. Preparation design for a Class II resin-based composite restoration is similar to the preparation design for Class II glass ionomer cement restorations described previously (Figure 3.12). The proximal box should ideally just break gingival contact, and the buccal and lingual walls should be within the line angles and converge toward the occlusal. There should be an occlusal extension from the proximal box with a dovetail into the occlusal surface to provide additional retention (Figure 3.13). All cavosurface margins should be beveled (Donly and Garcia-Godoy, 2002). "Slot" preparations, which basically only includes the proximal box is not appropriate in the primary dentition (Paquette et al., 1983).

A matrix band or T-band can be adapted interproximally and secured firmly with a wedge. This contains the restorative material during

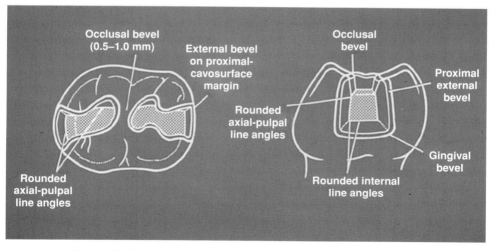

Figure 3.12   Schematic diagram of a Class II resin-based composite preparation.

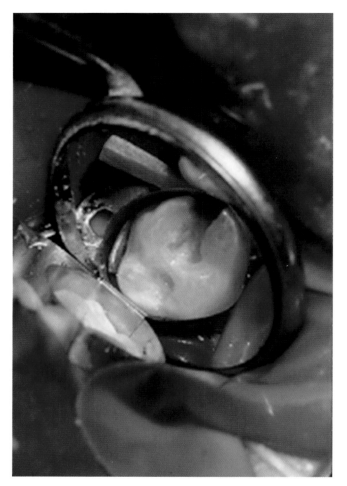

Figure 3.13   A Class II resin-based composite preparation in a primary molar.

placement and helps create an excellent proximal contact. Following the Class II preparation, glass ionomer cement base/liner can be placed over prepared dentin, or a dentin adhesive can be placed over prepared dentin according to manufacturer's instructions. Enamel cavosurface margins should be acid etched with 35–40% phosphoric acid for 15–30 s, and then rinsed with water thoroughly and dried. Adhesive should be placed and polymerized; then resin-based composite can be placed in increments of no more than 2 mm depth and polymerized (Caughman et al., 1995). If a "flowable" composite is utilized as the restorative material for a Class II restoration, filler of higher than 70% by weight should be used to minimize polymerization shrinkage and provide favorable wear characteristics. The wedge and matrix are removed, and the restoration is finished and

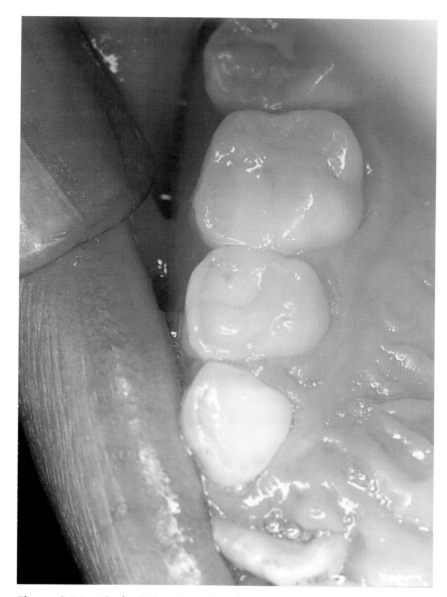

Figure 3.14   The final Class II resin-based composite restoration.

polished as described previously (Figure 3.14). Following finishing and polishing, placement and polymerization of an unfilled resin over the polished surface fills any imperfections created during finishing and achieves optimal surface polymerization, which can improve wear of the restoration (Simonsen and Kanca, 1986; Roberson et al., 1988; Dickinson and Leinfelder, 1993).

Strip crown restorations

Bonded resin-based composite strip crowns have been recommended as an effective restorative method for multiple-surface carious primary incisors (Lee, 2002; Waggoner, 2002). The longevity of resin-bonded crowns depends on the quantity and quality of sound dental structure, tooth position, technique and material used, and case selection (Kupietzky et al., 2003). A contraindication for a strip crown is minimal tooth structure, particularly enamel. The greater the overbite, the more stress expected for anterior teeth during mastication and protrusive movement. Gingival health is also an important factor. Gingivitis leads to bleeding on pressure contact. Placement of celluloid strip crown forms can easily place enough pressure on inflamed gingival tissue to cause bleeding. Risk assessment is an important factor in decision making, including the decision of whether to place composite strip crowns. Patients who have multiple caries and/or tooth demineralization exhibit poor oral hygiene and compliance with daily oral hygiene, and when maintenance is considered unlikely would not be good candidates for composite strip crown restorations.

Preparation design for strip crown restorations is straightforward (Webber et al., 1979). First, the incisal edge should be reduced 1.5 mm. Then, the proximal surfaces should be reduced, tapering the reduction slice toward the incisal edge (Figure 3.15). Approximately 1.0–1.5 mm proximal reduction, per proximal surface, is adequate. Care must be taken

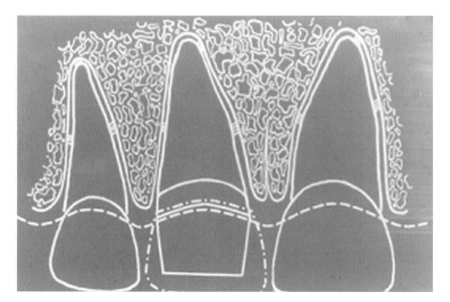

Figure 3.15   Schematic diagram of a primary maxillary anterior tooth preparation for a strip crown, stainless steel crown, or esthetic resin-faced stainless steel crown.

to avoid cutting gingival tissue, which causes bleeding and difficulty in isolating the tooth for a successful restoration. The final step in tooth preparation is placing a bevel on the labial-incisal and lingual-incisal of the prepared tooth. This makes the preparation take the form of the celluloid crown and will relieve the chance of the incisal edge of the prepared tooth to keep the celluloid crown form from properly seating.

The appropriate celluloid crown form is then selected. The natural mesiodistal width of the tooth is the easiest way to select the proper size. The gingival margin of the celluloid crown form can be cut with scissors so that it provides a nice free gingival margin adaptation and the natural position, including incisal height, of the tooth (Grosso, 1987). The prepared tooth structure is then acid etched with 35–40% phosphoric acid for 15–30 s. The tooth is rinsed and dried, and then the dentin and enamel bonding adhesive is applied, as recommended by the manufacturer. Filled resin-based composite is placed into the celluloid crown form, filling approximately half to two-thirds of the crown. This will usually provide an adequate amount of resin. Heavily filled resins (greater than 70% by weight) are encouraged to be used because light does not easily penetrate the resin and make restoration margins apparent. It is recommended to place a small hole in the incisal edge of the celluloid crown form so that excess resin can extrude through the hole. This relieves the creation of air voids within the strip crown resin. The celluloid crown form containing the resin is carefully placed onto the prepared tooth until it is completely seated. Excess resin at the free gingival margin and incisal edge can be easily removed with an explorer prior to polymerization of the resin. The resin is then polymerized, exposing both the facial and the lingual to the visible light-curing unit. The celluloid crown form is peeled away and there should be minimal finishing and polishing necessary. Any finishing and polishing that must be completed can be done with finishing burs and abrasives, as discussed previously (Croll, 1990). Checking the occlusion to see that the restoration is in normal occlusion is important.

Stainless steel crowns

Anterior

Esthetic SSC

There are a number of companies that provide esthetic anterior primary stainless steel crowns (SSCs) (Figure 3.16; Waggoner, 2002). These are referred to as preveneered SSCs (Croll and Helpin, 1996; Croll, 1998). These pre-veneered SSCs can be esthetically pleasing (Figure 3.17). The indications for placing esthetic SSCs are severe anterior caries, inability to isolate the tooth adequately for the placement of resin-based composite, and children diagnosed as high risk for caries (Seale, 2002; Waggoner, 2002). Due to the uncooperative behavior of many children of age 3 and less, the esthetic

Crown	Company	Phone #	Starter kit	Individual crowns	Additional information
NuSmile	Orthodontic Technologies	1-800-346-5133	16 crowns $260.00	Anterior $17.98 Posterior $34.50	Different lengths available Resin facing on an SSC Crimp only on lingual surface
Cheng Crowns	Peter Cheng Orthodontic Laboratory	1-800-288-6784	16 crowns $280.00	Anterior $19.00 Posterior $35.00	One length, one shade Resin facing on an SSC Crimp only on lingual surface
Kinder Krowns	Mayclin Dental Studios	1-800-522-7883	16 crowns $259.00	Anterior $17.95	Different lengths available 2 shades Resin facing on an SSC Crimp only on lingual surface
Dura Crowns	Space Maintainers Laboratory	1-800-423-3270	24 crowns $396.00	Anterior $16.50	May be crimped on labial and lingual 1 shade Flexible facing attached to SSC
New Millenium Crowns	Space Maintainers Laboratory	1-800-423-3270	24 crowns(ant) $290.00 12 crowns(post) $169.50	Anterior $9.95 Posterior $12.95	Lab-enhanced composite resin crown form
Pedo Jackets	Space Maintainers Laboratory	1-800-423-3270	96 crowns(ant) $219.00 24 first molars $64.50	Ant/post 5 for $12.50	Copolyester crown form 1 shade
Strip Crowns	Space Maintainers Laboratory	1-800-423-3270	96 crowns(ant) $210.00 48 first molars $116.00 48 second molars $116.00	Ant/post 5 for $11.00	Seamless plastic crowns form without long cervical collars Other strip crowns forms (3M) are also available through other major dental suppliers

Figure 3.16 Aesthetic crowns for primary dentition. Reprinted from the *Journal of Pediatric Dental Care* with permission from the Southeastern Society of Pediatric Dentistry (Lin, 2005).

SSCs can be the treatment of choice due to ease of placement and fact that perfect isolation of the tooth is not necessary.

The main problem associated with these pre-veneered SSCs is the potential for complete or partial fracture of the veneered facial surface. Manufacturers use different methods to bond resin to the SSC surface; however, the problem of potential fracture of the facing appears with all of the esthetic SSCs available. Due to the physical properties associated with the resin facing veneers, the resin has minimal flexure and can dislodge with the tensile and shear stress associated with day-to-day function (Lin, 2005).

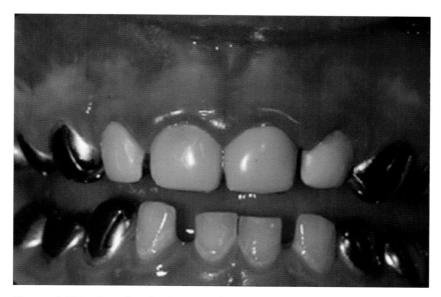

Figure 3.17   Resin-faced esthetic stainless steel crowns on the primary maxillary incisors.

When a single tooth needs to be restored, an esthetic SSC may look "bulky," due to the thickness of the resin facing. Additional facial tooth preparation can help create better esthetics, but the restoration may still appear to be positioned facially. When all four incisors are in need of restoration, this problem is minimal because all crowns can be positioned in a more esthetically pleasing manner.

SSC

Anterior SSCs have demonstrated clinical success as a restorative procedure (Seale, 2002; Waggoner, 2002). Although not esthetic, these crowns can be crimped on the facial and lingual gingival margins to obtain a well-adapted fit to tooth structure. In young children, where behavior frequently offers a challenging operating environment and where longevity of the restoration is a critical factor, SSCs can be quite effective as a restoration. As the child matures, the dentist can offer the option to have the SSC replaced with an esthetic SSC or to have the facial surface cut out of the SSC and place a resin-based composite for facial esthetics (Helpin, 1983). In these circumstances, a carbide bur can cut away the facial surface of the SSC and a mechanical undercut can be placed at crown margins created during removal of the crown facial surface. The underlying facial tooth surface and glass ionomer cement used to cement the SSC can be acid etched with 35–40% phosphoric acid for 15–30 s, a

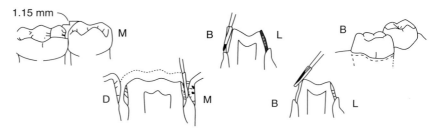

Figure 3.18   Schematic diagram of a stainless steel crown preparation.

bonding adhesive placed as recommended by the manufacturer, and a heavily filled resin-based composite is placed and polymerized.

Posterior

SSC

There are significant clinical data indicating the effectiveness of the posterior primary SSC (Randall, 2002; Seale, 2002). Indications include multiple surface caries, inability to isolate the tooth, expected longevity of multiple years, high caries risk, and posterior primary tooth restoration being provided under general anesthesia. Children less than 4 years of age frequently fall into one or more of these categories.

Tooth preparation begins with 1.5–2.0 mm of occlusal tooth reduction. Proximal surfaces are then reduced 1.0–1.5 mm, converging the preparation toward the occlusal surface. The line angles are rounded, and then a 45° bevel is placed at the occlusolabial and occlusolingual margins (Figure 3.18). It is important that no chamfer margin be created during preparation, which may prevent a crimped crown from being appropriately seated at the gingival crown extension. A SSC is then fit to the prepared tooth.

There are two types of SSCs available (Figure 3.19): precrimped (Ion, 3 M ESPE, St. Paul, MN) and noncrimped (Unitek, 3 M ESPE, St. Paul, MN). Either of these crowns should have the gingival margin cut so that it extends subgingivally, but not to the extent of causing blanching at the periodontal ligament attachment. The adapted crown margin is polished and crimped to snugly fit the tooth. Although some SSCs are precrimped, additional crimping may be necessary. The SSC is then cemented with glass ionomer cement, being sure the crown is seated (Figure 3.20).

Esthetic SSC

There are esthetic posterior primary SSCs available. Again, fracture or partial fracture of the resin is the main problem associated with these crowns. The need for additional tooth reduction, compared to a typical SSC, is usually necessary, and the free gingival margin adaptation of the crown can be difficult.

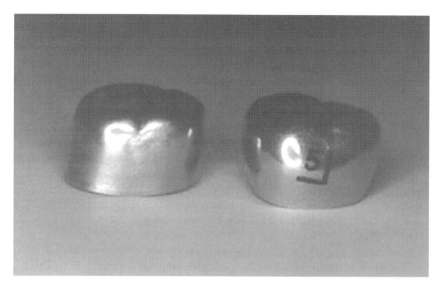

Figure 3.19   The two types of stainless steel crowns. The crown on the left does not have precrimped gingival margins, while the crown on the right does have precrimped gingival margins.

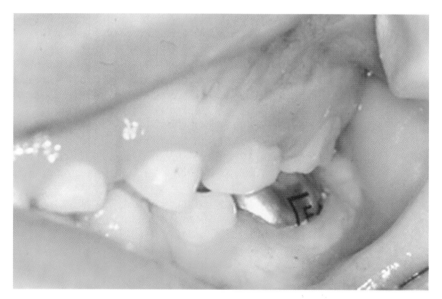

Figure 3.20   A stainless steel crown that has been cut and crimped to be adapted to the tooth just beneath the free gingival margin.

REFERENCES

Abadeer L, Donly KJ, and Ngo HC. 2005. What do we do with those at risk erupting molars? *J Pediatr Dent Care* 11:18–19.

Achong RA, Briskie DM, Hildebrandt GH, Feigal RJ, and Loesche WJ. 1999. Effect of chlorhexidine varnish mouthguards on the levels of selected oral microorganisms in pediatric patients. *Pediatr Dent* 21:169–75.

Adair SM. 2006. Evidence-based use of fluoride in contemporary pediatric dental practice. *Pediatr Dent* 28:133–42.

Adair SM, Piscitelli WP, and McKnight-Hanes C. 1997. Comparison of the use of an adult and a child dentifrice by a sample of preschool children. *Pediatr Dent* 19:99–103.

American Academy of Pediatric Dentistry. 2007a. Policy on use of a caries-risk assessment tool (CAT) for infants, children and adolescents. Reference manual 2006–7. *Pediatr Dent* 28(Suppl):24–8.

American Academy of Pediatric Dentistry. 2007b. Guideline on prescribing dental radiographs for infants, children, adolescents, and persons with special health care needs. Reference manual 2006–7. *Pediatr Dent* 28(Suppl):200–201.

American Academy of Pediatric Dentistry. 2007c. Fluoride therapy. Reference manual 2006–7. *Pediatr Dent* 28(Suppl):95–6.

American Dental Association. Council on Scientific Affairs and ADA Council on Dental Benefit Programs. Statement on posterior resin-based composites. 1998. *J Am Dent Assoc* 129:1627–8.

Anderson MH. 2003. A review of the efficacy of chlorhexidine on dental caries and the caries infection. *Can Dent Assoc J* 31:211–4.

Ando M, González-Cabezas C, Isaacs RL, Eckert GJ, and Stookey GK. 2004. Evaluation of several techniques for the detection of secondary caries adjacent to amalgam restorations. *Caries Res* 38:350–56.

Anttonen A, Seppä L, and Hausen H. 2003. Clinical study of the use of the laser fluorescence device DIAGNOdent for detection of occlusal caries in children. *Caries Res* 37:17–23.

Arends J, Dijkman GEHM, and Dijkman AG. 1995. Review of fluoride release and secondary caries reduction by fluoridating composites. *Adv Dent Res* 9:367–76.

Asboe-Jörgensen V, Attström R, Lang NP, and Löe H. 1974. Effect of chlorhexidine dressing on healing after periodontal surgery. *J Periodontol* 45:13–17.

Attin T, Hartman O, Hilgers RD, and Hellwig E. 1995. Fluoride retention of incipient enamel lesions after treatment with a calcium fluoride varnish in vivo. *Arch Oral Biol* 40:169–74.

Attin T, Opatowski A, Meyer C, Zingg-Meyer B, Buchalla W, and Monting JS. 2001. Three-year follow up assessment of Class II restorations in primary molars with a polyacid-modified composite resin and a hybrid composite. *Am J Dent* 14:148–52.

Barnes DM, Blank LW, Thompson VP, Holston AM, and Gingell JC. 1991. A 5- and 8-year clinical evaluation of a posterior composite resin. *Quintessence Int* 22:143–51.

Barr-Agholme M, Oden A, Dahllof G, and Modeer T. 1991. A 2-year clinical study of light-cured composite and amalgam restorations in primary molars. *Dent Mater* 7:230–33.

Beltran-Aguilar ED, Goldstein JW, and Lockwood SA. 2000. Fluoride varnishes: A review of their clinical use, cariostatic mechanism, efficacy and safety. *J Am Dent Assoc* 131:589–96.

Berg JH. 2002. Glass ionomer cements. *Pediatr Dent* 24:430–38.

Berkowitz R. 1996. Etiology of nursing caries: A microbiologic perspective. *J Public Health Dent* 56:51–4.

Berkowitz RJ and Jones P. 1985. Mouth-to-mouth transmission of the bacterium *Streptococcus mutans* between mother and child. *Arch Oral Biol* 30:377–9.

Berkowitz RJ, Turner J, and Green P. 1981. Maternal salivary levels of *Streptococcus mutans*: The primary oral infection in infants. *Arch Oral Biol* 26:147–9.

Burgess JO, Walker R, and Davidson JM. 2002. Posterior resin-based composite: Review of the literature. *Pediatr Dent* 24:465–79.

Burin C, Burin C, Loguercio AD, Grande RHM, and Reis A. 2005. Occlusal caries detection: A comparison of a laser fluorescence system and conventional methods. *Pediatr Dent* 27:307–12.

Caufield PW, Ratanapridakul K, Allen DN, and Cutter GR. 1988. Plasmid-containing strains of *Streptococcus mutans* cluster within family and racial cohorts: Implication in natural transmission. *Infect Immun* 56:3216–20.

Caughman W, Rueggeberg F, and Curtis J. 1995. Clinical guidelines for photocuring restorative resins. *J Am Dent Assoc* 126:1280–86.

Chestnut IG, Schafer S, Jacobsen APM, and Stephen KW. 1998. The influence of tooth-brushing frequency and postbrushing rinsing on caries experience in a caries clinical trial. *Community Dent Oral Epidemiol* 26:406–11.

Côrtes DF, Ekstrand KR, Elias-Boneta AR, and Ellwood RP. 2000. An in vitro comparison of the ability of, visual inspection and radiographs to detect occlusal caries and evaluate lesion depth. *Caries Res* 34:443–7.

Creanor SL, Russell JI, Strang DM, and Burchell CK. 1990. The prevalence of clinically undetected occlusal dentine caries in Scottish adolescents. *Br Dent J* 169:126–9.

Croll T and Helpin M. 1996. Preformed resin-veneered stainless steel crowns for restoration of primary incisors. *Quintessence Int* 27:309–13.

Croll TP. 1990. Bonded composite resin creowns for primary incisors: Technique update. *Quintessence Int* 21:153–7.

Croll TP. 1998. Primary incisor restoration using resin-veneered stainless steel crowns. *ASDC J Dent Child* 65:89–95.

Croll TP, Bar-Zion Y, Segura A, and Donly KJ. 2001. Clinical performance of resin-modified glass ionomer cement restorations in primary teeth. *J Am Dent Assoc* 132:1110–16.

Davies A. 1973. The mode of action of chlorhexidine. *J Period Res* 8(Suppl):68–75.

Davies RM, Jensen SB, Schiött CR, and Löe H. 1970. The effect of topical application of chlorhexidine on the bacterial colonization of teeth and gingiva. *J Period Res* 5:96–101.

Dickinson GL and Leinfelder KF. 1993. Assessing the long-term effect of a surface penetrating sealant. *J Am Dent Assoc* 124:68–72.

Donly KJ and Brown DJ. 2005. Identify, protect, restore: Emerging issues in approaching children's oral health. *Gen Dent* 53:106–10.

Donly KJ and Garcia-Godoy F. 2002. The use of resin-based composite in children. *Pediatr Dent* 24:480–88.

Donly KJ, Segura A, Wefel JS, and Hogan MM. 1999a. Evaluating the effects of fluoride-releasing dental materials on adjacent interproximal caries. *J Am Dent Assoc* 130:817–25.

Donly KJ, Segura A, Kanellis M, and Erickson RL. 1999b. Clinical performance and caries inhibition of resin-modified glass ionomer cement and amalgam restorations. *J Am Dent Assoc* 130:1459–66.

Donly KJ and Stookey GK. 2004. Topical fluoride therapy. In: Harris NO and Garca-Godoy F (eds), *Primary Preventive Dentistry*, 6th edn. Upper Saddle River, NJ: Pearson Prentice Hall, pp 241–83.

Ekstrand J, Koch G, and Petersson LF. 1980. Plasma fluoride concentration and urinary fluoride excretion in children following application of the fluoride-containing varnish Duraphat. *Caries Res* 14:185–9.

Ekstrand J, Koch G, and Petersson LG. 1983. Plasma fluoride concentration in pre-school children after ingestion of fluoride tablets and toothpaste. *Caries Res* 17:379–84.

Ekstrand K, Qvist V, and Thylstrup A. 1987. Light microscope study of the effect of probing in occlusal surfaces. *Caries Res* 21:368–74.

Featherstone JDB. 2006. Caries prevention and reversal based on the caries balance. *Pediatr Dent* 28:128–32.

Feigal RJ and Donly KJ. 2006. The use of pit and fissure sealants. *Pediatr Dent* 28:143–50.

Forgie AH, Paterson M, Pine CM, Pitts NB, and Nugent ZJ. 2000. A randomized controlled trial of the caries-preventive efficacy of a chlorhexidine-containing varnish in high-caries-risk adolescents. *Caries Res* 34:432–9.

Frencken JE, Makoni F, and Sithole WD. 1996. Atraumatic restorative treatment and glass-ionomer sealants in a school oral health programme in Zimbabwe: Evaluation after 1 year. *Caries Res* 30:428–33.

Frencken JE, Makoni F, and Sithole WD. 1998. ART restorations and glass ionomer sealants in Zimbabwe: Survival after 3 years. *Community Dent Oral Epidemiol* 26:372–81.

Frencken JE, Songpaisan Y, Phantumvanit P, and Pilot T. 1994. An atraumatic restorative treatment (ART) technique: Evaluation after 1 year. *Int Dent J* 44:460–64.

Garcia-Godoy F and Donly KJ. 2002. Dentin/enamel adhesives in pediatric dentistry. *Pediatr Dent* 24:462–4.

Grosso FC. 1987. Primary anterior strip crowns. *J Pedodont* 11:182–7.

Hayes C. 2001. The effect of noncariogenic sweeteners on the prevention of dental caries: A review of the evidence. *J Dent Educ* 65:1106–69.

Heinrich-Weltzien R, Weerheijm KL, Kühnisch J, Oehme T, and Stösser L. 2002. Clinical evaluation of visual, radiographic, and laser fluorescence methods for detection of occlusal caries. *ASDC J Dent Child* 69:127–32.

Helpin ML. 1983. The open-faced steel crown restoration in children. *ASDC J Dent Child* 50:34–8.

Hibst R and Gall R. 1998. Development of a diode laser-based fluorescence caries detector. *Caries Res* 32:294.

Hibst R and Paulus R. 2000. Molecular basis of red excited caries fluorescence. *Caries Res* 34:323.

Hicks J, Garcia-Godoy F, Donly KJ, and Flaitz C. 2003. Fluoride-releasing restorative materials and secondary caries. *Can Dent Assoc J* 31:229–45.

Holmgren CJ, Lo EC, Hu D, and Wan H. 2000. ART restorations and sealants placed in Chinese school children-results after 3 years. *Community Dent Oral Epidemiol* 28:314–20.

Kidd EA and Beighton D. 1996. Prediction of secondary caries around tooth-colored restorations: A clinical and microbiological study. *J Dent Res* 75:1942–6.

Kidd EAM, Joyston-Bechal S, and Beighton D. 1995. Marginal ditching and staining as a predictor of secondary caries around amalgam restorations: A clinical and microbiological study. *J Dent Res* 74:1206–11.

Kidd EAM, Naylor MN, and Wilson RF. 1992a. Prevalence of clinically undetected and untreated molar occlusal dentine caries in adolescents on the Isle of Wight. *Caries Res* 26:397–401.

Kidd EAM, Toffenetti F, and Mjör IA. 1992b. Secondary caries. *Int Dent J* 42:127–38.

Kohler B, Andreen I, and Jonsson B. 1988. The earlier the colonization by mutans streptococci, the higher the caries prevalence at 4 years of age. *Oral Microbiol Immunol* 3:14–7.

Kupietzky A, Waggoner WF, and Galea J. 2003. The clinical and radiographic success of bonded resin composite strip crowns for primary incisors. *Pediatr Dent* 25:577–81.

Lang NP and Brecx MC. 1986. Chlorhexidine digluconate—an agent for chemical plaque control and prevention of gingival inflammation. *J Period Res* 21(Suppl):74–89.

Lang NP and Briner WW. 1984. Chemical control of gingivitis in man. *J Am Dent Assoc* 109:223.

Le YL and Verdonschot EH. 1994. Performance of diagnostic systems in occlusal caries detection compared. *Community Dent Oral Epidemiol* 22:187–91.

Lee JK. 2002. Restoration of primary anterior teeth: Review of the literature. *Pediatr Dent* 24:506–10.

Levy SM, Maurice TJ, and Jakobsen JR. 1992. A pilot study of preschoolers' use of regular flavored dentifrices and those flavored for children. *Pediatr Dent* 14:388–91.

Lijima Y, Cai F, Shen P, Walker G, Reynolds C, and Reynolds EC. 2004. Acid resistance of enamel subsurface lesions remineralized by a sugar-free chewing gum containing casein phosphopeptide-amorphous calcium phosphate. *Caries Res* 38:551–6.

Lin B. 2005. Aesthetic crowns for the primary dentition. *J Pediatr Dent Care* 11:36–40.

Lindley MG, Birch GG, and Khan R. 1976. Sweetness of sucrose and xylitol. Structural considerations. *J Sci Food Agric* 27:140–44.

Löe H and Schiött CR. 1970. The effect of suppression of the oral microflora upon the development of dental plaque and gingivitis. In: McHugh, WE (ed.), *Dental Plaque*. Edinburgh: E&S Livingstone, pp 247–55.

Loesche WS, Svanberg ML, and Pape HR. 1979. Intraoral transmission of *Streptococcus mutans* by a dental explorer. *J Dent Res* 58:1765–70.

Longbottom C, Pitts NB, Lussi A, and Reich E. 1998. In vitro validity of a new laser-based caries detection device. *J Dent Res* 77:766.

Lopez L, Berkowitz R, Spiekerman C, and Weinstein P. 2002. Topical antimicrobial therapy in the prevention of early childhood caries: A follow-up report. *Pediatr Dent* 24:204–6.

Lopez L, Berkowitz RJ, Zlotnik H, Moss M, and Weinstein P. 1999. Topical antimicrobial therapy in the prevention of early childhood caries. *Pediatr Dent* 21:9–11.

Lussi A. 1993. Comparison of different methods for the diagnosis of fissure caries without cavitation. *Caries Res* 27:409–16.

Lussi A. 1996. Impact of including or excluding cavitated lesions when evaluating methods for the diagnosis of occlusal caries. *Caries Res* 30:389–93.

Lussi A and Francescut P. 2003. Performance of conventional and new methods for the detection of occlusal caries in deciduous teeth. *Caries Res* 37:2–7.

Lussi A, Imwinkelried S, Longbottom C, and Reich E. 1998. Performance of a laser fluorescence system for detection of occlusal caries. *Caries Res* 32:297.

Lussi A, Megert B, Longbottom C, Reich E, and Francescut P. 2001. Clinical performance of a laser fluorescence device for detection of occlusal caries lesions. *Eur J Oral Sci* 109:14–19.

Ly KA, Milgrom P, and Rothen M. 2006. Xylitol, sweeteners, and dental caries. *Pediatr Dent* 28:154–63.

Mallow PK, Durward CS, and Klaipo M. 1998. Restoration of permanent teeth in young rural children in Cambodia using the atraumatic restorative treatment (ART) technique and Fuji II glass ionomer cement. *Int J Paediatr Dent* 8:35–40.

Marinho VCC, Higgins JPT, Logan S, and Sheiham A. 2005. Fluoride toothpastes for preventing dental caries in children and adolescents. Cochrane Database Syst Rev 4.

Mendes FM, Nicolau J, and Duarte DA. 2003. Evaluation of the effectiveness of laser fluorescence in monitoring in vitro remineralization of incipient caries lesions in primary teeth. *Caries Res* 37:442–4.

Merrett MCW and Elderton RJ. 1984. An in vitro study of restorative dental treatment decisions and dental caries. *Br Dent J* 157:128–33.

Mjor IA. 1997. The reasons for replacement and the age of failed restorations in general dental practice. *Acta Odontol Scand* 55:58–63.

Morgan MV, Adams GG, Bailey DL, Tsao CE, and Reynolds EC. 2006. CPP-ACP gum slows progression and enhances regression of dental caries. *J Dent Res* 85(Special Issue B):2445.

Naccache H, Simard PL, Trahan L, Brodeur JM, Demers M, Lachapelle D, and Bernard PM. 1992. Factors affecting the ingestion of fluoride dentifrice by children. *J Public Health Dent* 52:222–6.

Nelson GV, Osborne JW, Gale EN, Norman RD, and Phillips RW. 1980. A 3-year clinical evaluation of composite resin and a high copper amalgam in posterior primary teeth. *ASDC J Dent Child* 47:414–18.

Oldenburg TR, Vann WF, and Dilley DC. 1987. Composite restorations for primary molars: Results after 4 years. *Pediatr Dent* 9:136–43.

Paquette D, Vann WF, Oldenburg TR, and Leinfelder KF. 1983. Modified cavity preparations for composite resin in primary molars. *Pediatr Dent* 5: 246–51.

Peers A, Hill FJ, Mitropoulos CM, and Holloway PJ. 1993. Validity and reproducibility of clinical examination, fiber-optic transillumination, and bitewing radiology for the diagnosis of small approximal carious lesions: An in vitro study. *Caries Res* 27:307–11.

Phantumvanit P, Songpaisan Y, Pilot T, and Frencken JE. 1996. Atraumatic restorative treatment (ART): A 3-year community field trial in Thailand-survival of one-surface restorations in the permanent dentition. *J Public Health Dent* 56(Special Issue):141–5, 161–3 (discussion).

Pine CM and ten Bosch JJ. 1996. Dynamic of and diagnostic methods for detecting small carious lesions. *Caries Res* 30:381–8.

Pretty IA, Edgar WM, and Higham SM. 2002. Detection of in vitro demineralization of primary teeth using quantitative light-induced fluorescence (QLF). *Int J Peadiatr Dent* 12:158–67.

Pretty IA, Smith PW, Hall AF, Edgar WM, and Higham SM. 2001. The intra- and inter-examiner reliability of QLF analyses. *Caries Res* 35:269–70.

Randall RC. 2002. Preformed metal crowns for primary and permanent molar teeth: Review of the literature. *Pediatr Dent* 24:489–500.

Redford DA, Clarkson BH, and Jensen M. 1986. The effect of different etching times on the sealant bond strength, etch depth and pattern in primary teeth. *Pediatr Dent* 8:11–15.

Reynolds EC. 1997. Remineraliztion of enamel sub-surface lesions by casein phosphopeptide-stabilized calcium phosphate solutions. *J Dent Res* 76:1587–95.

Reynolds EC. 1998. Anticariogenic complexes of amorphous calcium phosphate stabilized by casein phosphopeptides: A review. *Spec Care Dent* 8: 8–16.

Ripa LW. 1989. Review of the anticaries effectiveness of professionally applied and self-applied topical fluoride gels. *J Public Health Dent* 49(Special Issue):297–309.

Roberson TM, Bayne SC, Taylor DF, Sturdevant JR, Wilder AD, Sluder TB, Heymann HO, and Brunson WD. 1988. Five-year clinical wear analysis of 19 posterior composites. *J Dent Res* 67(abstract # 63):120.

Roberts JF and Longhurst P. 1987. A clinical estimation of the fluoride used during application of a fluoride varnish. *Br Dent J* 162:463–6.

Roberts MC, Riedy CA, Coldwell SE, Nagahama S, Judge K, Lam M, Kaakko T, Castillo JL, and Milgrom P. 2002. How xylitol-containing products affect cariogenic bacteria. *J Am Dent Assoc* 133:435–41.

Rocha RO, Ardenghi TM, Oliveira LB, Rodrigues CRMD, and Ciamponi AL. 2003. In vivo effectiveness of laser fluorescence compared to visual inspection and radiography for the detection of occlusal caries in primary teeth. *Caries Res* 37:437–41.

Rölla G and Melsen B. 1975. On the mechanism of the plaque inhibition by chlorhexidine. *J Dent Res* 54(Special Issue B):57–62.

Schneiderman A, Elbaum M, Shultz T, Keem S, Greenebaum J, and Driller J. 1997. Assessment of dental caries with digital imaging fiber-optic transillumination (DIFOTI™): In vitro study. *Caries Res* 31:103–10.

Seale NS. 2002. The use of stainless steel crowns. *Pediatr Dent* 24:501–5.

Seppä L. 1988. Effects of a sodium fluoride solution and a varnish with different fluoride concentrations on enamel remineralization in vitro. *Scand J Dent Res* 96:304–9.

Sheehy EC, Brailsford SR, Kidd EAM, Beighton D, and Zoitopoulos L. 2001. Comparison between visual examination and a laser fluorescence system for in vivo diagnosis of occlusal caries. *Caries Res* 35:421–6.

Shen P, Cai F, Nowicki A, Vincent J, and Reynolds EC. 2001. Remineralization of enamel subsurface lesions by sugar-free chewing gum containing casein phosphopeptide-amorphous calcium phosphate. *J Dent Res* 80:2066–70.

Siegrist BE, Gusberti FA, Brecx MC, Weber HP, and Lang NP. 1986. Efficacy of supervised rinsing with chlorhexidine digluconate in comparison to phenolic and plant alkaloid compounds. *J Periodontol Res* 16(Suppl):60–73.

Simonsen RJ. 1980. Preventive resin restorations: 3-year results. *J Am Dent Assoc* 100:535–9.

Simonsen RJ and Kanca J. 1986. Surface hardness of posterior composite resins using supplemental polymerization after simulated occlusal adjustment. *Quintessence Int* 17:631–3.

Söderling E, Isokangas P, Pienihäkkinen K, and Tenovuo J. 2000. Influence of maternal xylitol consumption on acquisition of mutans streptococci by infants. *J Dent Res* 79:882–7.

Söderling E, Isokangas P, Pienihäkkinen K, Tenovuo J, and Alanen P. 2001. Influence of maternal xylitol consumption on mother-child transmission of mutans streptococci: 6-year follow-up. *Caries Res* 35:173–7.

Swift EJ. 2002. Dentin/enamel adhesives: Review of the literature. *Pediatr Dent* 24:456–61.

Tabak LA. 2006. In defense of the oral cavity: The protective role of the salivary secretions. *Pediatr Dent* 28:110–17.

Tinanoff N and Douglass JM. 2002. Clinical decision making for caries management in children. *Pediatr Dent* 24:386–92.

Tonn EM and Ryge G. 1988. Clinical evaluations of composite resin restorations in primary molars: A 4-year follow-up study. *J Am Dent Assoc* 117:603–6.

Trahan L. 1995. Xylitol: A review of its action on mutans streptococci and dental plaque—its clinical significance. *Int Dent J* 45:77–92.

Twetman S, Axelsson S, Dahlgren H, Holm AK, Kallestal C, Lagerlof F, Lingstrom P, Mejare I, Nordenram G, Norlund A, Petersson L, and Soder B. 2003. Caries preventive effect of fluoride toothpaste: A systematic review. *Acta Odontol Scand* 61:347–55.

Van Der Veen MH, and de Josselin de Jong E. 2000. Application of quantitative light-induced fluorescence for assessing early caries lesions. *Monogr Oral Sci* 17:144–62.

Van Dorp CSE, Exterkate AM, and ten Cate JM. 1988. The effect of dental probing on subsequent enamel demineralization. *ASDC J Dent Child* 55:343–7.

Van Wuyckhuyse BC, Perinpanayagam HE, Bevacqua D, Raubertas RF, Billings RJ, Bowen WH, and Tabak LA. 1995. Association of free arginine and lysine concentrations in human parotid saliva with caries experience. *J Dent Res* 74:686–90.

Verdonschot EH, Bronkhorst EM, Burgersduk RCW, König KG, Schaeken MJM, and Truin GJ. 1992. Performance of some diagnostic systems in examinations for small occlusal carious lesions. *Caries Res* 26:59–65.

Vilkinis V, Horsted-Bindslev P, and Baelum V. 2000. Two-year evaluation of class II resin-modified glass ionomer cement/composite open sandwich and composite restorations. *Clin Oral Investig* 4:133–9.

Waggoner WF. 2002. Restoring primary anterior teeth. *Pediatr Dent* 24:511–6.

Walsh LJ. 2007. Clinical applications of Recaldent products: Which ones to use where. *Aust Dent Pract* 18(3):144–6.

Wan AKL, Seow WK, Purdie DM, Bird PS, Walsh LJ, and Tudehope DI. 2003. The effects of chlorhexidine gel on *Streptococcus mutans* infection in 10-month-old infants: A longitudinal, placebo-controlled, double-blind trial. *Pediatr Dent* 25:215–22.

Webber DL, Epstein NB, Wong JW, and Tsamtsouris A. 1979. A method of restoring primary anterior teeth with the aid of a celluloid crown form and composite resins. *Pediatr Dent* 1:244–6.

Weerheijm KL, Groen HJ, Bast AJJ, Kieft JA, Eijkman MAJ, and van Amerongen WE. 1992a. Clinically undetected occlusal dentine caries: A radiographic comparison. *Caries Res* 26:305–9.

Weerheijm KL, Gruythuysen RJM, and van Amerongen WE. 1992b. Prevalence of hidden caries. *ASDC J Dent Child* 59:408–12.

Welbury RR, Shaw AJ, Murray JJ, Gordon PH, and McCabe JF. 2000. Clinical evaluation of paired compomer and glass ionomer restorations in primary molars: Final results after 42 months. *Br Dent J* 189:93–7.

Wenzel A, Larsen MJ, and Fejerskov O. 1991. Detection of occlusal caries without cavitation by visual inspection, film radiographs, xeroradiographs, and digitized radiographs. *Caries Res* 25:365–71.

Wenzel A, Verdonschot EH, Truin GJ, and König KG. 1992. Accuracy of visual inspection, fiber-optic transillumination, and various radiographic image modalities for the detection of occlusal caries in extracted non-cavitated teeth. *J Dent Res* 71:1934–7.

Zickert I, Emilson CG, and Krasse B. 1982. Effect of caries preventive measures in children highly infected with *Streptococcus mutans. Arch Oral Biol* 27:861–8.

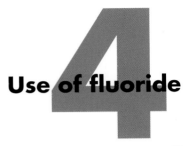

Use of fluoride

Norman Tinanoff

INTRODUCTION

The use of fluoride supplements and topical fluoride therapy in preschool children is complex and controversial. Since the introduction of water fluoridation, fluoride supplements, and topical fluoride therapies in the late 1940s, the mechanisms of actions and dosages have been debated and have evolved, especially with regard to preschool children. Originally, the mechanisms of water fluoridation and fluoride supplements were ascribed to changes of enamel mineral formation during the development of unerupted teeth. Although these initial concepts were insufficient, recent reports dismissing systemic mechanisms of fluoride also may be an over-simplification of the pre and posteruptive effects of fluoride.

Similarly, the initial dosage of fluoride supplements was empirical, based on simulating fluoride exposure from optimally fluoridated (1 ppm) water. Because of epidemiological studies showing mild fluorosis in some children with the original dosage, the fluoride supplement dosage has been altered several times over the past 30 years. However, complexities with fluoride supplement dosing remain as a result of the fact that fluoride is now a ubiquitous part of a preschool child's diet. Children consume processed foods and drinks that may have different fluoride concentrations than their home water, swallow fluoride from toothpastes, and may receive infant formula diluted with fluoridated or nonfluoridated water. These complex issues of dosage are further compounded by epidemiological studies showing changing prevalence of caries and fluorosis, as well as difficulties with dentists or physicians incorrectly prescribing fluoride and patients not complying with fluoride prescriptions.

Topical fluoride use in preschool children has also evolved. New modalities, such as fluoride varnishes, have become more prevalent for office treatment because of the safety of premeasured doses, reduced ingestion, and better acceptance by children. Overlaying both the issues of topical fluoride therapy and fluoride supplement use is the current focus on caries risk and cost versus benefit. One should no longer prescribe fluoride supplements or perform a professionally applied topical fluoride treatment without considering a child's caries risk. Recent recommendations suggest limited use of fluoride for low-risk children, but significantly more intensive regimes for high-risk children.

This chapter addresses both systemic and topical fluoride therapy for preschool children in the context of the changes in exposure to systemic fluoride, benefits in an era of less caries, and new modalities of delivery. Because of the age group involved, the issue of fluoride supplements and dietary intake of fluoride will be covered in detail. The chapter also gives recommendations regarding use of fluoride supplements, fluoridated toothpaste, and professional applications based on a child's caries risk.

SYSTEMIC FLUORIDE

Mechanisms

The original belief regarding how fluoride inhibited dental caries was based exclusively on a systemic theory in which developing teeth exposed to fluoride would undergo replacement of hydroxyapatite with a more acid-insoluble fluorapatite within the mineral lattice. Over the years it has become clear that the original notion of systemically produced fluorapatite could not fully explain the clinical caries reduction because only small amounts of fluorapatite were formed in developing enamel. This led to speculation that the systemic route of fluoride administration may be unimportant and that posteruptive fluoride effects outweigh the preeruptive effects (Beltran and Burt, 1988; Thylstrup, 1990; Clarkson et al., 1996). These posteruptive topical effects are based on fluoride altering enamel demineralization and remineralization patterns, as well as inhibiting bacterial metabolism. Thus, in recent years the emphasis has been on the topical effects of fluoride, even with regard to water fluoridation that has traditionally been considered to act systemically.

However, there is little data to determine the exact mechanisms, or the percent of the effect, that can be attributed to a systemic route or a topical route. Indeed, there is data that suggest that the systemic effect cannot be ruled out. Teeth of children who reside in a fluoridated community have higher fluoride content than those of children who reside in suboptimal fluoridated communities (Aasenden et al., 1971; Weatherell et al., 1977). Additionally, there are reports showing that both pre- and posteruption fluoride exposures are necessary to maximize the caries preventive effect of water fluoridation (Backer Dirks et al., 1961; Lemke et al., 1970; Marthaler, 1979; Singh et al., 2003).

To add further complications to the issue of systemic versus topical effects, it may be an oversimplification to designate fluoride simply as "systemic" or "topical" because fluoride that is swallowed may contribute to a topical effect on erupted teeth, and conversely swallowed fluoride may exert a topical effect on unerupted teeth. Perhaps, it is easier to understand the mechanisms of systemic and topical fluoride in the context of preeruptive and posteruptive effects of fluoride (Figure 4.1). The preeruptive effects, are based not only on deposition of fluoride in teeth during the mineralization of enamel, but also on fully formed teeth that remain unerupted for a considerable time acquiring significant amounts of fluoride on the surface enamel from the crypt fluid. Thus, fully formed unerupted teeth are topically exposed to fluoride in plasma for several years, producing a fluoride-rich zone on the enamel surface before eruption (Weatherell et al., 1977). In contrast, fluoride that is swallowed increases the plasma fluoride levels, and subsequently the salivary and gingival crevicular fluoride levels, to produce a topical effect on erupted teeth via a systemic route (Rolla and Ekstrand, 1996). Early studies by Bowen showed that primates given doses of fluoride by gastric intubation were found to have elevated levels of plaque fluoride derived from salivary secretions and gingival crevicular fluids. This clearly demonstrated a topical effect from the systemic route (Bowen, 1973).

Body uptake of fluoride

The major route for fluoride absorption is by the gastrointestinal tract. Fluoride is rapidly absorbed, primarily in the intestine, producing a rise in plasma fluoride concentrations minutes after ingestion. Prior to ingestion, plasma fluoride levels are approximately 0.02 ppm in individuals residing

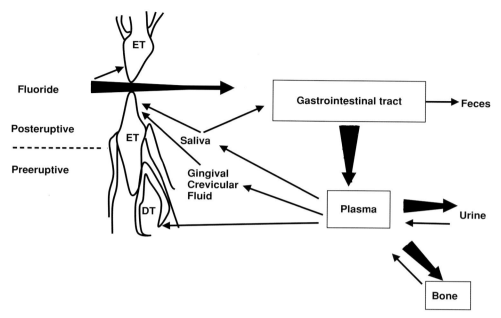

Figure 4.1   The metabolic route and target of fluoride that is swallowed in preschool child with erupted teeth (ET) and developing teeth (DT).

in communities with optimally fluoridated water (Ekstrand, 1996). After ingestion, fluoride levels in plasma will peak in the plasma during the first hour and subsequently rapidly decline due to the continuing uptake by bone, teeth, and urinary excretion (Whitford, 1996) (Figure 4.1). Elevation of the plasma fluoride levels depend on the fluoride dose ingested, dose frequency, and plasma half-life. The plasma half-life, which is the time required for the plasma fluoride concentration to fall by one-half, is typically 4–10 h. However, the ingestion of fluoride with foods, especially those containing metal ions, such as calcium, magnesium, or aluminum inhibits absorption. Decreased absorption up to 60% has been associated with calcium-rich breakfast foods (Ekstrand et al., 1978; Ekstrand and Ehrnebo, 1979). When fluoride is not absorbed, it will be excreted by the fecal route.

Fluoride is an avid mineralized tissue seeker. During the growth phase of the skeleton, a relatively high proportion of an ingested fluoride dose will be deposited in the skeleton. Studies of metabolism in infants show that 80% of a 0.25 mg fluoride dose will be retained in mineralized tissue (Ekstrand et al., 1994). The fluoride concentration of bone becomes a reservoir for fluoride and reflects the net balance between uptake and release. As bone is reorganized, fluoride is released and can enter the circulatory system or be redeposited back into forming bone. The percentage of excretion versus bone uptake varies depending on the patient's age, past exposure to fluoride, and activity level. Ultimately, if ingested fluoride is not

Table 4.1   Recommended total dietary fluoride intake[a].

Age	Reference weight (kg)	Adequate intake (mg/day)	Tolerable upper intake (mg/day)
0–6 months	7	0.01	0.7
6–12 months	9	0.5	0.9
1–3 years	13	0.7	1.3
4–8 years	22	1.1	2.2
≥9 years	40–76	2.0–3.8	10.0

[a] Adapted from Institute of Medicine (1997).

taken up by mineralized tissues, it will be excreted in the urine. Acid–base conditions in the urine affect fluoride excretion. At lower pH values, more fluoride is reabsorbed into the nephron, consequently with less fluoride excretion (Ekstrand, 1996).

Dietary consumption of fluoride

Optimally fluoridated water

Water is the predominant source of fluoride for most children living in communities where the fluoride concentration in water supplies is between 0.7 and 1.2 ppm. The optimum daily fluoride consumption can be calculated by body weight (Table 4.1), generally based on the formula of 0.05 mg/kg/day (IOM, 1997). This level has been extrapolated from the theoretical consumption of 1 L of 1 ppm F/day for a 20 kg child. In some countries, such as the United States, where the majority of food and drink processing is done in cities with optimally fluoridated water supplies, children living in low-fluoride areas also receive some of the benefits of fluoridated water from consumption of processed foods. This has been termed the "halo effect" and is believed to be a major factor in caries reduction in children residing in nonfluoridated areas. Complicating the dietary consumption of fluoride for preschool children is the fact that they often spend considerable time outside their homes at baby sitters or preschools, which may have different levels of water fluoridation than their residences. The Iowa Longitudinal Fluoride study, which examined patterns of fluoride intake in children from birth to 36 months, found considerable variation in children's fluoride uptake over time. Surprisingly, between 20 and 50% of the children exceeded the ideal daily level of fluoride consumption of 0.05 mg/kg (Levy et al., 2001).

Fluoride supplements

Fluoride supplements were introduced in the late 1950s to give anticaries benefits to populations that resided in areas where optimally fluoridated water was not available. Fluoride supplementation programs were based on the premise that the cariostatic effect of fluoride was predominately systemic rather than topical and that systemic doses of fluoride should be equivalent to those ingested from optimally fluoridated water. Summaries of trials of the effect of systemic fluoride supplements on dental caries showed a 50–80% caries reduction in primary teeth where the age of initiation was 2 years or younger (21 trials), and a 39–80% reduction in permanent teeth (34 trials) (Murray and Naylor, 1996). However, one must be cautious of the conclusions of these investigations since they were reported at a time of much greater caries incidence than the present, and methods and analysis of some studies weaken confidence in the findings.

In 1960 the dose of supplements was suggested to provide 1 mg F/day in children over the age of 3 and between 0.4–0.6 mg F/day in children less than 3 (Arnold et al., 1960). While this original dose was shown to be highly effective against caries, this supplementation regimen was associated with the development of enamel fluorosis (Aasenden and Peebles, 1974). The result of the Aasenden and Peeples trial was influential in reevaluating the fluoride supplementation guidelines; and in 1979 the American Academy of Pediatrics (AAP) recommended that, for communities with drinking water with less than 0.3 ppm F, children from birth to 2 years should receive 0.25 mg/day, children 2–3 years of age should receive 0.5 mg/day, and children 3–16 years should receive 1 mg/day (AAP, Committee on Nutrition, 1979).

In 1994 a committee of the American Dental Association (ADA) further recommended that supplements not be given to children under 6 months of age, and adjusted the dose to 0.5 mg/day for children between the ages of 3 and 6 years (Meskin, 1995). This recommendation was subsequently endorsed by the American Academy of Pediatrics (AAP, 1995) and the American Academy of Pediatric Dentistry (AAPD reference manual, 1995). Part of this recommendation was the requirement that the child's drinking water should be analyzed if the fluoride content is unknown. The Centers for Disease Control and Prevention in 2001 further recommended that fluoride supplements be administered only to children at high risk for dental caries, and stated that, for children under age 6, practitioners and parents should weigh the risks for caries with and without fluoride supplements versus the potential for enamel fluorosis (MMWR, 2001). Thus, current recommendations for fluoride supplementation are based on fluoride content of the water, the child's age, and the child's caries risk (Table 4.2). Examples of fluoride prescriptions are shown in Table 4.3.

Irrespective of efficacy, there are issues associated with administration of fluoride supplements that make supplementation not the first-line approach for caries prevention in preschool children. Concerns with fluoride supplementation include the following:

- Children, whether living in a fluoridated or nonfluoridated area, ingest sufficient quantities of fluoride from toothpaste, beverages, and foods (Levy and Guha-Choudhury, 1999).

Table 4.2 Current dietary fluoride supplement schedule[a].

	Fluoride concentration in community drinking water		
Age	<0.3 ppm	0.3–0.6 ppm	>0.6 ppm
0–6 months	None	None	None
6 months to 3 years	0.25 mg/day	None	None
3–6 years	0.5 mg/day	0.25 mg/day	None
6–16 years	1.0 mg/day	0.50 mg/day	None

[a] For children at caries risk (MMWR, 2001).

- There is confusion among practitioners and parents regarding supplementation for children who spend time away from home where water fluoride levels may differ from their home.
- There is an association of dental fluorosis in the permanent teeth with fluoride supplement use (Burt and Eklund, 1999; Ismail and Bandekar, 1999; Pendrys, 2000).
- Parents of high-risk children often do not comply with a fluoride supplement regimen (Levy et al., 1998).
- Many practitioners prescribe fluoride supplements without testing the child's water supply for fluoride content; without considering the caries-risk status of a child (Sohn et al., 2007); and without weighing the potential benefits of caries reduction versus the risk of mild fluorosis.

In addition to the issues of fluoride supplements for children, there was a period when physicians and dentists prescribed fluoride supplements to pregnant women with the goal of imparting caries resistance to their unborn child. Although fluoride crosses the placenta, there is little evidence that fluoride provided to the mother during pregnancy reduces caries prevalence in the offspring (Leverett et al., 1997). This practice of prenatal fluoride supplementation is no longer recommended (MMWR, 2001).

Table 4.3 Examples of fluoride prescriptions for children at caries risk that reside in a fluoride-deficient area.

Eight-month old
  Prescription: Fluoride solution (0.5 mg/mL)
  Dispense: 50 mL
  Instructions: In evening before bed, dispense $1/2$ mL into child's mouth

Six-year old
  Prescription: NaF tablets (1 mg)
  Dispense: 120 tablets
  Instructions: Before bed, chew 1 tablet, swish and swallow

Infant formula

The fluoride intake of infants may vary due to consumption patterns of milk and infant formula. Human breast milk and undiluted milk from other mammals is extremely low in fluoride. Additionally, since 1978 manufacturers of infant formula have removed fluoride from the water incorporated into infant formulas. Consequently, the fluoride content of ready-to-use formulas in the United States and Canada now generally ranges from 0.1 mg to 0.3 mg/L, which provides only a modest source of fluoride (Fomon and Ekstrand, 1996). However, non-milk-based formulas have higher fluoride content because the calcium that is added to formulas contains fluoride.

The more important issue is the fluoride content of concentrated or powdered formulas when reconstituted with fluoridated water. For example, a 1-year-old infant consuming 1 L of powdered formula that was reconstituted with optimally fluoridated water will receive twice the recommended daily dose of fluoride (Table 4.4, example 1). Therefore, use of fluoridated water for reconstituting powdered formulas should be avoided. The ADA now recommends that if concentrated liquid or powdered infant formula is the primary source of nutrition, it should be mixed with water that is fluoride free or contains low levels of fluoride to reduce the risk of fluorosis (ADA, 2006). Commercially bottled water generally is low in fluoride, but only a few companies list the fluoride content on their

Table 4.4 Examples of calculations critical to fluoride consumption.

Example 1. Use of optimally fluoridated water in powdered infant formula
The optimal dose of fluoride per day is 0.05 mg/kg/day (Institute of Medicine, 1997)

A 1-year-old child, who weighs 10 kg, consumes an average of 32 ounces (1 L) of infant formula a day. The formula is powdered formula that is reconstituted with optimally fluoridated water:
   1 L of formula at 1 ppm F = 1 mg F/day
   1 mg F/10 kg body weight = 0.1 mg F/kg

Example 2. Use of too much toothpaste
The optimal dose of fluoride per day is 0.05 mg/kg/day (Institute of Medicine, 1997).

A 3-year-old child, who weighs 14 kg, swallows half of a ribbon of toothpaste (0.5 g) each time he brushes, twice a day:
   0.5 g of toothpaste × twice a day × 1,000 ppm F = 1 mg F
   1 mg F/14 kg body weight = 0.07 mg/kg

Example 3. Caution when using professional topical fluoride in preschool children
The probable toxic dose of fluoride is 5 mg/kg (Whitford, 1996)

A 3-year-old child, who weights 14 kg, swallows 10 mL of professional strength acidulated phosphate fluoride gel
   10 mL × 1.23% F (1.23 g/100 mL) = 123 mg F
   123 mg F/14 kg = 8.8 mg F/kg

labels (Johnson, 2003). One can be sure that bottled water is fluoride free if the label states that the water has been distilled or has undergone reverse osmosis.

A study of children in North Carolina, aged 2–6 years, found that milk and water amount to 40% of total liquids consumed per day. Fluoride intake from liquids other than water and milk averaged 0.36 mg/day in 2- and 3-year-olds and 0.54 mg/day in 4- to 6-year-olds (Pang et al., 1992).

Toothpaste

There are fluorosis risks associated with swallowing of fluoridated toothpaste by preschool children (Pendrys, 1995). Nearly all toothpaste sold in the United States and Canada contains between 1,000 and 1,100 ppm F. A full ribbon of toothpaste on an adult toothbrush weighs approximately 1 g, which is equivalent to 1 mg of fluoride in toothpaste containing 1,000 ppm F. Various studies indicate that children under age 6 swallow between 24 and 60% of the toothpaste on their brush. This ingestion varies with age and is directly related to the amount applied to the brush (Fomon and Ekstrand, 1996). Thus, preschool children who use unregulated amounts of fluoride toothpaste are at risk for fluorosis (Table 4.4, example 2).

Supervised use of a pea-sized amount of toothpaste (approximately 1/4 g) on the toothbrush in children under age 6 has been shown to be helpful in regulating the amount of toothpaste swallowed (Davies et al., 2003), and sharply reduces the risk of fluorosis (Pendrys, 1995). Since 1991, manufactures of fluoride toothpaste in the United States state this recommendation on the toothpaste package labels. Furthermore, toothpaste labeling mandated by the U.S. Food and Drug Administration in 1996 directs parents of children under age 2 to seek advice from a dentist or physician before introducing their child to fluoride toothpaste. A recent recommendation, however, suggests that children under age 2 may brush with a "smear" of fluoridated toothpaste and children over 2 years should brush with a pea-sized amount (SIGN, 2005). The Maternal and Child Health Bureau also recommends a smear of fluoridated toothpaste for high caries–risk children under the age of 2 (MCHB, 2007) (Figure 4.2).

Fluorosis

Fluoride ingested during tooth development can result in a range of visual changes to the enamel, referred to as fluorosis. The mild form of fluorosis appears as chalk-like, lacy markings across the tooth's enamel surface that generally is not apparent to the affected person. Mild fluorosis affects neither cosmetic appearance nor dental function (Figure 4.3). The prevalence of mild fluorosis has increased due to an increase in total intake of fluoride from all sources. It was found that 25% of children in Iowa from birth to 36 months of age were ingesting an estimated 0.8 mg F/day, and 10% were ingesting more than 1 mg/day, resulting in 25% of the children

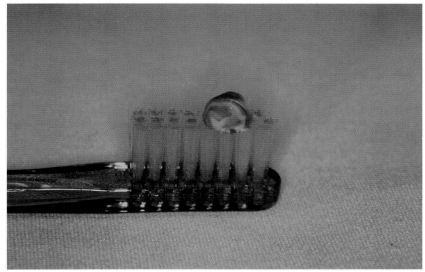

(a)

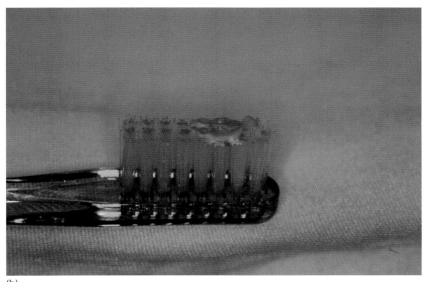

(b)

Figure 4.2   Pea-sized (for children between the ages of 2 and 6 years) or smear (for children under age 2) amount of fluoridated toothpaste on the brush (SIGN, 2005).

ingesting more than double the recommended daily dose of fluoride (Levy et al., 2001). Moderate fluorosis is defined as opaque white areas on more that 50% of the enamel surface. The rare, severe form of fluorosis manifests as pitted and brittle enamel (MMWR, 2001).

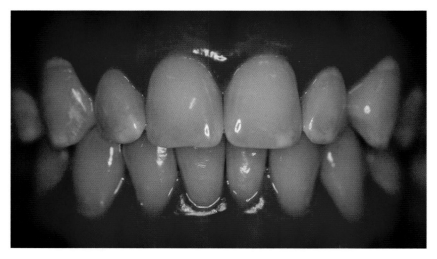

Figure 4.3 Mild fluorosis on maxillary incisors and canines due to elevated levels of fluoride in water supplies.

Although both primary and permanent teeth may be affected by fluorosis, fluorosis tends to be greater in permanent teeth perhaps because mineralization of primary teeth occurs before birth. The placenta may serve as a partial barrier to the transfer of high concentration of plasma fluoride from a pregnant mother to her developing fetus.

Concerns regarding the risk for enamel fluorosis due to systemic intake of fluoride are limited to children under age 7. The transitional and early maturation stages of enamel development appear to be most susceptible to the effects of fluoride. For fluorosis of the maxillary central incisors, the most sensitive period of excess fluoride ingestion is between 1 and 2 years (DenBesten and Thariani, 1992).

Thus, fluorosis is related to dose, duration, and timing of the fluoride intake. As stated above, the main fluoride sources for preschool children are drinking water, infant formula reconstituted with fluoridated water, fluoride supplements, and toothpaste. A low prevalence of mild fluorosis has been accepted as a reasonable and minor consequence of fluoride intake, balanced against the substantial protection from dental caries (MMWR, 2001).

TOPICAL FLUORIDES

Toothpaste

Without question the most widely used method of applying fluoride topically is by means of toothpaste. In countries where toothpastes are used, over 95% of the products contain a fluoride compound (Murray and Naylor, 1996). Fluoridated toothpaste studies of 2- to 3-year duration have been shown to reduce caries experience by approximately 15–30% (MMWR, 2001), and several have shown that in 3- to 6-year-olds daily toothbrushing with fluoride toothpaste significantly reduces caries incidence (Holtta and Alaluusua, 1992; Sjögren et al., 1995; Schwarz et al., 1998).

Most persons report brushing their teeth at least once per day, but more frequent use may offer additional protection. Brushing twice a day is a social norm that is generally accepted. Additionally, having greater contact with fluoride toothpaste during brushing may have advantages. A child instructed in a modified brushing technique consisting of applying toothpaste evenly on the teeth, brushing for 2 min and refraining from rinsing, has been found to reduce caries by an average of 26% compared to children who also brushed with fluoridated toothpaste, but received no instructions on use or rinsing (Sjögren and Birkhed, 1993). Other studies have confirmed that rinsing after brushing with fluoride toothpaste should be kept to a minimum or eliminated altogether in order to maximize the beneficial effect of the fluoride in the toothpaste (Sjögren and Birkhed, 1994; Sjögren et al., 1994).

Professional topical

Topical fluoride exposure has several mechanisms of action to prevent dental caries. More concentrated professional topical fluoride products, such as fluoride gels or varnishes, leave a temporary layer of calcium fluoride on the enamel surface. The calcium fluoride is subsequently released to the plaque fluid when the plaque pH drops due to bacterial metabolism. The released fluoride primarily affects caries by remineralizing partially demineralized enamel and by altering bacterial metabolism (Rolla and Ekstrand, 1996). Low levels of fluoride may affect bacterial metabolism by interfering with the glycolytic and sugar transport enzymes that alter the ability of bacteria to degrade simple sugars to acid. High levels of fluoride (above 0.1%) may also have bactericidal effects (Hamilton and Bowen, 1996). (Table 4.5 compares the fluoride concentration of professional topical fluoride products to the concentration of fluoride in brush-on gels, rinses, and toothpaste.)

Professional topical fluoride applications performed semiannually reportedly reduce caries by approximately 30% (Ripa, 1991). The recommended application time for these treatments is 4 min, and the efficacy of shorter application periods has not been tested in human clinical trials. Proper application techniques that reduce the swallowing of the fluoride are essential to reducing the potential for acute symptoms (Table 4.4, example 3).

Fluoride varnish, as a means of delivering fluoride at professional topical strengths, has been widely used in Canada and Europe since the 1970s, but was not introduced into the United States until 1991. At present,

Table 4.5   Percentage of fluoride ion concentration compared to the concentration of sodium fluoride in common topical fluoride preparations.

	F ion concentration	NaF concentration
Acidulated phosphate fluoride professional topical	1.23%	2.7%
Sodium fluoride professional topical	0.9%	2%
Sodium fluoride varnish	2.3%	5%
Tray or brush-on gel	0.5%	1.1%
Weekly rinse	0.09%	0.2%
Daily rinse	0.02%	0.05%
Toothpaste	0.1%	0.22%

fluoride varnishes are approved in the United States as a cavity liner (Food and Drug Administration, 1999), but are primarily used "off-label" for topical fluoride treatments (Figure 4.4). As of 2007 there were at least 10 commercially available fluoride varnish products in the United States. All of the products contained 5% sodium fluoride in a resin base, except for one that is 1% difluorosilane in a polyurethane base. The most referenced fluoride varnish products in 2007 were Duraphat, DuraFluor, Fluor Protector, and Cavity Shield (Pub Med, 2007, National Library of Medicine/National Institutes of Health, http://www.pubmed.gov).

Fluoride varnish is ideal for preschool children because of ease of use and its safety due to single-dose dispensers. Products that are available now come in containers of either 0.25, 0.4, or 0.6 mL of varnish, corresponding to 12.5, 20, or 30 mg fluoride, respectively. The caries-preventive

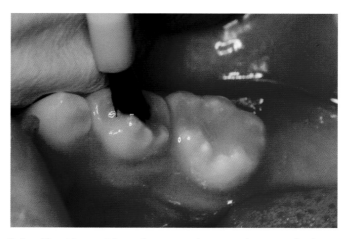

Figure 4.4   Fluoride varnish application to the entire dentition of a 3-year-old.

Table 4.6 Summary recommendations regarding dietary supplement and topical fluoride for preschool children, based on caries risk.

	Low caries risk	Moderate caries risk	High caries risk
Dietary supplements[a]	May not have additional benefit	6 months to 3 years = 0.25 mg F 3–6 years = 0.5 mg F	6 months to 3 years = 0.25 mg F 3–6 years = 0.5 mg F
Toothpaste	Twice daily[b] Smear under 2 years; pea-sized over 2 years	Twice daily[b] Smear under 2 years; pea-sized over 2 years	Twice daily[b] Smear under 2 years; pea-sized over 2 years
Professional topical	May not have additional benefit	F varnish at 6-month interval[c]	F varnish at 3- to 6-month interval[c]
Brush-on high-potency F gel	Not recommended	Not recommended	Caution when prescribing
Daily rinse	Not recommended	Not recommended	Not recommended

[a] Fluoride levels in drinking water considerations.
[b] Direct parental supervision; do not rinse after brushing.
[c] Modified from American Dental Association, Council on Scientific Affairs (2006).

efficacy of fluoride varnishes generally is equal to that of other topical fluoride vehicles (Beltran-Aguilar et al., 2000), and their efficacy to reduce caries in primary teeth has been demonstrated in numerous studies (Holm, 1979; Frostell et al., 1991; Twetman et al., 1996; Petersson et al., 1998; Weintraub et al., 2006). The ADA has recommended that fluoride varnish be administered twice a year for preschool children at moderate caries risk and 4 times a year for children at high caries risk (ADA, Council on Scientific Affairs, 2006). Table 4.6 summarizes recommendations regarding dietary supplement and topical fluoride for preschool children, based on caries risk. Caries-risk factors for preschool children are extensively reviewed in Chapter 8.

An interesting report on fluoride varnish specific to preschool children with early childhood caries was reported in 2001. This study examined children treated with 5% NaF varnish every 3 months versus untreated children. After 18 months those children treated with varnish had half the number of new carious and one-third more arrested caries on the maxillary anterior teeth than the control group (Lo et al., 2001). Such an approach may be an alternative to or allow postponement of restorative treatment on maxillary anterior teeth in selected young children.

CONCLUSIONS

(1) In preschool children, both pre- and posteruptive effects of fluoride appear to reduce caries.

(2) Fluoride sources for preschool children include fluoridated drinking water, infant formula reconstituted with fluoridated water, toothpaste, foods/drinks produced in fluoridated areas, and fluoride supplements.

(3) Irrespective of efficacy, there are concerns associated with the use of fluoride supplements including lack of compliance, inaccurate dosing, risk of fluorosis, and prescribers not considering a child's caries risk or fluoride level of water supplies.

(4) Mild fluorosis has been accepted as a reasonable and minor consequence of fluoride intake balanced against the substantial protection from dental caries.

(5) Supervised use of a "pea-sized" amount of fluoridated toothpaste in children under age 6 has been shown to be effective in regulating the amount of fluoride swallowed. Children under age 2 may brush with a "smear" of fluoridated toothpaste.

(6) Brushing instructions consisting of applying fluoridated toothpaste evenly on the teeth, brushing for 2 min, and refraining from rinsing reduce caries more than no instructions.

(7) Fluoride varnish is a safe and easy way to administer professional topical fluoride treatment in preschool children.

(8) The issues to be considered for dietary fluoride supplements are a child's age, fluoride content of water supplies, caries risk and compliance; the issue for professional topical fluoride treatments is caries risk.

REFERENCES

Aasenden R, Allukian M, Brudevold F, and Wellock WD. 1971. An in-vivo study on enamel fluoride in children living in a fluoridated and in a non-fluoridated area. *Arch Oral Biol* 16:1399–11.

Aasenden R and Peebles TC. 1974. Effects of fluoride supplementation from birth on human deciduous and permanent teeth. *Arch Oral Biol* 19:321–6.

ADA Positions and Statements. 2006. *Interim Guidance on Fluoride Intake for Infants and Young Children*. Available at http://www.ada.org/prof/resources/pubs/adanews/adanewsarticle.asp?articleid=2212 (accessed November 8, 2006).

American Academy of Pediatric Dentistry. 1995. Reference Manual 1994–1995. *Pediatric Dentistry*. 16(Special Issue):1–96.

American Academy of Pediatrics, Committee on Nutrition. 1979. Fluoride supplementation: Revised dosage schedule. *Pediatrics* 63:150–52.

American Academy of Pediatrics, Committee on Nutrition. 1995. Fluoride supplementation for children: Interim policy recommendations. *Pediatrics* 95:777.

American Dental Association, Council on Scientific Affairs. 2006. Professionally applied topical fluoride. *J Am Dent Assoc* 137:1151–9.

Arnold FA, McClure FJ, and White CL. 1960. Sodium fluoride tablets for children. *Dent Prog* 1:8–12.

Backer Dirks O, Houwink B, and Kwant GW. 1961. The results of 6½ years of artificial fluoridation of drinking water in the Netherlands—the Tiel Cumemborg experiment. *Arc Oral Biol* 5:284–300.

Beltran ED and Burt BA. 1988. The pre- and posteruptive effects of fluoride in the caries decline. *J Public Health Dent* 48:233–40.

Beltran-Aguilar ED, Goldstein JW, and Lockwood SA. 2000. Fluoride varnishes: A review of their clinical use, cariostatic mechanism, efficacy and safety. *J Am Dent Assoc* 131:589–96.

Bowen WH. 1973. The effect of single daily doses of fluoride on saliva, plaque and urine in monkeys (*Macaca fascicularis*). *J Int Dent Assoc Child.* 4:11–14.

Burt BA and Eklund SA. 1999. *Dentistry, Dental Practice, and the Community*, 5th edn. Philadelphia: W.B. Saunders Company.

Clarkson BH, Fejerskov O, Ekstrand J, and Burt BA. 1996. Rational use of fluoride in caries control. In: Fejerskov O, Ekstrand J, and Burt BA (eds), *Fluorides in Dentistry*, 2nd edn. Copenhagen, Denmark: Munksgaard, pp 347–57.

Davies RM, Davies GM, and Ellwood RP. 2003. Prevention. Part 4: Toothbrushing: What advice should be given to parents? *Br Dent J* 195:135–41.

DenBesten PK and Thariani H. 1992. Biological mechanisms of fluorosis and level and timing of systemic exposure to fluoride with respect to fluorosis. *J Dent Res* 71:1238–43.

Ekstrand J. 1996. Fluoride metabolism. In: Fejerskov O, Ekstrand J, and Burt BA (eds), *Fluoride in Dentistry*, 2nd edn. Copenhagen, Denmark: Munsgaard. pp 55–68.

Ekstrand J and Ehrnebo M. 1979. Influence of milk products on fluoride bioavailability in man. *Eur J Clin Pharmacol* 16:211–15.

Ekstrand J, Ehrnebo M, and Boreus LO. 1978. Fluoride bioavailability after intravenous and oral administration: Importance of renal clearance and urine flow. *Clin Pharmacol Ther* 23:329–37.

Ekstrand J, Fomon S, Ziegler EE, and Nelson S. 1994. Fluoride pharmacokinetics in infancy. *Pediatr Res* 35:157–63.

Fomon SJ and Ekstrand J. 1996. Fluoride intake. In: Fejerskov O, Ekstrand J, and Burt BA (eds), *Fluoride in Dentistry*, 2nd edn, Copenhagen, Denmark: Munsgaard, pp 40–52.

Food and Drug Administration. 1999. US Department of Health and Human Services. 21 CFR Part 355. *Anticaries Drug Products for Over-the-Counter Human Use*. Code of Federal Regulation 280–85.

Frostell G, Birkhed D, and Edwardsson S. 1991. Effect of partial substitution of invert sugar for sucrose in combination with Duraphat treatment on caries development in preschool children: The Malmo study. *Caries Res* 25:304–10.

Hamilton IR and Bowen GHW. 1996. Fluoride effects on oral bacteria. In: Fejerskov O, Ekstrand J, and Burt BA (eds), *Fluorides in Dentistry*, 2nd edn. Copenhagen, Denmark: Munksgaard, pp 230–51.

Holm AK. 1979. Effect of a fluoride varnish (Duraphat) in preschool children. *Community Dent Oral Epidemiol* 7:241–5.

Holtta P and Alaluusua S. 1992. Effect of supervised use of a fluoride toothpaste on caries incidence in preschool children. *Int J Paediatr Dent* 2:145–9.

Institute of Medicine. 1997. Fluoride. In: *Dietary Reference Intakes for Calcium, Phosphorus, Magnesium, Vitamin D, and Fluoride*. Washington, DC: National Academy Press, pp 288–313.

Ismail AI and Bandekar RR. 1999. Fluoride supplements and fluorosis: A meta-analysis. *Community Dent Oral Epidemiol* 27:48–56.

Johnson SA. 2003. Concentration levels of fluoride in bottled drinking water. *J Dent Hyg* 77:161–7.

Lemke CW, Doherty JM, and Arra MC. 1970. Controlled fluoridation: The dental effects of discontinuation in Antigo, Wisconsin. *J Am Dent Assoc* 80: 782–6.

Leverett DH, Adair SM, Vaughan BW, Proskin HM, and Moss ME. 1997. Randomized clinical trial of the effect of prenatal fluoride supplements in preventing dental caries. *Caries Res* 31:174–9.

Levy SM and Guha-Chowdhury N. 1999. Total fluoride intake and implications for dietary fluoride supplementation. *J Public Health Dent* 59:211–23.

Levy SM, Kiritsy MC, Slager SL, and Warren JJ. 1998. Patterns of dietary fluoride supplement use during infancy. *J Public Health Dent* 58:228–33.

Levy SM, Warren JJ, Davis CS, and Kirchner L. 2001. Patterns of fluoride intake from Birth to 36 months. *J Public Health Dent* 61:70–77.

Lo EC, Chu CH, and Lin HC. 2001. A community-based caries control program for pre-school children using topical fluoride: 18-month results. *J Dent Res* 80:2071–2074.

Marthaler TM. 1979. Fluoride supplements for systemic effects in caries prevention. In: Johansen E, Taves DR, and Olsen TO (eds), *Continuing Evaluation of the Use of Fluorides*. Washington DC: AAAS, pp 33–59.

Maternal Child Health Bureau. 2007. *Topical Fluoride Recommendations for High-Risk Children*. Expert Panel. October 22–3.

Meskin LH (ed.) 1995. Caries diagnosis and risk assessment: A review of preventive strategies and management. *J Am Dent Assoc* 126(Suppl): 1S–24S.

Murray JJ and Naylor MN. 1996. Fluorides and dental caries. In: Murray JJ (ed.), *Prevention of Oral Disease*. Oxford: Oxford University Press, pp 32–67.

Morbidity and Mortality Weekly Report (MMWR). 2001. National Library of Medicine. 2007. National Institutes of Health. *Recommendations for Using Fluoride to Prevent and Control Dental Caries in the United States*, Vol. 50/No. RR-14, August 17.

Pang DTY, Phillips CL, and Bawden JW. 1992. Fluoride intake from beverage consumption in a sample of North Carolina children. *J Dental Res.* 71:1382–8.

Pendrys DG. 1995. Risk of fluorosis in a fluoridated population: Implications for the dentist and hygienist. *J Am Dent Assoc* 126:1617–24.

Pendrys DG. 2000. Risk of enamel fluorosis in nonfluoridated and optimally fluoridated populations: Considerations for the dental professional. *J Am Dent Assoc* 13:746–55.

Petersson LG, Twetman S, and Pakhomov GN. 1998. The efficiency of semi-annual silane fluoride varnish applications: A two-year clinical study in preschool children. *J Public Health Dent* 58:57–60.

Ripa LW. 1991. A critique of topical fluoride methods (dentifrice, mouthrinses, operator-, and self-applied gels) in an era of decreased caries and increased fluorosis prevalence. *J Public Health Dent* 51:23–41.

Rolla G and Ekstrand J. 1996. Fluoride in oral fluids and dental plaque. In: Fejerskov O, Ekstrand J, Burt BA (eds), *Fluorides in Dentistry*, 2nd edn. Copenhagen, Denmark: Munksgaard, pp. 215–29.

Schwarz E, Lo ECM, and Wong MCM. 1998. Prevention of early childhood caries—results of a fluoride toothpaste demonstration trial on Chinese preschool children after three years. *J Public Health Dent* 58:12–18.

Scottish Intercollegiate Guideline Network (SIGN). 2005. *Prevention and Management of dental decay in the pre-school child*. Available at http://www.sign.ac.uk/pdf/sign83.pdf (accessed April 30, 2008).

Singh KA, Spencer AJ, and Armfield JM. 2003. Relative effects of pre- and posteruption water fluoride on caries experience of permanent first molars. *J Public Health Dent* 63:11–19.

Sjögren K and Birkhed D. 1993. Factors related to fluoride retention after tooth-brushing and possible connection to caries activity. *Caries Res* 27:474–7.

Sjögren K and Birkhed D. 1994. Effect of various post-brushing activities on salivary fluoride concentration after toothbrushing with a sodium fluoride dentifrice. *Caries Res* 28:127–31.

Sjögren K, Birkhed D, and Rangmar B. 1995. Effect of a modified tooth-paste technique on approximal caries in preschool children. *Swed Dent J* 110(Suppl):1–10.

Sjögren K, Ekstrand J, and Birkhed D. 1994. Effect of water rinsing after tooth-brushing on fluoride ingestion and absorption. *Caries Res* 28:455–9.

Sohn W, Ismail AI, and Taichman LS. 2007. Caries risk-based fluoride supple-mentation for children. *Pediatr Dent* 29:23–31.

Thylstrup A. 1990. Clinical evidence of the role of preeruptive fluoride in caries prevention. *J Dent Res* 69(Special Issue):742–50.

Twetman S, Petersson LG, and Pakhomov GN. 1996. Caries incidence in re-lation to salivary mutans streptococci and fluoride varnish applications in preschool children from low- and optimal-fluoride areas. *Caries Res* 30:347–53.

Weatherell J, Deutsch D, Robinson C, and Hallsworth AS. 1977. Assimilation of fluoride by enamel throughout the life of the tooth. *Caries Res* 11:85–115.

Weintraub, JA, Ramos-Gomez F, and June B. 2006. Fluoride varnish efficacy in preventing early childhood caries. *J Dent Res* 85:172–6.

Whitford GM. 1996. *The Metabolism and Toxicity of Fluoride*, 2nd edn. Basel: Karger.

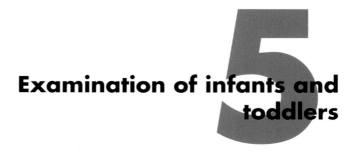

Examination of infants and toddlers

Adriana Segura

The American Academy of Pediatric Dentistry recommends a child's first visit to occur 6 months after the eruption of the first tooth or at 1 year of age. The objectives of the first visit are to educate the parent, introduce prevention modalities, and assess the risk for oral disease.

Access to care for the populations ages 0–5 years provides the ultimate challenge. Previous research from the Medical Expenditures Panel Survey in 1996 showed that 38% of U.S. children had a preventive visit (Watson et al., 2001). Preschool children from families with income at least 3 times below the poverty level are 4.8 times more likely to have to decay (Vargas et al., 1998; Edelstein, 2002). The Centers for Disease Control and Prevention (CDC) (2007) released a report stated that caries had increased among children from ages 2 to 5 years. Results like these clearly indicate that parents need to be counseled and assisted in obtaining early preventive visits.

Certain factors do affect the access to preventive care. Lewis et al. (2007) investigated specific issues that contributed to the prevalence of early preventative visit. They analyzed the National Survey of Children Health data and determined that 72% of children were reported to have had a preventive visit in 2003 (van Dyck et al., 2004; Lewis et al., 2007). A contributing factor was the creation of the Title XXI, State Children's Health Insurance Program in 1997. The creation of this program assisted families who were not eligible for Medicaid. Disparities were still evident. The ratio of the dental care uninsured to the health care uninsured was 2.6. Lewis et al. (2007) concluded that children who were 5 years old and younger that were of nonwhite/ethnicity, lacked dental insurance, and lacked care from a physician were less likely to have received a preventive dental visit.

An increased awareness of the detrimental effects of early childhood caries has prompted the involvement of different types of health professionals to address the access to care issue. The potential of changing behavioral attitudes is the basis of the early preventive visit. As advocates of oral health the American Academy of Pediatric Dentistry, American Academy of Pediatrics, and the American Dental Association have a standing policy for children to have a dental home by age 1 (American Academy of Pediatrics 2003; American Academy of Pediatric Dentistry, 2006). The recognition of the disease has led to a paradigm shift in prevention strategies and the implementation of policies for early examination.

Many factors limit the access to care in the underserved population. Several models and innovative strategies have been started to improve oral health in children. Washington State's Access to Baby and Child Program focused on four areas to improve access to preventive services: (1) outreach to the community, (2) training and certification for oral health providers, (3) improved dental benefits, and (4) increased the fee for service reimbursement (Milgrom et al., 1997). The program is expanded to training pediatricians and family physicians. Families that have used the program have increased the use of preventive services and the numbers of dentists treating Medicaid children had more than doubled (Nagahama et al., 2002).

North Carolina into the Mouth of Babes Programs aimed to train primary care providers and staff in order to access children from ages 0 to 3 who were not receiving regular dental care (Rozier et al., 2003). In order for physicians to be eligible for reimbursement, they were required to attend an education/training course. This program exemplifies the role primary health care professionals can play in oral health.

These two programs are just an example of how dental and nondental professionals can interact and collaborate to increase access to care. Education, screening, and referral are part of these programs and thus can provide increased collaboration with the dental provider in the community.

The source and referral from the WIC Program is also an important collaboration to foster in the community (McCunniff et al., 1998). Evidence supports that early intervention, including intervention with mothers, benefits the young child.

The establishment of the dental home allows for early intervention and optimal care for the young child (Thomas, 1997; Nowak and Casamassimo, 2002). The establishment of the dental home is modeled after the medical home. The medical home was proposed by the Academy of Pediatrics in 1992. The policy stated that all children can receive better care when there is an established relationship with the physician, the child, and the child's family (American Academy of Pediatrics, 1992). The home should be accessible, family centered, continuous, comprehensive, coordinated, compassionate, and culturally centered.

Providing a dental home by age 1 allows the practitioner to complete a risk assessment, provide an introduction to dentistry, and provide anticipatory guidance to the parent. The dental anticipatory guidance is replicated after the medical anticipatory guidance model (Nowak and Casamassimo, 1995). The initial appointment gives the health professional an opportunity to guide the parent through important oral health information. The areas of discussion are dental developmental milestones, oral hygiene, diet, oral habits, trauma, and fluoride in its systematic and topical uses, and expectations of behavior during dental appointments. These are modified at each appointment to be age appropriate for the child.

The first part of the appointment is obtaining information from the parent. This should be conducted prior to the actual examination. Information gathering should include questions in regard to medical history, social history, prenatal, natal and neonatal history, cognitive and development history, and dental history. After obtaining all pertinent information, anticipatory guidance topics are discussed and then the actual knee-to-knee examination is conducted.

MEDICAL HISTORY

The medical history should be thorough and all inclusive of perinatal and natal history. The history will be critical when assessing risk factors. A child who receives primary care from a physician on a regular care is indicative that the child's has had access to health care. Knowledge of compliance of the recommended the immunization schedule also gives an insight to the parent's perception of health beliefs and the access to this type of medical preventive care. Frequency of illnesses can expose the child to frequent intake of sweetened medications. Sugar-based medications can place a child at higher risk for caries.

SOCIAL HISTORY

Family environment has key influences on oral health. Recent research has emphasized the medical and nonmedical determinants of health (Kindig and Stoddart, 2003; Spencer, 2003). At the same time Population Health Research has also investigated the dental and nondental determinants of oral health (Crall et al., 1990; Fejerskov, 2004). A conceptual model includes determinants that are nonmedical and nondental. This model is modified from Keyes and Jordan. Keyes and Jordan (1963) postulated the etiologic factors necessary for the caries diseases process to be initiated. Components necessary are (1) cariogenic bacteria, (2) susceptible tooth or host, and (3) substrate—fermentable carbohydrates.

The conceptual model modifies the Keyes model and adds other determinants that affect oral health (Fisher-Owens et al., 2007). Different domains at different levels affect the child's health. The domains are genetic, biologic factors, social environment, physical environment, health behaviors, dental care, and medical care. These influential factors can be at an individual, family, and community level. Examples of individual determinants are having dental insurance or the use of dental care. Family-level influences can be social support, culture, and family function. Community-level determinants can be health care system characteristics and community oral health environment.

Questions can be structured in such a manner to obtain some of this information. A lot of information can be obtained by simply asking who is with the child during the daytime, who brushes the child's teeth, does the child receive regular pediatric checkups, are there other siblings in the family household, and what types of food are eaten at home. Cultural practices can greatly affect dietary practices and health beliefs. These are also determinants in the conceptual model.

PRENATAL, NATAL, AND NEONATAL HISTORY

Implications of preterm birth

Complications during pregnancy are of significance in an infant's health. Diabetes, hypertension, and preeclampsia are all risk factors for possible enamel hypoplasia (Noren et al., 1978). Premature infants are exposed to varieties of physical stresses. Infants with a gestational age under 37 weeks are susceptible to metabolic disorders, pulmonary disorders, jaundice, and nutritional deficiencies. Mineralization of primary central incisors begins at the twelfth and sixteenth gestational age. Any deprivation of calcium, phosphate, fluoride, and vitamins A, C, and D can lead to hypoplastic enamel (Pimlott et al., 1985; Seow et al., 1989). Investigators have also researched the association of premature, low birth weight of infants, and enamel hypoplasia (Seow et al., 1987). Chandra et al. (1977) found an association with infants' low birth weight and deficiency in the cell-mediated immunity. Caufield et al. (1993) postulated that a weaker immune response may predispose the infant to an earlier window of infectivity. Initial acquisition of *mutans streptococci* is usually between 1 and 2 years of age.

Prolonged intubation during the neonatal period can exert the alveolar pressure and cause a disruption of amelogenesis (Seow, 1991). It is difficult to conclude a complete association or correlation with low birth weight and caries in the primary dentition (Burt and Satishchandra, 2001; Shulman, 2005). Shulman did conclude certain correlations in the 2005 study: there was higher Decayed, Filled Surfaces in children whose mothers had low education, infants that were not breast-fed, infants that had bottle use after 1 year of age, and mothers who had less than two prenatal visits. Prenatal history will help explain any dental abnormalities found during the examination.

COGNITIVE HISTORY

The health professional should be familiar with general developmental milestones of the young child (Table 5.1). The advent of language skills usually begins at 1 year of age. The vocabulary of an 18-month-old consists of about 10 words and a 3-year-old should have a vocabulary close to 1,000 words.

Infant and childhood fears need to be taken into consideration when examining the child. Crying is a form of communication for the infant. Fear of strangers begins usually around 7–12 months of age (Pinkham, 2005). Separation anxiety initiates around 6 months of age. Children under the age of 3 are considered to be in the precooperative stage or lacking the ability to cooperate (Wright, 1994). Due to lack of ability to cooperate at this age, the parent is never separated from the child during the examination. Any variation from the expected milestones should be explained to parent and informed of the need for further evaluation. Knowledge of these milestones will assist the health provider to adapt the anticipatory guidance to an age-appropriate level.

DENTAL HISTORY

Certain question should address any teething difficulties, previous dental trauma, dietary practice, eruption times, fluoride exposures, and oral hygiene practices. Previous caries experience is still the most important

Table 5.1 Speech and language milestones.

Hearing and understanding	Talking
Birth to 3 months • Startles to loud sounds. • Quiets or smiles when spoken to. • Seems to recognize your voice and quiets if crying. • Increases or decreases sucking behavior in response to sound.	**Birth to 3 months** • Makes pleasure sounds (cooing, gooing). • Cries differently for different needs. • Smiles when sees you.
4–6 months • Moves eyes in direction of sounds. • Responds to changes in tone of your voice. • Notices toys that make sounds. • Pays attention to music.	**4–6 months** • Babbling sounds more speech-like with many different sounds, including p, b, and m. • Vocalizes excitement and displeasure. • Makes gurgling sounds when left alone and when playing with you.
7 months to 1 year • Enjoys games like peek-o-boo and pat-a-cake. • Turns and looks in direction of sounds. • Listens when spoken to. • Recognizes words for common items like "cup," "shoe," and "juice." • Begins to respond to requests ("Come here," "Want more?").	**7 months to 1 year** • Babbling has both long and short groups of sounds such as "tata upup biblbibi." • Uses speech or noncrying sounds to get and keep attention. • Imitates different speech sounds. • Has one or two words (bye-bye, dada, mama) although they may not be clear.
1–2 years • Points to a few body parts when asked. • Follows simple commands and understands simple questions ("Roll the ball," "Kiss the baby," "Where's your shoe?"). • Listens to simple stories, songs, and rhymes. • Points to pictures in a book when named.	**1–2 years** • Says more words every month. • Uses some one- to two-word questions ("Where kitty?" "Go bye-bye?" "What's that?"). • Puts two words together ("more cookie," "no juice," "mommy book"). • Uses many different consonant sounds of the beginning of words.
2–3 years • Understands differences in meaning ("go-stop," "in-on," "big-little," "up-down"). • Follows two requests ("Get the book and put it on the table.").	**2–3 years** • Has a word for almost everything. • Uses two- to three-word "sentences" to talk about and ask for things. • Speech is understood by familiar listeners most of the time. • Often asks for or directs attention to objects by naming them.
3–4 years • Hears you when call from another room. • Hears television or radio at the same loudness level as other family members.	**3–4 years** • Talks about activities at school or at friends' homes. • People outside family usually understand child's speech.

Table 5.1 *(Continued)*

Hearing and understanding	Talking
• Understands simple, "who?" "what?" "where?" "why?" questions.	• Uses a lot of sentences that have four or more words. • Usually talks easily without repeating syllables or words.
4–5 years • Pays attention to a short story and answers simple questions about it. • Hears and understands most of what is said at home and in school.	**4–5 years** • Voice sounds clear like other children's. • Uses sentences that give lots of details (e.g., "I like to read my books"). • Tells stories that stick to topic. • Communicates easily with other children and adults. • Says most sounds correctly except a few like *l, s, r, v, z, ch, sh, th.* • Uses the same grammar as the rest of the family.

predicative factor of future risk for caries (Demers et al., 1990). These questions will help formulate the individualized prevention plan.

PREPARATION

The armamentarium for the actual examination is simple and inexpensive. A source of light, two chairs, and a dental mirror need to be available. The examination can be done with or without the use of dental chair. The examination is done with the assistance of the parent.

The practitioner sits in front of the parent. Both the parent and the practitioner are facing each other. The knees are in very close proximity (Figure 5.1). The infant is placed on the parent's lap facing the parent. The child's legs should be wrapped around the parent's waist. This type of positioning allows the parent to hold the hands if necessary and permits the child to directly visualize the parent for comfort (Figure 5.2). The child's head is then cradled in the practitioner's knees. The cognitive development of a child under 3 is not developed enough for the practitioner to expect cooperation or that the child will able to comprehend the tell-show-do behavior management technique. As part of the anticipatory guidance, the parents should be reassured that crying is a normal behavioral response. A crying response will facilitate the examination. If the child does not open the mouth, the practitioner can facilitate this by placing the finger in between the lips. The finger is slid along the buccal surface of the maxillary teeth and gentle pressure is applied on the retromolar pad. This will cause an automatic reflex for the child to open the mouth. The knee-to-knee position facilitates a clear path for the parent to visualize any oral findings (Figure 5.3).

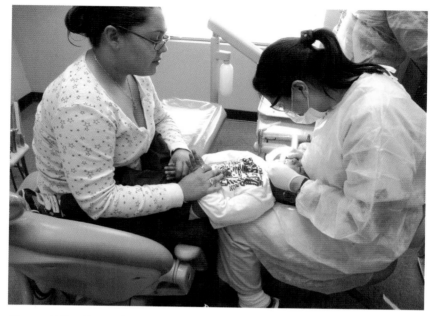

Figure 5.1   Knee-to-knee position: The practitioner and the parent sit facing each other in chairs, with knees touching.

During the positioning process of a child, the practitioner should begin a general appraisal of the child. The general appraisal can be done throughout the examination. The purpose of the appraisal is to evaluate the physical well-being of the child. Any peculiar or nonexplanatory bruising or trauma should be further investigated. Critical judgment is necessary on the part of the practitioner. da Fonseca et al. (1992) noted that in 1,248 cases of child abuse two-thirds of all cases had involvement of the craniofacial region.

EXAMINATION

Extraoral

The examination should be done in systematic and orderly fashion. The examination should assess for any facial asymmetry assessing face, ears, head, and the neck. The lip commissures should be evaluated for the presence of dryness and any ulceration. Infants and toddlers frequently will continually moisten their lips with their tongue or the moisture of milk/liquids on the corners of their lips can harbor a *Candida albicans* infection.

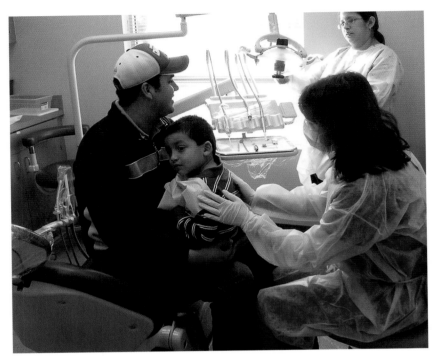

Figure 5.2   The child is placed on the parent's lap and facing the parent.

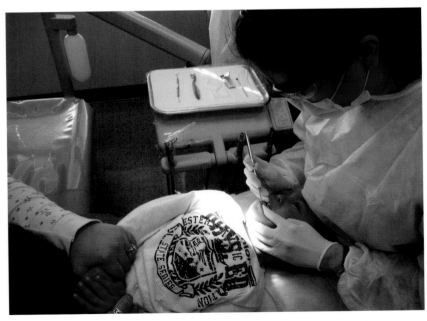

Figure 5.3   The parent is able to hold the child's hand if necessary in this position.

Palpation of the cervical lymph nodes should be palpated for any tenderness, mobility, or any enlargement. These are significant as they are part of the lymphatic systems for the oral cavity, throat, pharynx, and tonsils. The anterior cervical nodes are positioned beneath the sternocleidomastoid muscles. The posterior cervical nodes are in front of the trapezius muscle. The submandibular nodes are below the mandible on each side and are related to the floor of the mouth. The submental nodes are below the chin area and are also in relation to the oral cavity. The enlargement of any of these nodes would indicate an infection of the oral cavity, tonsillar, or the posterior pharyngeal regions.

Intraoral

The examination should be done with an aid pen light or a dental operatory light. The salivary flow or the moisture should be evaluated. Certain medications can have xerostomic side effects.

The intraoral examination should begin with the palpation of all soft tissues. The examination should assess the pharyngeal area including the evaluation of the tonsillar tissue. The size of the tonsils should be noted. The estimation of the size is based on a scale: 1, normal size; 2, absent because of surgery; 3, moderate enlargement, not beyond the pillars; and 4, marked enlargement, meeting the uvula (Corbo et al., 2001). The documentation of the size of tonsillar tissue becomes important if restorative treatment has to be rendered under conscious sedation.

The dorsum of the tongue should be evaluated for color, coatings, and any textural abnormalities. Mobility of tongue should be assessed in order to determine the presence of ankyloglossia or tongue tie. Ankyloglossia is characterized by a short frenulum. In young infants that are being breast-fed, there might be difficulty in latching on to the breast, thus not allowing adequate milk to be transferred. Controversary exists on whether ankyloglossia interferes with breast-feeding (Ballard et al., 2002). The Hazelbaker assessment lingual tool categorizes the severity of ankylosia based on appearance and function (Hazelbaker, 1993). Surgical intervention is only indicated when there is a tight lingual frenulum and there is interference in latching and causing maternal pain (Amir et al., 2005; Kupietsky and Botzer, 2004).

Soft tissue examination

White subsurface lesions can be noted at birth or during the neonatal period (Flaitz, 2005). These cysts are characterized by their position in the oral cavity. They are usually present as solitary, discrete papules, 1–3 mm in size and are asymptomatic. Bohn's nodules are located on the soft and hard palate. Epstein pearls are located on the mid-palatine raphe. Dental palatal lamina cysts are located on the alveolar ridge. These are asymptomatic and require no treatment.

Often early in the eruption sequence a localized swelling may be present. It is usually amber, red, or blue in color and overlying an erupted tooth. This is termed eruption hematoma or cyst. There might be an associated delay of the eruption of the tooth. Treatment is usually not indicated, as it resolves with the tooth eruption.

The child's periodontal tissue varies from the adult periodontium (Casamassimo, 1999). The gingival tissue is more vascular. The tissue is redder and lacks stippling. The interdental papilla is flatter because of the increased spacing in the primary dentition.

Gingivitis is the most common disease entity affecting the periodontium in the young child. Signs of gingivitis are bleeding and inflammation. Inflammation of the free gingiva will be present if there is generalized plaque accumulation. Gingivitis is reversible with proper oral hygiene.

Alveolar bone loss is very rare in the young child. If there are any signs of mobility or loss of alveolar bone, a differential diagnosis of a systemic disorder should be considered. Entities such as hypophosphatasia, cyclic neutropenia, prepubertal periodontal disease and Langerhans' cell histiocytosis should be part of the differential (Henry and Sweeney, 1996). A medical consult should be obtained.

Hypophosphatasia is an autosomal recessive disorder that is due to a deficiency in the enzyme alkaline phosphatase. The result is abnormal calcification process of bones and increased urinary excretion of phosphoethanolamine. Research has shown that the Langerhans' cell histiocytosis is characterized by infiltration of tissues and organs by histiocytosis. The histiocytosis displays a neoplastic feature (Willman, 1994). The classic presentation is lytic lesions of the bone. Prepubertal periodontal disease is characterized by the proliferation of the microorganisms *Actinobacillus actinomycetemcomitans* and can result in tooth mobility before the age of 3. Cyclic neutropenia is the result of periods of reduced or absence of neutrophils. Oral features are significant gingival inflammation and alveolar bone loss.

Hard tissue examination

Primary teeth begin to form around 7 weeks in utero (Full, 2005). The enamel of the primary teeth is completely formed by the first year of age. The first tooth general erupts by 6 months of age. The primary mandibular central incisor is usually the first tooth to erupt.

All primary teeth should erupt between the ages of 24 and 36 months (Figure 5.4).

Certain variations in the eruption pattern may occur. One of these variations can manifest itself as neonatal or natal teeth. Although these are rare occurrences, it is important to inform parents of their significance. Presence of teeth at birth is termed natal teeth. The eruptions of teeth after birth have been termed neonatal teeth. Several factors have been studied as possible explanations for these occurrences: superficial positioning of the tooth germ, infection, malnutrition, febrile incidents, hormonal stimulation, and

Primary teeth eruption chart

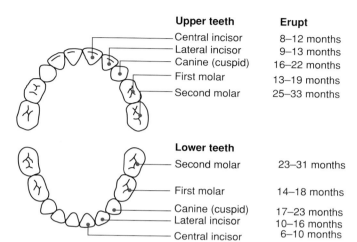

Upper teeth	Erupt
Central incisor	8–12 months
Lateral incisor	9–13 months
Canine (cuspid)	16–22 months
First molar	13–19 months
Second molar	25–33 months

Lower teeth	
Second molar	23–31 months
First molar	14–18 months
Canine (cuspid)	17–23 months
Lateral incisor	10–16 months
Central incisor	6–10 months

Figure 5.4   Eruption pattern of the primary dentition.

osteoblastic activity (Cunha et al., 2001; Leung and Robson, 2006). Histological differences have been noted on these teeth. Polarized and microradiography studies have shown variation in the enamel structure: hypomineralization, hypomaturation, and hypoplastic enamel (Soni et al., 1967). Bigeard et al. (1996) noted natal teeth have reduced enamel thickness and having an outer prism free layer. The early eruption of these teeth may be due to remodeling activity that occurs in close proximity to the tooth germ area (Uzamis et al., 1999). A differential diagnosis is important to discern whether these teeth are part of the primary dentition or they are supernumerary. Factors to consider before extraction are (1) extent of mobility and possibility of aspiration, (2) severe maternal pain when breast-feeding, and (3) evidence of ulcerations (Riga-Fede) on the infants tongue.

The classification of primary teeth is designated with letters. The upper case letter "A" begins with the upper right second primary molar follows around to the left second primary molar, tooth "J." Then the lettering continues to the left mandibular primary second molar, tooth "K," and then the mandibular right second primary molar is designated as "T." The primary dentition is complete by age 3 (Figure 5.5).

Once the primary dentition is complete there is general spacing between the teeth. Primate spaces are spaces between the cuspids and primary molars in the mandible. In the maxilla it is present between the cuspids and laterals spaces. The remaining general spacing between the primary teeth is called developmental spaces.

The structural integrity of the teeth needs to be appraised. Developmental defects are of clinical significance when it pertains to assessing the

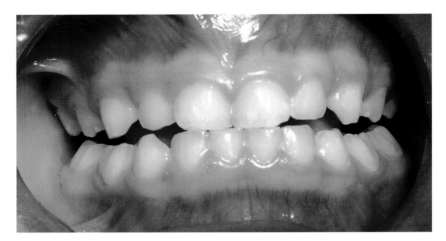

Figure 5.5   Complete primary dentition.

risk of caries. Certain defects may place the child at higher risk for caries. Primary enamel is formed in utero beginning at 15–19 weeks. Enamel hypoplasia is a defect in the mineralization process. Ameloblasts are derived from the ectoderm. The formation of enamel is dependent on the ectodermal and mesodermal interaction. Genetic diseases and environmental factors can be attributed to the disturbance in the mineralization process.

Genetic diseases as amelogenesis imperfecta (AI) and dentigenesis imperfecta affect the structure of the enamel and dentin respectfully. The extent of the defect in the structural entity is noted in the difference in the ultrastructural analysis. There are four types of AI (Seow, 1991). AI hypoplastic is characterized by the presences of pits arranged in rows and columns, and insufficient enamel formation. This is autosomal dominant inherited. Teeth affected with AI hypocalcification presents with normal thickness of enamel, but poorly mineralized. The enamel manifests a yellow brown color. The enamel is very soft and fragile. AI hypomaturation presents with normal thickness of enamel, which has a low mineral content. The enamel is mottled and easily chips away. AI hypomaturation and hypocalcification can be inherited autosomal recessive or dominant. AI hypomaturation/hypoplastic is characterized with taurodontism. The enamel is mottled, yellow brown in color, and pitted. The fourth type is inherited autosomal dominant.

Dentgenesis imperfecta involves a defect in the predentin matrix, resulting in amorphous, a tubular dentin (Dummitt, 2005). There are three types of dentigenesis imperfecta. Shield type I occurs in conjunction with osteogenesis imperfecta. The teeth appear to have bulbous crowns and obliterated pulp chambers. This is characterized by the presence of brittle bones and the teeth appear to have a translucent tooth color. Shield type II appears to have opalescent dentin. Shield type III is rare and the predominant feature is a bell-shaped crown.

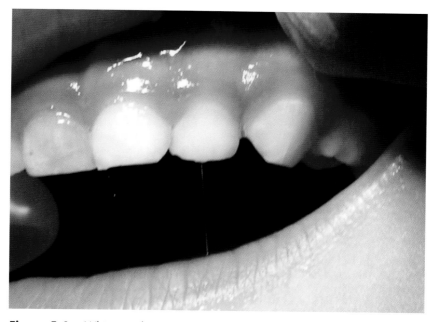

Figure 5.6   White spot lesion present on tooth H (left primary cuspid).

Other components can also affect the mineralization process: hypoparathyroidism, defects in enzymes that are linked with vitamin D metabolism, and inherited disorders of calcium metabolism.

IDENTIFICATION OF CARIES

The dentition needs to be evaluated for stains, white spot lesions, or actual cavitations. In order to properly visualize the surfaces of the teeth many times it will be necessary to wipe of any plaque present on the surface. This may be done gently with gauze. The white spot lesion appears to have a very chalky appearance (Figure 5.6). White spots are signs of early demineralization. If the pH stays below 5.5 and the saliva is not able to buffer, the demineralization process will continue until cavitation occurs. Early intervention will prevent frank cavitations. The application of fluoride varnish is indicated if the surface is intact. If the surface has already a cavitation, restorative treatment will be necessary (Figure 5.7).

OCCLUSION ASSESSMENT

Infants are usually not sufficiently cooperative to analyze or classify the occlusion. General evaluation can be done of the anterior-posterior

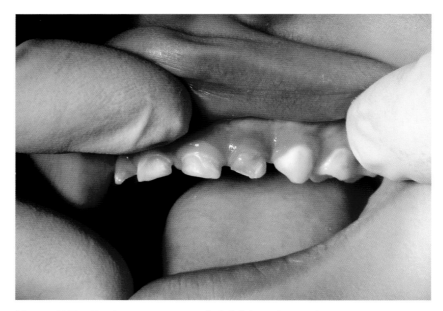

Figure 5.7 Frank cavitation on tooth G (left lateral incisor).

dimension, transverse relationships, and the vertical dimension. The anterior-posterior dimension can be assessed by measuring the overjet. This will help determine any effects of an oral habit. This is determined by estimating the horizontal overlap of the maxillary incisor. Vertical dimension is the overbite (vertical overlap) of the incisors and this will also help determine any effects of an oral habit. An anterior open bite can be indicative of an oral habit. Assessing the transverse relationship will determine the presence of any anterior or posterior crossbite. Any deviation of the norm should be charted, but the age of the young child usually precludes any treatment.

Signs of prolonged nonnutritive sucking (NNS) may be exhibited from visualizing the position of anterior teeth (Nowak and Warren, 2000). NNS is part of the natural rooting reflex and a part of normal development. Psychoanalytical theory and learning theory postulate different rationale for the presence NNS (Johnson and Larson, 1993). Psychoanalytical theory arises on the belief that pleasure is arrived from oral stimulation. The learning theory is based on that NNS is an adaptive response that becomes a learned response (Palermo, 1956). Effects of prolonged NNS by either a pacifier or a digit sucking are determined by three factors: intensity, duration, and frequency of the habit (Modeer et al., 1982). Adair et al. (1995) noted that the children who had a history of having a pacifier had a significantly larger mean overjet. Ogaard et al. (1994) noted a statistical significance in maxillary protrusion in infants who had prolonged pacifier past 24 months of age. The American Academy of Pediatrics has policy recommending the continuation of a pacifier to age 1 (American Academy of Pediatrics, 2005). This policy was changed due to research associating less sudden infant syndrome with the use of the pacifier. The American Academy of Pediatric Dentistry recommends discontinuation of the pacifier habit at 24 months of age or earlier (American Academy of Pediatric Dentistry, 2006).

TREATMENT PLANNING

The history, information gathering, and examination will give the practitioner adequate information to decide the risk factors that place a child at risk for caries. The caries-risk assessment tool of the American Academy of Pediatric Dentistry can be used to classify the child's risk for caries at a high, moderate, or low level (American Academy of Pediatric Dentistry, Council on Clinical affairs, 2002). The mode of transmission from mother to child has to be emphasized during the examination process (Berkowitz et al., 1975). After the examination is complete, the practitioner can demonstrate oral hygiene to parent. A toothbrush prophylaxis and fluoride varnish can be completed in the knee-to-knee position.

The information obtained will help determine the frequency of recall schedule. Parents should be counseled and educated on the significance of each risk factor. Parents should be encouraged to brush their child's teeth twice a day. The anticipatory guidance information will assist the parent in making healthy choices for the child's diet.

This chapter has provided the objectives and procedure for the knee-to-knee examination. The examination itself does not require a lot time. The rationale for the infant oral examination is preventing oral disease. An infant program can be integrated into any dental and medical office.

REFERENCES

Adair SM, Milano M, Lorenzo I, and Russell C. 1995. Effects of current and former pacifier use on the dentitions of 24 to 59-month-old children. *Pediatr Dent* 17:437–44.

American Academy of Pediatric Dentistry. 2006. Policy of oral habits. Reference manual 2006–2007. *Pediatr Dent* 28:43–4.

American Academy of Pediatric Dentistry. Council on Clinical Affairs. 2002. Policy on use of a caries-risk assessment tool (CAT) for infants, children and adolescents. *Pediatr Dent* 25:18.

American Academy of Pediatrics. 1992. Ad hoc task force on definition of the medical home. The medical home. *Pediatrics* 90:774.

American Academy of Pediatrics. 2003. Policy statement: Oral health risk assessment timing and establishment of the dental home. *Pediatrics* 111:1113–10.

American Academy of Pediatrics. 2005. Task force on sudden infant death syndrome. The changing concept of sudden infant death syndrome: Diagnostic coding shifts, controversies regarding the sleeping environment, and new variables to consider in reducing risk. *Pediatrics* 116:1245–55.

Amir LH, James JP, and Beaty J. 2005. Review of tonque-tie release at a tertiary maternal hospital. *J Paediatr Child Health* 41:243–5.

Ballard JL, Auer CE, and Khoury JC. 2002. Ankyloglossia: Assessment, incidence, and effect of frenuloplasty on the breastfeeding dyad. *Pediatrics* 110:e63.

Berkowitz RJ, Jordan HV, and White G. 1975. The early establishment of *Streptococcus mutans* in the mouth of infants. *Arch Oral Biol* 20:1–6.

Bigeard L, Hemmerle J, and Sommermater JI. 1996. Clinical and ultrastructural study of natal tooth: Enamel and dentin assessments. *J Dent Child* 63:23–31.

Burt BA and Satishchandra P. 2001. Does low birth weight increase the risk of caries? A systematic review. *J Dent Educ* 65:1024–7.

Casamassimo P. 1999. Periodontal considerations. In: Pinkham JR, Casamassimo PS, McTigue DJ, Fields HW, and Nowak AJ (eds), *Pediatric Dentistry. Infancy through Adolescence*, 2nd edn. Philadelphia, PA: Elsevier Saunders, pp 353–7.

Caufield PW, Cutter GR, and Dasanayake AP. 1993. Initial acquisition of mutans streptococci by infants: Evidence for a discrete window of infectivity. *J Dent Res* 72:37–45.

CDC. 2007. *Trends in Oral Health Status: United States, 1988–1994 and 1999–2004*, Series 11, Number 248. 104.

Chandra RK, Ali SK, Kutty KM, and Chandra S. 1977. Thymus-dependant lymphocytes and delayed hypersensitivity in low birth weight infants. *Biol Neonate* 31:15–18.

Corbo GM, Forastiere F, Agabiti N, Pistelli R, Dell'Orco V, Perucci CA, and Valente S. 2001. Snoring in 9- to 15-year-children: Risk factors and clinical relevance. *Pediatrics* 108:1149–54.

Crall JJ, Edelstein B, and Tinnanoff N. 1990. Relationship of microbiological, social and environmental variables to caries status in young children. *Pediatr Dent* 12:233–6.

Cunha RF, Baer FAC, Torriani DD, and Frossard WTG. 2001. Natal and neonatal: Review of the literature. *Am Acad Pediatr Dent* 23:158–65.

da Fonseca MA, Feigal RJ, and ten Bensel RW. 1992. Dental aspects of 1,248 cases of child maltreatment on file at a major county hospital. *Pediat Dent* 14:152–7.

Demers M, Brodeur JM, Simard PL, Mouton C, Veilleux G, and Frechette S. 1990. Caries: Predictors suitable for mass-screenings in children: A literature review. *Community Dent Health* 7:11–21.

Dummitt C. 2005. Anamolies of the developing dentition. In: Pinkham JR, Casamassimo PS, McTigue DJ, Fields HW, and Nowak AJ (eds), *Pediatric*

Dentistry. Infancy through Adolescence, 5th edn. Philadelphia, PA: Elsevier Saunders, pp 61–73.

Edelstein BL. 2002 Disparities in oral health and access to care: Findings of national surveys. *Ambul Pediatr* 2(Suppl):141–7.

Fejerskov O. 2004 Changing paradigms in concepts on dental caries: Consequences for oral health care. *Caries Res* 38:182–91.

Fisher-Owens SA, Gansky SA, Platt LJ, Weintraub JA, Soobader M, Bramlett M, and Newacheck PW. 2007. Influences on children's oral health: A conceptual model. *Pediatrics* 120:510–20.

Flaitz CM. 2005. Differential diagnosis of oral lesions and developmental anomalies. In: Pinkham JR, Casamassimo PS, McTigue DJ, Fields HW, and Nowak AJ (eds), *Pediatric Dentistry. Infancy through Adolescence*, 5th edn. Philadelphia, PA: Elsevier Saunders, pp 9–73.

Full CM. 2005. Dynamics of change: Dental changes. In: Pinkham JR, Casamassimo PS, McTigue DJ, Fields HW, and Nowak AJ (eds), *Pediatric Dentistry. Infancy through Adolescence*, 5th edn. Philadelphia, PA: Elsevier Saunders, pp 172–92.

Hazelbaker AK. 1993. *The Assessment Tool for Lingual Frenulum Function (ATLFF): Use in a Lactation Consultant Private Practice*. Thesis. Pasadena, CA: Pacific Oaks College.

Henry RJ and Sweeney EA. 1996. Langerhans' cell histocytosis: Case reports and literature review. *Pediatr Dent* 18:11–16.

Johnson ED and Larson BE. 1993. Thumb-sucking: Literature review. *J Dent Child* 60:385–91.

Keyes PH and Jordan HV. 1963. Factors influencing the initial transmission and inhibition of dental caries. In: Harris RS (ed.), *Mechanisms of Hard Tissue Destruction*. New York, NY: Academy Press, pp 261–83.

Kindig D and Stoddart G. 2003. What is population health? *Am J Public Health* 93:380–83.

Kupietsky A and Botzer E. 2004. Ankyglossia in the infant and young child: Clinical suggestions for diagnosis and management. *Pediatr Dent* 27: 40–46.

Leung AKC and Robson WL. 2006. Natal teeth: A review. *J Natl Med Assoc* 98:226–8.

Lewis CW, Johnston BD, Linsenmeyar KA, Williams A, and Mouradian W. 2007. Preventive dental care for children in the United States: A national perspective. *Pediatrics* 119:e544–53.

McCunniff MD, Damiano PC, Kanellis MJ, and Levy SM. 1998. The impact of WIC dental screenings and referrals on utilization of dental services among low-income children. *Pediatr Dent* 20:181–7.

Milgrom P, Hujoel P, Grembowski D, and Ward JM. 1997. Making medicaid child dental services work: A partnerships in Washington State. *J Am Dent Assoc* 128:753–63.

Modeer T, Odernrick L, and Lindner A. 1982. Sucking habits and their relation in posterior-crossbites in 4-year-old children. *Scandinavia J Res* 90: 323–8.

Nagahama SI, Fuhriman SE, Moore CS, and Milgrom P. 2002. Evaluation of a dental society-based ABCD Program in Washington State. *J Dent Assoc* 133:1251–7

Noren J, Grahnen H, and Magnusseon BO. 1978. Maternal diabetes and changes in hard tissues of primary teeth. III: A histological and microradiographic study. *Acta Odontol Scand* 36:127–35.

Nowak AJ and Casamassimo PJ. 2002. The dental home. The primary care oral health concept. *J Am Dent Assoc* 133:93–8.

Nowak AJ and Casamassimo PS. 1995.Using anticipatory guidance to provide early dental intervention. *J Am Dent Assoc* 126:1156–63.

Nowak AJ and Warren JJ. 2000. Infant oral health and oral habits. *Pediatr Clin North Am* 47:1043–66.

Ogaard B, Larsson E, and Lindsten R. 1994. The effects of sucking habits, cohort, sex, intercanine widths, and breast or bottle feeding on posterior crossbite in Norwegian and Swedish 3-year-old children. *Am J Orthod Dentofacial Orthop* 106:161–6.

Palermo DS. 1956. Thumbsucking: A learned response. *Pediatrics* 17:392–9.

Pimlott JF, Howley TP, Nikiforuk G, and Fitzhardinge PM. 1985. Enamel defects in prematurely born, low birth-weight infants. *Pediatr Dent* 7: 218–23.

Pinkham JR. 2005. The dynamics of change: Emotional changes. In: Pinkham JR, Casamassimo PS, McTigue DJ, Fields HW, and Nowak AJ (eds), *Pediatric Dentistry. Infancy through Adolescence*, 5th edn. Philadelphia, PA: Elsevier Saunders, pp 166–205.

Rozier RG, Sutton BK, Bawden JW, Haupt K, Slade GD, and King RS. 2003. Prevention of early childhood caries in North Carolina medical practices. *Implications Res Pract* 67:876–85.

Seow WK. 1991. Enamel hypoplasia in the primary dentition: A review. *J Dent Child* 58:441–52.

Seow WK, Humphrys C, and Tudehope DI. 1987. Increased prevalence of developmental defects in low-birth-weight children: A controlled study. *Pediatr Dent* 9:221–5.

Seow WK, Masel JP, Weir C, and Tudehope DI. 1989. Mineral deficiency in the pathogenesis of enamel hypoplasia in prematurely born, very low birth-weight children. *Pediatr Dent* 11:297–301.

Shulman JD. 2005. Is there an association between low birth weight and caries in the primary dentition? *Caries Res* 39:161–7.

Soni NN, Siberkweit M, and Brown CH. 1967. Polarized light and microradiographic study of natal teeth. *J Dent Child* 49:300–303.

Spencer N. 2003. Social, economic and political determinants of child health. *Pediatrics* 112:704–6.

Thomas HF. 1997. First dental visit, first birthday: A rationale and protocol for infant oral health care. *Tex Dent J* 114:15–19.

Uzamis M, Olmez S, Ozturk H, and Celik H. 1999. Clinical and ultrastructural study of natal and neonatal teeth. *J Clin Pediatr Dent* 23:173–7.

van Dyck P, Kogan MD, Heppel D, Blumberg SJ, Cynamon ML, and Newacheck PW. 2004. The national survey of children's health: A new data source. *Matern Child Health* 8:1360–66.

Vargas CH, Crall JJ, and Schneider DA. 1998. Sociodemographic distribution of pediatric dental caries: NHANES III, 1988–1994. *J Am Dent Assoc* 129:1229–1238.

Watson MR, Manski RJ, and Macek MD. 2001. The impact of income on children's and adolescents' preventative dental visits. *J Am Dent Assoc* 132:1580–87.

Willman C. 1994. Detection of clonal histiocytosis in Langerhans' cell: Biology and clinical significance. *Br J Cancer* 70:29–33.

Wright GZ. 1994. Psychologic management of children's behaviors. In: McDonald RE and Avery DR (eds), *Dentistry for the Child and Adolescent*, 6th edn. St Louis, MO: Mosby, pp 32–51.

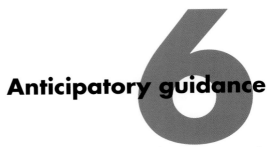

Anticipatory guidance

Paul S. Casamassimo and Arthur J. Nowak

WHY ANTICIPATORY GUIDANCE

Preventive maintenance is routinely recommended by manufacturers for all newly purchased equipment. Data support the routine maintenance of automobiles, appliances, the kitchen floor, and the lawns, and landscaping that surround our homes and offices. We spend a lot of money to make those purchases, yet even when reminded by salespersons or printed instructions that preventive maintenance will extend life and optimize performance, many people do not heed the advice.

It is not surprising then that too often we deal with our body and its health in a similar manner. Presently, obesity is a major health issue; in fact it is an epidemic, in spite of studies demonstrating that if we reduce our caloric intake, select healthful foods, and exercise regularly, we can maintain our recommended weight. We can enjoy similar positive outcomes in oral health if we follow the recommendations of early intervention, optimal use of fluoride, daily plaque removal, controlling our diets and eating habits, and periodically visit our oral health professional.

Historically, oral health has been neglected or taken for granted, especially with children and the primary dentition. Although an early examination between 18 and 24 months was recommended by the authors of early pedodontic texts such as those authored by Sidney Finn and Ralph McDonald (1963), the driving force for the first asymptomatic examination was the entry into kindergarten or first grade and that was when it was most often, unless pain or a traumatic event intervened. Toothbrushing may or may not have been practiced at home. Age-appropriate brushes were not available until the 1960s. Fluoridated dentifrices made their appearance about the same time. Fluoridation of community water started in the 1950s, but dental insurance was almost nonexistent before the 1950s and only began to be offered by industry and labor unions a decade later.

Prevention as we know it today in dentistry was uncommon before the 1960s, except in a few dental practices. The first national voice of concern was from a small group of practitioners, fed up with the lack of support by organized dentistry. They banded together and formed the American Society for Preventive Dentistry in the 1960s, and sponsored the first "prevention convention" that reported on innovative and revolutionary departures from the mainly reparative practice methods used in dentistry at the time. Suddenly, we learned about early intervention, a first dental visit by age 1, optimal prescription of fluorides, reduction of fermentable carbohydrates in foods and liquids, personalized recall schedules, and the use of sealants on caries-susceptible tooth surfaces. But progress was slow. In a report that summarized the number of prevention-related articles published in the *Journal of Dentistry for Children* from 1968 to 1988, the authors reported that only 16% of the over 1,000 articles published had a preventive theme (Nowak, 1990). This report epitomized the fact that the dental profession was still not embracing prevention as well as treatment.

THE SEEDS OF ANTICIPATORY GUIDANCE

The basis for prevention of early childhood caries has been with us for a while. The bacterial strain, *Streptococcus mutans*, was isolated from a cavity by Clark in 1924, and Keyes, in the 1960s, reported the transmissibility and infectious properties of dental caries. It was not until the 1980s that Berkowitz and others reported that *Streptococcus mutans* caused the primary infection in infants (Berkowitz et al., 1975). This discovery was followed in 1993 by Caufield and coworkers who reported a "window of infectivity" when the infant was most susceptible to the disease (Caufield et al., 1993). Evidence of a controllable infection was mounting.

Further evidence to support optimal prevention was the concept of remineralization reported by Silverstone and others in the 1980s (Silverstone et al., 1981). We learned that dental caries is a dynamic process where loss of enamel mineral content (demineralization) and its replacement, or remineralization, is ongoing at the tooth surface on a molecular level. Under normal conditions, a state of equilibrium is reached, but is challenged by accumulation of plaque, increase in acid production, and, in the absence of topical fluorides and saliva, dissolution of enamel surfaces occurs.

With these concepts, early childhood caries is easy to explain. The healthy equilibrium is severely disturbed in the infant who consumes fermentable carbohydrates (especially at sleep times) continuously and whose teeth are not cleaned, causing often a dramatic demineralization of enamel of maxillary anterior teeth. The cavitation of these teeth was once called nursing bottle caries and is now known as early childhood caries (ECC) or severe early childhood caries (S-ECC) and is devastating to the infant and parents.

Today, government, health advocacy organizations, the American Academies of Pediatric Dentistry and Pediatrics as well as the American Dental Association define early childhood caries as the presence of one or more decayed (noncavitated or cavitated lesions), missing (due to caries), or filled tooth surfaces in any primary tooth in a child 71 months of age or younger (CDC, 1997). ECC can be further diagnosed based on the age of the child and the dmf score (Table 6.1).

The literature has established unequivocally that ECC leads to higher risk of caries in the remaining primary dentition and the developing permanent dentition (Johnsen et al., 1986). This disease can alter the quality of life of the growing child because of growth and development problems, increased dental treatment costs, loss of school days, increased days with restricted activity, modified diets, delays in speech development, and finally behavioral and learning problems at both school and home (Acs et al., 1999; Filstrup et al., 2003; Williamson et al, 2008).

Table 6.1 Diagnosis of ECC and dmfs score.

Age	dmfs score
Less than 3 years	1
3 years	≥ 4
4 years	≥ 5
5 years	≥ 6

BACKGROUND OF THE CONCEPT OF ANTICIPATORY GUIDANCE

For generations, new parents depended on their own parents or other family members to provide information on child rearing. With societal change that began in the mid-1960s, multigenerational families became separated because of employment opportunities or upward mobility. In addition, everyday living was becoming more difficult with increasing choices about where to live, whether to rent or buy a home, where to send children to school, and even where to buy food.

Access to health care became more complex and often frustrating. The neighborhood general practice family physician gave way to doctors or clinics controlled by insurers, often specialists in family medicine or pediatrics. Health supervision rather than problem-based care entered our lexicon. Following birth of the child, a prescribed series of follow-up appointments were required for the asymptomatic infant/toddler, including immunizations and then finally the physical examination mandated prior to school entry. Diagnostics continually improved with the development of tests based on study evidence. No longer were pharmaceuticals limited to a few choices. The demand for well-child care for all young children made appointments hurried and frequently managed by physician extenders to aid the overscheduled practice. To facilitate communication, handouts were developed and distributed to parents to improve understanding and compliance. Commercially available books and manuals were promoted to assist parents and answer those more difficult and complex questions. Studies reported that many illnesses could be prevented and health promotion and disease prevention became exciting possibilities. The earliest examples included the polio vaccine, but recommendations for lifestyle changes began to be promoted widely, such as the Surgeon General's report on the negative implications on the use of tobacco products (U.S. Public Health Service, 1964).

Throughout this period it became increasingly evident that care of children could vary from one physician to another. Parents wanted more information and to be more involved in treatment decisions. Guidelines were needed that would assist physicians on what was needed to be accomplished at each age-related visit. The American Academy of Pediatrics responded by publishing its first preventive pediatrics "periodicity table" in 1967. The "Suggested Schedule for Preventive Child Health Care" emphasized that each child is unique, but with competent parenting, no manifestations of health problems and normal development, these recommendations should be followed (AAP, 1967).

Now that a schedule of recommended visits was available, a need arose for effective health promotion to coordinate efforts between diverse medical and nonmedical professionals and agencies and to keep pace with changes in rearing practices, family structure, communities, and society.

In 1990, with funding from Health Resources and Services Administration's Maternal and Child Health Bureau and the Health Care Financing Administration's Medical Bureau, an initiative called *Bright Futures* was formed (Green and Palfrey, 1994). Supported by thirty-one organizations, the *Bright Futures* mission was to, "promote and improve the health, education and well-being of infants, children, adolescents, families and communities." The goal was to develop comprehensive health supervision guidelines with the collaboration of four interdisciplinary panels of experts in infant, toddler, school-age child, and adolescent health. The guidelines were to be a practical developmental approach to provide health supervision for children from birth through adolescence. In 1994, *Bright Futures: Guidelines for Health Supervision of Infants, Children and Adolescents* was published and updated in 2000 and again in 2007.

The foundation of *Bright Futures* is health promotion, which means to-do behaviors that actively support the physical, emotional, mental, and social well-being of children, adolescents, and their families. Families must participate as full partners in the health interview, physical examinations, and screening procedures, by providing information on the sibling and parent's health, social history, employment status, community support, child care, educational, and recreational activities.

In a medical home (AAP, 2002), families establish long-term trusting relationships with doctors and staffs. In a medical home, the services tend to be continuous, coordinated, comprehensive, and cost-effective. In addition they are family centered, community based, and compassionate. An important component to *Bright Futures* and the medical home is anticipatory guidance (AG) (Nowak and Casamassimo, 1995). AG helps families understand what to expect during their child's current and approaching stage of development. It provides personalized instruction and family education. In pediatric health supervision time-limited visits, topics that should be considered include healthy habits, prevention of illness and disease, nutrition, oral health, sexuality, social development, family relationships, parental health, community interactions, self-responsibility, and school/vocational achievements. These are covered differentially, based on a child's needs.

APPLICATION OF ANTICIPATORY GUIDANCE TO PEDIATRIC DENTISTRY

A number of publications and oral health policies and clinical guidelines were being developed and promoted in the 1990s and early 2000 that greatly modified the traditional concepts of disease/treatment toward oral health promotion. These promotions emphasized early intervention, risk assessments, optimal fluoride use and occlusal sealants, and personalized recall schedules based on the child's risk:

• American Academy of Pediatric Dentistry (AAPD) guideline on periodicity of examination, preventive dental services, anticipatory guidance, and oral treatment for children. This outlines a health supervision paradigm with preventive interventions, approved by the pediatric dentistry specialty. It was created in 1991 and revised in 1992, 1996, 2000, 2003, and 2007 (AAPD, 2007a).

- An article entitled, "Using Anticipatory Guidance to Provide Early Dental Intervention," by Nowak and Casamassimo, is the first entry into the dental literature using the term (Nowak and Casamassimo, 1995).
- *Bright Futures in Practice: Oral Health* is one of the first attempts in pediatric dentistry to provide a comprehensive risk-based health supervision paradigm for oral health from birth through adolescence (Casamassimo, 1996).
- A review paper by Nowak entitled "Rationale for the Timing of the First Oral Evaluation" provides a comprehensive justification for seeing a child at 1 year of age rather than at 3 years, which was the prevailing standard at the time (Nowak, 1997).
- "The Dental Home: A Primary Oral Health Concept" was the first appearance of the application of the medical concept to pediatric dentistry (Nowak and Casamassimo, 2003).
- "AAPD Policy on the Dental Home" is another professionally derived statement about the child's relationship with the dentist and was first published in 2001 and revised 2004 (AAPD, 2007b).
- AAPD policy on use of a caries-risk assessment tool for infants, children, and adolescents takes state-of-the-art science and the principles of risk assessment and provides a clinically useful tool for rating a child's susceptibility to dental caries. It was first released in 2002 and revised in 2006, incorporating experience with its application and new science (AAPD, 2007c).

DEFINITION OF ANTICIPATORY GUIDANCE

In pediatric health care delivery, AG is the process of providing practical, developmentally appropriate health information about children to parents/caretakers in anticipation of significant physical, emotional, and psychological milestones. By providing this information, parents/caretakers will be alerted and prepared to manage these changes to maximize development and minimize anxieties and concerns.

Anticipatory guidance as applied to oral health care can be easily introduced to the dentist's protocol for managing a child's first and subsequent visits. Its structure begins to be developed initially from the responses of the parents to the child's health history, continues during the interview with the parents, is further influenced by the findings of the oral examination, and is finalized during the discussion with the parents of the child's treatment needs and follow-up. Anticipatory guidance can be applied throughout childhood to account for lifestyle and developmental changes, well into young adulthood.

Interactive communications between the dentist and parents/caretakers are paramount to have a successful professional visit. Parents become engaged in the process and participate in decision making with the dentist. They can question recommendations and seek assistance on how they might be integrated into the busy family schedules. This will shape individualized strategies to implement recommendations that are personalized for the child, to accomplish the treatment goals within the structure of the parent's ability to cooperate and facilitate their execution.

ANTICIPATORY GUIDANCE TOPICS

Changing advice for the changing child

The following sections describe the content of the six areas of anticipatory guidance: oral and dental development, fluoride use, diet and nutrition, oral hygiene, habits, and injury prevention. We use the term, "pre-three" to describe children in the first 36 months of age throughout this chapter. Application of these topics to a child at any particular age in the pre-three period requires an assessment of lifestyle, child development, family function, and parental ability. Feeding illustrates this dynamism of transition with a child primarily fed from birth by mother with bottle or breast with limited food choices and a fledgling dentition. The child may quickly transition into a day care setting and will begin solid foods at some point, so feeders and food may increase in complexity. The maxillary primary incisors historically present the first caries risk from excessive bottle use, but as the dentition matures and the diet changes, the posterior teeth become most susceptible to caries. The ambulatory child may have access to foods at his or her discretion and food may be used as a motivator or behavioral control rather than just for nutrition.

The tables in this chapter are organized to allow the clinician to fix a snapshot in time of the life of the child, with those aspects of life most commonly associated with an age, like tooth eruption, at the midpoint of that age. Children who are new to a dental home may need to have all elements of anticipatory guidance to the left of their age line provided because the dentist cannot assume the behaviors or risk have already been dealt with.

The principles of anticipatory guidance should be remembered in the context of the other three overall goals of health supervision that are disease detection, disease prevention, and health promotion. Anticipatory guidance should be seen as the hands-on, direct application of preventive strategies.

General developmental stages of the pre-three child

Dentists traditionally have not seen children at this age and are often not familiar with the limitations and characteristics of the pre-three child. This section offers a window of what the dentist can expect to see in the child under 36 months of age who is a rapidly developing human, but one who is still limited in all areas and dependent on parents for survival. The latter part of the first year of life has the infant with minimal gross motor skills. At 9 months of age, the child can sit upright briefly with support, can grasp large objects, and can squirm. Speech is limited to polysyllabic sounds and this child's main method of communication is crying. At 12 months of age, a child may be walking with a little assistance and by 24 months can walk alone easily and is running with abandon in the third year of life. Motor skills move from a primitive ability to hold large objects in the first year of life to development of pincer grasp. By 36 months, the child can stack objects and play games that mimic life activities like feeding dolls.

Language grows from the polysyllabic sounds that a dentist would hear at an ideally placed first visit to a few words beside mama and dada at age 12 months. By 2 years of age the vocabulary has grown to perhaps 50 words, mainly those used to negotiate life and satisfy wants. Linguistic growth is significant in the second year of life. The child will emerge at 5 years of age with a working vocabulary of about 2,000 words.

Emotional development has import for oral health. Stranger anxiety begins with object permanence and persists throughout the pre-three phase of life. Few pediatric health practitioners would ever try to separate the child from the parent during this period. Even at 18 months of age, a child clings to mother. In cases in which parents must surrender a child to day care, a transitional object like a blanket or stuffed animal may be given to the child. It is important to recognize the importance of these objects in comfort of the child, and oral habits may fulfill this role as well. Cooperative play emerges by this same age, but temper tantrums are also a part of the later phases of the pre-three period.

Implications of development for dental intervention

The perceptive reader will understand that certain principles of pre-three care will probably hold true and should be incorporated into oral health care in this period:

(1) It is almost impossible to communicate with these children until the later part of their third year of life, so behavior management success will be limited,

(2) Instruction of the child on oral hygiene is a wasted effort due to poor motor skills, so energy should be devoted to parental instruction,

(3) Children will cry during these visits and this coping and communication tool should not be discouraged,

(4) Habits that seem to console the child are beneficial and in the absence of compelling reasons to stop them, should be allowed to continue,

(5) Due to stranger anxiety, children will be reluctant to separate and cooperate so parental presence is mandatory.

Of course, some children will exceed expectations with cooperation and ability, but the normal distribution of development suggests these will be few. Further development includes physical, emotional, and intellectual areas, and while one area may be accelerated, another may be normal or delayed, trumping any positive benefit for oral health care. Each child should be evaluated as an individual and anticipatory guidance tailored to that child's particular skill sets and characteristics, as well as those of the parent.

Orofacial and dental development applied to the pre-three child

Body awareness is a growing concept in health. Understanding the form and function of one's body may lead one to seek early intervention by a health professional or to recognize that self-help options are more effective in certain situations. The infant oral health visit offers the opportunity to review the child's anatomy and oral facial development with parents. The objective of this aspect of anticipatory guidance should be to enable the parent to measure change against a normal healthy oral cavity. This can be used to relate changes in tissue from traumatic injury, infection, growth delays, and application of oral hygiene practices.

Tooth eruption is the primary change that needs to be reviewed. Using a chronology of tooth development and eruption, the clinician can place the child within a range of normal or discuss the implications of delay or acceleration of tooth emergence. Environmental and systemic effects can be discussed and shown to parents as relevant to an individual child's enamel and tooth morphology. Tooth position, spacing, and intercuspation emerge throughout the first 3 years of life as concepts that should be reviewed. These will pay off later when decisions need to be made for orthodontic intervention because parents will understand them. Even within the preschool period, concerns related to the effect of pacifiers and minor traumatic injuries can be dealt with over the telephone rather than with an additional visit.

It is beyond the scope of this chapter to go into depth on all of the potential issues that might alter or affect dental anatomy, function, and physiology. Table 6.2 shows the instructional issues often arising with parents that can have implications for anticipatory guidance on oral and dental development as well as the other topics in AG.

Fluoride

General effects and issues of fluoride in the pre-three child

There is no question that appropriate fluoride use contributes to reduction in dental caries. Historically, it was thought that the primary effect of fluoride was systemic. More recent investigations suggest that the effect is topical by increasing the resistance of tooth structure to demineralization,

Table 6.2 Anticipatory guidance knowledge base for pre-three care.

Area of anticipatory guidance	Knowledge base for area
Oral and dental development	
Eruption	• Normal range, delay, acceleration and potential etiologies, sequence, occlusion, and exfoliation • Eruption problems including malposition, cyst formation, teething, Riga-Fede disease, and bruxing
Teeth	• Color, shape, staining causes, role in speech, and chewing
Soft tissue	• Mucosal color, ulceration, alveolar anatomy, and congenital abnormalities
Anatomy	• Structures, integrity, and color
Fluorides	
Systemic	• Water fluoridation procedures, supplementation, fluoride vehicles, timing, storage safety, fluorosis risk, bottled water, breast milk, formula, prenatal fluorides, and halo effect in diet
Topical	• Role of dentifrice, storage safety, caries and fluorosis risks, swallowing, amounts of dentifrice for age, and supplementation issues (if indicated)
Nonnutritive habits	
Assessment	• Frequency, duration, and intensity • Thumbs, fingers, pacifiers, toys, or blankets • Perceived emotional benefit to child • Effects on oral cavity • Interventions currently being used
Management	• Interventions to discontinue the habit • Techniques, effectiveness, and safety of interventions • Life cycle of habits • Systemic effects of habits
Diet and nutrition	
Feeding	• Food in caries paradigm • Breast-feeding, weaning, and effect(s) on teeth and jaws • Formula feeding, frequency, and content of formulas • Development of feeding skills
Snacking	• Snacking frequency and contents • Food choices • Safety and general health benefits
Diet	• Infant food choices and evolution of pre-three diet
Problems and issues	• Obesity concerns, picky eating, ethnic variations, and food aspiration

(Continued)

Table 6.2 (Continued)

Area of anticipatory guidance	Knowledge base for area
Oral hygiene	
Science	• Role of plaque (caries paradigm) • Plaque removal goals • Developmental issues
Activity	• Type of cleaning currently performed • Parental involvement • Frequency and duration • Devices • Dentifrice
Problems and issues	• Positioning difficulties • Child resistance and behavior • Taste of dentifrice, choices • Technical skills of parents • Role of flossing, injury
Injury prevention	
General issues	• Accidental injury awareness • Car safety • Choking risks and toys and food • Matching skills with activity • Child proofing and poisoning safety
Oral health issues	• Normal anatomy • Trauma assessment and management • Dental home access numbers for emergency management • Snacking safety • Fluoride safety • Medication use for oral problems • Signs of child abuse • Helmet safety

enhancing the process of remineralization, and reducing the cariogenic potential of dental plaque.

Contemporary decision making about the optimal use of fluoride should be based on the age of the child, history of dental disease, perceived risk of future disease, and the availability of water that is optimally fluoridated. Present evidence-based recommendations are from the Center for Disease Control and Prevention (2001). The recommendations for the use of fluoride to prevent and control dental caries state that only community water fluoridation and fluoride-containing toothpastes should be included in a preventive program for all children. All other fluoride modalities are recommended only for children at risk for dental caries, including fluoride supplements, mouth rinses, gels, and varnishes.

With increased use of bottled and filtered waters to replace tap water, the amount of fluoride from drinking waters available to children is questionable. Most bottled waters contain less then 0.3 ppm fluoride. FDA regulations require listing fluoride content on the label only if fluoride was added by the bottler. Very few bottled waters list fluoride concentration, which complicates recommendations to parents on the need for additional fluoride. In homes where water-filtering systems are used, a reverse osmosis system can remove up to 95% of fluoride from the water, while carbon-based systems remove very little.

Use of fluoride supplements by a pregnant woman is of no benefit to the infant, with most of it going to maternal and fetal skeletal tissue or being excreted. The risk of prenatal fluoride supplementation has not been investigated in humans. Breast milk contains little if any fluoride and should not be considered a source.

Today, concern is over excess fluoride due to its omnipresence in the environment, in our nutritional intake of food and beverages, and because of the widespread use of fluoridated toothpaste, some of which is inadvertently swallowed. Although clinically identifiable fluorosis and treatable fluorosis affects a very small percentage of people, much attention is given to control of fluoride intake, often to the detriment of topical anticaries benefit.

In summary, optimal use of an appropriate amount of fluoride throughout life can help to prevent and control dental caries. Fluoride supplementation should be based on the child's risk for dental caries development, the fluoride content of water consumed by the child, and the child's age. In most cases, there is no need for fluoride supplementation from birth to 6 months of age. If on a professional examination it is noted that there are areas of enamel decalcification or discoloration, a program of fluoride varnish application may be recommended.

Fluoride AG in the pre-three child

Fluoride remains one of the three most critical areas of anticipatory guidance because of its known benefits for oral health and the potential risks of misuse. The use of fluorides is covered in depth in Chapter 4 but the content of discussion in all phases of anticipatory guidance is the same. Is systemic intake optimal? Is the child using fluoride toothpaste and doing so appropriately? Is the presence of fluoride products in the home safe? At every supervision visit, fluoride needs to be reviewed because of the dynamic nature of exposure. A good way to approach fluoride in this age period is as one would a medication. Indications, benefits, dosages, route of administration, side effects, and refill information should all be covered.

Prior to age 3, a review of the child's caries-risk status will determine if supplementation is indicated. This is done at each health supervision visit. Once teeth begin to erupt and if the child is at high risk, a "smear" of fluoridated toothpaste 2 times a day with supervision is recommended.

Between ages 2 and 6 years, a "pea-sized" amount of fluoridated toothpaste is recommended twice a day with supervision (Hagan et al., 2008).

Diet and nutrition

Pre-three dietary and nutritional considerations

By the time a dentist sees a pre-three child, the diet is likely a combination of breast milk or formula and some solid food. By 1 year of age, the formula-fed child should be having four feedings per day. The breast-fed child may be in the process of weaning or may still have access to the breast. At 1 year of age, the child should be learning to feed himself, although parents may not give the child free rein to do this because of the inherent messiness. By the end of the second year of life, most children are feeding themselves. It seems that much of the dietary formation for life occurs in the pre-three period. Between the first and second year of life, the child self-selects food and by 2 years of age, the child's diet is essentially that of the family. By the second year of life, eating habits are firmly fixed and difficult to change. Snacking is encouraged in the second year of life, most commonly one small snack that will not interfere with meals between each of the three major meals of the day. Aspiration of food is a risk well into the preschool years, so food size is important. The 2-year-old can be a picky eater, so food selection may be unpredictable. Most authorities agree that it takes about 10 exposures to a food to get a child to take that food routinely. The recommendation for juice is 4–6 ounces per day well into the school years. These stages of dietary change may be altered by food allergies and ethnic influences, which can only be identified in a thorough history.

Application of dietary and nutritional development to oral health

Perhaps more than any other area, diet and nutrition exhibit the dynamic between development and function. Exclusive breast-feeding to 6–12 months of age is recommended by many agencies and health advocates. Breast-feeding requires more time, limited to the mother, and requires support from spouses and health care providers.

Children transition from the breast and bottle to a sippy cup or regular cup or glass. In addition, food goes from liquid to solid, from few to multiple choices, and from drinking to chewing. Bottle-feeding should be stopped at 9–12 months of age and the child switched to a cup. A sippy cup or transitional capped vessel is often used to assist in the change. The caries risk associated with a bottle is continued with a sippy cup if the contents are sugared. The one advantage of the sippy cup is that it is not as conveniently given to a child at night. Parents may alternate bottle and sippy cup for some time and should be questioned in detail on their practices.

Bottle-feeding ad lib and nocturnally continues to occur with frequency, and has been documented in a large number of working families well into the third year of life (Hammer and Bryson, 1999), so in the 3-year anticipatory guidance paradigm, entry at any age demands the dentist ask about the bottle. Clinicians can no longer assume that simple admonition about the risk of nocturnal bottle use will result in behavior change. The pressures of work, single parenting, and caretaking multiple children may make ad lib and nocturnal bottle or sippy cup feeding a convenient behavior modification tool for parents. Reasonable and workable alternatives need to be offered to families to break the habit.

Poor sugar control looms large as a reason for the early childhood epidemic. The amount of sugar in the pre-three child population has grown in the form of carbonated beverages and sweetened juices, displacing milk as the beverage of choice. The transition from bottle to solid food should be the latest point at which consideration of sugar intakes is done in anticipatory guidance and in many instances delaying until then can result in dental caries. At an initial anticipatory guidance visit, sugar intake should be screened and if needed, a more detailed diet history done to identify amount, frequency and type of sugar consumed. The dentist needs to have a thorough awareness of the pre-three diet to be able to make realistic recommendations for alternatives. This may require the assistance of a dietician. A simple mandate to reduce sugar intake without workable alternatives is doomed to failure.

A final consideration is the safety of dental-friendly diet alternatives. Traditionally, these have been nutritious but also high in fat and salt. The negative contribution of dietary fat and sodium in dental snacks at this age is not well understood, but concerns about obesity stem from our understanding that dietary habits are fixed in the first 2 years of life. Dental personnel cannot recommend high-sodium, fatty snacks to benefit oral health if they contribute to obesity and systemic problems such as elevated blood pressure and diabetes. In addition, choking on nuts or chunks of hot dogs is a real risk and parents need to be instructed on how to prepare and serve these tooth-friendly food alternatives.

Oral hygiene

Oral hygiene goals and issues

The removal of plaque and debris from teeth and surrounding tissues is an essential hygiene activity that must be performed daily. Plaque provides the foundation for bacteria to multiply and metabolize food to produce acids that initiate the caries process. Daily interruption of plaque and flushing away of its products has to be included in a preventive program for optimal outcomes. Repeated studies point to plaque in infancy as a predictor of dental caries later in the preschool years. Tooth cleaning can be best accomplished with an age-appropriate brush for use by the parent.

Although brushing is usually associated with the presence of teeth, the cleaning process can be included with the infant's daily bath, prior to the eruption of teeth. Including toothbrushing/mouth cleaning with other bathing activities may assist in the development of a lifelong habit.

For the pre-three child, the parent/caretaker assumes major responsibility for daily hygiene. As with bathing, brushing hair and clipping fingernails, tooth cleaning cannot be performed by pre-three children. It is difficult for the pre-three child to conceptualize the steps of oral hygiene operation, the three-dimensional nature of the oral cavity and tooth surfaces or accomplish the act safely with the stage of developed motor coordination.

Application of oral hygiene to the pre-three child

Once teeth erupt, an age-appropriate brush should be used. Because parents will be performing the cleaning, the appropriate brush is one with a long handle easy for an adult to grasp and a small head to fit comfortably in the pre-three's mouth. An appropriate location to perform the cleaning would be a place where the parent can stabilize the child and have good access to and visualization of the mouth. In today's busy world, this is often the bathroom in conjunction with other hygiene activity. Most likely the pre-three child will "fuss" with brushing. Parents need to be creative and innovative to create a "fun" time. This may include distraction with music, singing, or an egg timer watched by the child.

Other than with the at-risk infant, a fluoridated dentifrice before age 2 is not indicated. If you feel it would reduce the child's risk, then a fluoride-containing dentifrice can be recommended, but used sparingly. Pre-three children's ability to expectorate is limited and messy at best. Flossing is generally not recommended for the pre-three child until the interdental contacts have been established and even then it will be the parent's responsibility. Flossing may introduce an additional unnecessary and burdensome step that has little support from evidence as to its anticaries benefit.

In providing anticipatory guidance to parents for oral hygiene procedures, it is important to demonstrate application of dentifrice, a full "round" of tooth cleaning, and positioning. Do not assume that a parent can effect plaque removal without some instruction. Critical to a successful home hygiene program is its integration into the lifestyle of the family. Considerations must include location, timing, selection of devices and their expense, positioning, and problem solving relative to other needs of the child.

Nonnutritive habits

Habits in the pre-three child

Most infants and children will have a habit associated with the oral cavity. Although most of these habits may have an effect on orofacial structures, there are few associations with general health. Exceptions would be prolonged pacifier use and an increased risk for acute otitis media and early cessation of breast-feeding. A positive effect of pacifier use is reduction in occurrence of sudden infant death syndrome. Infants have an inherent biologic drive to suck. If not satisfied through feeding, they will resort to nonnutritive sucking to satisfy the need. Fingers, thumbs, toys, and blankets are easily available and quickly discovered by the child, although often not socially acceptable. Therefore, parents resort to pacifiers that are available in many shapes, sizes, and colors. Some manufacturers claim that their pacifier design has a "therapeutic" advantage, but studies have not verified these claims. Safety is a critical issue and pacifiers should never be attached to the child with a cord to prevent loss since suffocation can occur.

Application of habit management to the pre-three child

The effects of habits associated with the oral cavity were first reported over 100 years ago. Most studies were retrospective questionnaires and associated habits with open bites, crossbites, and excessive overjet. It is important that dentists ask questions on early feeding methods when interviewing parents. Habits become a problem and can affect normal orofacial development when the balance between the teeth and oral musculature is disrupted. Therefore, the dentist must determine the frequency, duration, and intensity of the habit in the interview. Once assessed and a problem or risk noted, depending on the age of the child and the determination of the parents, interventions may be indicated.

Current prospective studies report a higher prevalence of malocclusion associated with persistent nonnutritive sucking habits. It is no longer felt that the effects on the primary dentition are reversible if the habit is halted by 6 years of age. Therefore, discussions on nonnutritive sucking should be initiated by both physicians and dentists as early as 6–12 months. The goal is to cease nonnutritive sucking by 2 years of age. This discussion should address the positive benefits of the habit and potential changes to the oral structures if the habit becomes too intense. Parents should be shown their child's normal anatomy so they can assess and understand any effects of habits (Rivara and Grossman, 2007).

If habits persist beyond the third year, interventions to assist the child and parents should be instituted, beginning with gentle reminders to the child, distraction of the child from the habit when it occurs, and positive reinforcement of attempts by the child to stop the habit.

Injury prevention

Pre-three injury prevention

Experts would maintain that accidental injury is not prevented but controlled by proper education, modification of the environment, giving specific advice about particular childhood dangers at a particular age in a specific environment rather than general advice (e.g., telling a parent to avoid dangerous situations or offering cute stickers to remind parents about the dangers of poisoning), and avoiding a mismatch of a child's skills with environment (AAPD, 2007d). A starting toddler's parents would be counseled on the risks inherent in falls, for example, as the child begins to ambulate. A child's life is a series of windows of vulnerability to particular types of injuries.

All primary care professionals share responsibility to counsel families about unintentional injury. Morbidity and mortality statistics in the pre-three population are sobering, with motor vehicle accidents the primary cause of death in 1-year-old children. Fifty percent of deaths of children under 1 year of age can be related to suffocation, usually from foods. Almost half of the deaths of children under 4 years of age are accidental.

Application of injury prevention to the pre-three child

Provision of general health advice to families is not new in dentistry. Tobacco cessation and blood pressure monitoring are two examples of general health issues that cross over into oral health delivery and which have come under the shared purview of many primary health care providers. In the pre-three population, the dentist can offer guidance in both general terms and related to oral health issues. Advice regarding the use of car seats should be offered to all families from the first visit. Similarly, control of access to medications and assurance that these are all capped with childproof lids are other generalized messages that can be given to parents. Further, dentists should provide medications with these instructions as well as a review of child-appropriate doses.

Injury prevention really permeates all of the anticipatory guidance topics. Under dietary recommendations, the risk of aspiration needs to be addressed in practical terms as parents seek to implement snacking recommendations. In the area of fluoride, control of dose and storage are important topics often assumed or seen as secondary to proper therapeutic use of the drug. For both diet and fluoride, management of negative side effects like overdose or allergy needs to be reviewed. Oral hygiene is still another area that requires some thought, matching the child's skills with the environment we seek to create for tooth cleaning. Few if any pre-threes are capable of brushing effectively and can in fact induce injury if left alone to clean their teeth. Flossing is often recommended for this age group, without much supporting evidence of its benefit, but with clear risk of intraoral injury by children without the manual skills to manipulate floss.

The injury control principle of specific advice includes directions to parents about how to assess oral injury and the steps to take to obtain care quickly. Think of the dental home as a part of the emergency management system. Telephone numbers for after-hours access to the dentist, emergency departments, and poison control centers are useful ways to direct parents. An important building block of the dental home is accessible health care.

APPLYING ANTICIPATORY GUIDANCE IN THE DENTAL OFFICE

The mastery of the topical areas of anticipatory guidance is the first step in its application to care of the pre-three child. Office preparation is necessary to create a smooth-flowing process for infant oral health. The following sequence is suggested for instituting a preventive/promotional practice using anticipatory guidance:

(1) Mastery of topical areas by all members of the dental staff. This should involve training together and development of an office-specific manual on all aspects of AG for the pre-three child. Texts or policies of professional organizations are useful reference tools to include. Table 6.2 provides an outline for development of an office's reference library and policies.

(2) Development of age-specific forms for AG history-taking and preventive therapeutic prescribing. These may be available from professional groups, but should be tailored toward the population seen by the office, which might include versions in several languages and relating to particular cultural norms common to that population. It may be helpful to consolidate the data collection instrument with a checklist of AG recommendations, which can be provided to parents as both a history of their child's visit and your recommendations. Copies kept in the child's dental record can serve to remind the provider of the preventive advice given and findings from the previous examination that can be reviewed when the family returns.

(3) Development or securing of age-specific educational material. Many organizations provide this type of material, but few are divided into appropriate age ranges or topical areas in the detail needed. For conciseness, practices may want to develop handouts that are based on AG topics and which cover the first 3 years of life in some type of developmental format. This approach allows only those areas that need addressing to be covered (Tables 6.3–6.5).

Table 6.3 Anticipatory guidance (birth to 12 months).

	0–1 month	1–2 months	2–3 months	3–4 months	4–5 months	5–6 months	6–7 months	7–8 months	8–9 months	9–10 months	10–11 months	11–12 months
General developmental milestones												
							Gross motor • Sits alone 4–8 months and steadily 5–9 months • Stands alone 9–16 months **Fine motor** • Pincer grasp at 9–12 months **Cognitive** • Object permanence at 4–8 months **Language** • Responds to name at 6 months • Babbles with intonation at 9–12 months **Social** Stranger anxiety at 9–12 months					
Dental and oral development												
			Infant is edentulous				Lower incisor erupts	Upper incisor erupts	Lower lateral erupts (to 16 months)	Upper lateral erupts (to 13 months)		
Fluoride												
					Optimal systemic supplementation according to availability of fluoride in drinking water							
							Use fluoridated dentifrice based on risk					
Nonnutritive habits												
	All nonnutritive sucking habits are considered beneficial to the infant in this period Safety issues related to pacifier use should be reviewed as well as avoidance of sweeteners on pacifiers											
Diet and nutrition												
	Breast-feeding is encouraged according to guidelines of the American Academy of Pediatrics											

Table 6.3 (*Continued*)

0–1 month	1–2 months	2–3 months	3–4 months	4–5 months	5–6 months	6–7 months	7–8 months	8–9 months	9–10 months	10–11 months	11–12 months
										Wean from bottle	
										Advice on use of sippy cup	
						Educate parent on role and control of sugars in diet and dental caries process					
Oral hygiene											
				Provide instruction and begin oral/tooth cleaning							
					Address parental/caretaker oral health						
		Educate parent/caretaker on role of microflora in caries process and purpose of plaque removal									
Injury prevention											
		Encourage general safety behaviors including car seat use, safety at day care, and child proofing the home									
		Educate about the signs of child abuse									
		Provide 24 hour telephone contact for oral injury management in dental home									
							Instruct parent on dental injury as child begins to walk				
Perform caries-risk assessment at each health supervision interval											

Use of this chart: Place a vertical rule on the table at the child's current age and relevant areas of anticipatory guidance will be those nonshaded areas. On a first visit, beyond the age of 6 months, inclusion of earlier topics may be advisable.

Table 6.4 Anticipatory guidance (13–24 months).

	12–13 months	13–14 months	14–15 months	15–16 months	16–17 months	17–18 months	18–19 months	19–20 months	20–21 months	21–22 months	22–23 months	23–24 months
General developmental milestones												
Gross motor: Child walking with support and then independently at 12 months (median)												
Fine motor: Child manipulates objects and can use spoon to replace finger feeding												
Cognitive: Child can manipulate objects to create effects and begin knowing cause-effect												
Language: Child may develop up to 50 words during this period												
Social • Child may initiate separation from parent but return quickly • Child engages parent in social play												
Dental and oral development												
Upper first molar												
Lower first molar												
Upper canines												
Lower canines												
Discuss function of primary teeth in speech and chewing												
Discuss occlusion												
Fluoride												
Reassess fluoride status												
Use fluoridated dentifrice – smear amount												
Review sources of fluoride in daycare settings												
Review safety issues of fluoride and fluorosis												
Nonnutritive Habits												
All nonnutritive sucking habits are considered beneficial to the infant in this period												
Safety issues related to pacifier use should be reviewed as well as avoidance of sweeteners on pacifiers												
Discuss the effects of habits on teeth in anticipation of eliminating the habit in the next two years												
Diet and nutrition												
Insure bottle use has stopped												
Wean from sippy cup if still used												
Assess and manage dietary intake of sugar												
Oral hygiene												
Parent continues to brush allowing child to participate in some manner but not to achieve plaque removal												
Injury prevention												
Discuss electric cord safety												
Review management of traumatic injury												
Perform caries-risk assessment at each health supervision interval												

Use of this chart: Place a vertical rule on the table at the child's age at the time of visit and relevant areas of anticipatory guidance will be those nonshaded areas. On a first visit, beyond the age of 6 months, inclusion of earlier topics may be advisable, including those from Table 6.3.

Table 6.5 Anticipatory guidance (25–36 months).

24–25 months	25–26 months	26–27 months	27–28 months	28–29 months	29–30 months	30–31 months	31–32 months	32–33 months	33–34 months	34–35 months	35–36 months
General developmental milestones											
Gross motor: By the end of this period, can run and balance on one foot											
Fine motor: Can stack 6 blocks at 24 months and copy a circle by 36 months											
Cognitive: Develops sense of self during this period and has cooperative play at 36 months											
Language: Can make six word sentences and count 3 objects by 36 months											
Social: Plays simple games by 36 months, helps put things away											
Dental and oral development											
(To 23 months)				Lower second molar							
					Upper second molar						
					Discuss spacing, occlusion, overjet and overbite						
Fluoride											
		Review fluoride intake						Review fluoride intake			
Nonnutritive habits											
				Begin to discuss the cessation of habits							
				Instruct parents in identification of anatomic changes from habits							
Diet and nutrition											
						Review sugar in diet					
Oral hygiene											
					Review oral hygiene procedures based on risk and lifestyle						
Injury prevention											
						Review safety related to lifestyle					
Perform caries-risk assessment at each health supervision interval											

Use of this chart: Place a vertical rule on the table at the child's age at the time of visit and relevant areas of anticipatory guidance will be those nonshaded areas. On a first visit, beyond the age of 6 months, inclusion of earlier topics may be advisable, including those from Tables 6.3 and 6.4.

(4) Creation of a site or procedure for early intervention. In its purest form, AG is provided during the child's dental examination visit. If this is most conveniently done in a traditional operatory, then outfit it for the occasional knee-to-knee examination and easy access to the armamentarium needed such as fluoride varnish. If a separate "baby room" is preferred, it should be designed to allow examination and provision of AG in a simple seamless fashion. The site should provide easy access to demonstration devices and educational materials.

(5) Determine office procedures such as charting, record contents, billing codes, and recall mechanisms that relate to these patients, if they are managed differently from the main patient population.

REFERENCES

Acs G, Shulman R, Ng MW, and Chussid S. 1999. The effect of dental rehabilitation on the body weight of children with early childhood caries. *Pediatr Dent* 21:109–13.

American Academy of Pediatric Dentistry (AAPD). 2007a. Guidelines on periodicity of examinations, preventive dental services, anticipatory guidance and oral treatment for children. *Pediatr Dent* 29(7) Reference Manual, 2007–2008. Available at http://www.aapd.org/media/Policies_Guidelines/G_Periodicity.pdf (accessed April 30, 2008).

American Academy of Pediatric Dentistry (AAPD). 2007b. Policy on the dental home. *Pediatr Dent* 29(7) Reference Manual 2007–2008. Available at http://www.aapd.org/media/Policies_Guidelines/P_DentalHome.pdf (accessed April 30, 2008).

American Academy of Pediatric Dentistry (AAPD). 2007c. Policy on use of a caries risk assessment tool (CAT) for infants, children and adolescents. *Pediatr Dent* 29(7) Reference Manual 2007–2008. Available at http://www.aapd.org/media/Policies_Guidelines/P_CariesRiskAssess.pdf (accessed April 30, 2008).

American Academy of Pediatric Dentistry (AAPD). 2007d. Policy on oral habits. *Pediatr Dent* 29(7) Reference Manual 2007–2008. Available at http://www.aapd.org/media/Policies_Guidelines/P_OralHabits.pdf (accessed April 30, 2008).

American Academy of Pediatrics. 1967. Suggested schedule for preventive child health care. In: *Standards of Child Health Care*. Evanston, IL: American Academy of Pediatrics.

American Academy of Pediatrics. 2002. The medical home. *Pediatrics* 110:184–6.

Berkowitz RJ, Jordan HV, and White G. 1975. The early establishment of *Streptococcus mutans* in the mouths of infants. *Arch Oral Biol* 20:171–4.

Casamassimo P. 1996. *Bright Futures in Practice: Oral Health*. Arlington, VA: National Center for Education in Maternal and Child Health.

Caufield PW, Cutter GR, and Dasanayake AP. 1993. Initial acquisition of mutans streptococci by infants: Evidence for a discrete window of infectivity. *J Dent Res* 72:37–45.

Center for Disease Control and Prevention. 1997. Conference on early childhood caries. Bethesda, MD. October. *Comm Dent Oral Epidemiol* 1998(Suppl):26.

Center for Disease Control and Prevention. 2001. Recommendations for using fluoride to prevent and control dental caries in United States. *MMWR* 50(RR14):1–42.

Filstrup SL, Briskie D, da Fonseca M, Lawrence L, Wandera A, and Inglehart MR. 2003. Early childhood caries and quality of life: Child and parent perspective. *Pediatr Dent* 25:431–40.

Green M and Palfrey JS (eds). 1994. *Bright Futures: Guidelines for Health Supervision of Infants, Children and Adolescents*. Arlington, VA: National Center for Education in Maternal and Child Health.

Hagan JF, Shaw JS, and Duncan P. 2008. *Bright Futures: Guidelines for Health Supervision of Infants, Children and Adolescents*, 3rd edn. Elk Grove, IL: American Academy of Pediatrics, pp 155–69.

Hammer LD and Bryson S. 1999. Development of feeding practices during the first 5 years of life. *Arch Pediatr Adolesc Med* 153:189–94.

Johnsen DC, Gerstenmaier TA, and DiSantis RJ. 1986. Susceptibility of nursing caries children to future approximal molar decay. *Pediatr Dent* 8:168–70.

McDonald RE. 1963. *Pedodontics*. St Louis, MO: The C.V. Mosby Company.

Nowak AJ. 1997. Rationale for the timing of the first oral evaluation. *Pediatr Dent* 19:8–11.

Nowak AJ and Anderson JC. 1990. Preventive dentistry for children: A review from 1968 to 1988. *J Dent Child* 57:31–7.

Nowak AJ and Casamassimo P. 1995. Using anticipatory guidance to provide early dental intervention. *JADA* 126:1156–63.

Nowak AJ and Casamassimo P. 2003. The dental home: A primary care concept. *JADA* 133:93–8.

Rivara FP and Grossman D. 2007. Injury control. In: Kliegman RM, Behrman RE, Jenson HB, and Stanton BF (eds), *Nelson's Pediatrics*, 18th edn. Philadelphia: Saunders-Elsevier.

Silverstone LM, Johnson NW, Hardie JM, and Williams RAD. 1981. *Dental Caries: Aetiology, Pathology and Prevention*. London: Macmillan Press Ltd.

U.S. Public Health Service. 1964. *Smoking and Health*. Report of the Advisory Committee to the Surgeon General of the Public Health Service. Washington: U.S. Department of Health, Education, and Welfare, 387 pp.

Williamson R, Oueis H, Casamassimo PS, Rashid R, and Thikkurissy S. 2008. Association between early childhood caries and child behavior. *Pediatr Dent*, 30(6);505–9.

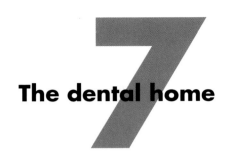

The dental home

Arthur J. Nowak and Paul S. Casamassimo

EMERGENCE OF THE DENTAL HOME CONCEPT

In the beginning of this century, the recognition of a long-standing, ongoing, and seemingly intractable early childhood caries epidemic in the United States focused attention on traditional approaches to oral health promotion and prevention. In spite of decades of declining permanent tooth caries, early childhood caries rates remained static for the last part of the twentieth century and began to worsen (Dye et al., 2007). Those elements that seemed to contribute to a reduction in dental caries in older children, such as fluoride, were not effective in abating the disease in the primary dentition.

On further examination of the patterns of disease and oral health care, preventive behaviors, and cultural shifts in the preschool population, it became clear that early childhood caries was a multifactorial disease quite different from the condition affecting older children and adults. Prenatal influences on tooth structure, variable fluoride availability, parental

transmission of cariogenic microflora, profound shifts in dietary carbohydrate ingestion in early life, absence of professionally supervised
preventive care, and cultural influences on oral health were some of
the many factors believed to contribute to the early childhood caries
epidemic. What also became clear was the need to reset the timing of the
first dental visit with its introduction of essential oral health promotion
and prevention services. The concept of the dental home was created,
inextricably tied to the age-one dental visit, borrowing from two decades
of health promotion of the medical home by pediatricians to overcome
similar problems of access, disparities, prevention, and early intervention
related to general health of very young children.

In 2002, Nowak and Casamassimo introduced the concept of the dental
home as a primary health concept to address the early childhood caries
epidemic and other aspects of oral health to the general dental profession
(Nowak and Casamassimo, 2002). The justification for the dental home and
moving the dentist–patient relationship from 3 years of age to 6 months of
age includes the following:

- *The early childhood caries epidemic's resistance to traditional therapeutic timing.* In addition to the seeding of very young children with early childhood caries, the problem encompasses a burden of disease that by age
  3 years becomes so severe in many children that it requires hospitalization, and even in its less severe forms is beyond the management skills
  of the general dentist.
- *The recognition of systemic influences on oral health and vice versa, including maternal health and increasing numbers of children with special
  needs.* Growing research supports the role of caretaker's oral health
  in early childhood caries. Less robust evidence points to a role for
  factors such as second-hand smoking and trace element ingestion
  in early childhood caries, with a logical conclusion of altering these
  environmental factors early rather than later in life. As the number of
  children with special health care needs increases and as they will be
  seeking care in private practices, prevention of difficult-to-treat oral
  disease becomes paramount. The implications of early childhood caries
  on systemic health are as yet not fully understood, but quality-of-life
  studies in children with early childhood caries suggest a negative
  effect. Weight gain, learning, behavioral aberration, and suffering are
  among the morbidities attributed to dental caries and its attendant
  pain.
- *Changes in dietary, behavioral, care seeking, and other aspects of parenting,
  many of which are reflected in increased caries risk.* The concept of caries-
  risk assessment and its corollary of preventive anticipatory guidance,
  health supervision, and continuity of care are all best supervised in
  a comprehensive and prepared care environment, by professionals
  who understand the biologic nature of dental caries and its natural
  progression.

- *Better understanding of health disparities and the cultural, ethnic, and systemic influences responsible for them.* Newer models of dental caries initiation built on the classic three-part biologic infectious disease model extend into the family and community, demanding a better understanding of factors beyond the patient. It makes sense that a dental home that is characterized by a community should be able to provide focused prevention better than a haphazard or one-size-fits all approach.
- *A changing health care system, increasing in complexity and access challenges.* In the case of Medicaid, for example, many states propagate rules for enrollment and dental care that are complicated for enrollees. Treatment planning with limited choice of procedures often challenges both patients and professionals. Commercial health insurance poses its own set of challenges. At this writing, the dental care system lacks the sophistication to assign individualized therapies aimed at specific outcomes in the context of reimbursement and health plan structure, but the dental home offers the best opportunity to investigate these issues.

The concept of the dental home is an evolving one, with many conceptual elements borrowed from the definition of the medical home propagated by the American Academy of Pediatrics (American Academy of Pediatrics, 2002), but a working definition, according to the American Academy of Pediatric Dentistry (AAPD) (American Academy of Pediatric Dentistry, 2008–2009) is as follows:

> The dental home is the ongoing relationship between the dentist and the patient, inclusive of all aspects of oral health care delivered in a comprehensive, continuously accessible, coordinated and family centered way. Establishment of a dental home happens no later than 12 months of age and includes referral to dental specialists when appropriate.

The characteristics of the dental home as characterized by the AAPD (Academy of Pediatric Dentistry, 2008–2009) are listed in Table 7.1. Definitions of the dental home may vary and will likely change to meet the dynamics of disease occurrence, population shifts, scientific advances, and changes in the health care system. Some aspects of the dental home are rudimentary to health care such as physical and fiscal access and cultural effectiveness in providing care to families with diverse backgrounds and with children with special needs. Other aspects of the dental home address elements of the oral health care system that are somewhat new such as family-centeredness and care coordination. This chapter provides some insight into what the dental home encompasses and what dental practices need to do to develop the concept into a working system.

Table 7.1 Characteristics of the dental home and rationale supporting them.

Characteristic	Rationale
Comprehensive care including both acute and preventive services	Prevention of early childhood caries is the primary driver for a dental home, but the need for acute trauma management and early detection and management of developmental issues are important corollaries
Comprehensive assessment of oral health needs	As evidence grows regarding the impact of factors on oral health, the need for a wider consideration of biologic and social factors along with a caries-risk assessment becomes evident. An example would be the effect of prematurity on oral development, dental care behavior, and competing systemic needs
Individualized preventive plan	The recognition of individualized disease susceptibility and the cost of one-size-fits-all preventive strategies will make targeted prevention both the rule and a necessary skill of practitioners
Anticipatory guidance	Anticipatory guidance pairs individualized prevention with a developmental schema for patients
Trauma and emergency plan	With a significant percentage of children under school age experiencing dental pain and with the recognition of the extent of dental trauma in this same population, the dental home will need to both prevent problems and handle those that emerge
Personal self-preventive information	The role of personal prevention is yet to be fully understood in the epidemic of early childhood caries, but what is known is that fluoride presents both an advantage and a risk, and children of this age cannot provide their own plaque removal
Dietary counseling	Perhaps the two most profound diet-related discoveries of the early childhood caries epidemic are the early introduction of massive amounts of sugar into the diet beginning as early as 1 year of age and the prolonged bottle or sippy cup feeding into the preschool years
Referral to specialists	The general dentist may not be able to manage all the needs of the child, and help from dental and other specialists may be required and the facility with which a practice can deliver a broad array of services will define the dental home
Care transition	The burden of an additional early-aged population to most practices will require that pediatric dental practices have plans to transfer the health care of teens and young adults to general dental offices
Individualized/ personalized recall schedule	Return visits are used to monitor oral health and assess the effectiveness of prevention, make recommendations to parents, check on their compliance, and reassess risk

EVIDENCE IN SUPPORT OF THE DENTAL HOME

The medical community arrived at the concept of the medical home after a thorough review of the patterns of health care and disease in the child population. Evidence supported the need to establish a relationship between the child and family and a health provider in order to accomplish necessary vaccinations, intercept developmental problems early, and to minimize use of emergency departments for routine care. The medical home concept proved effective in minimizing inappropriate care seeking, improving compliance, and enhancing well child care (St Peter et al., 1992; Baker et al., 1994; Christakis et al., 1999).

The dental literature lacks the richness of support for a dental home, most likely due to the novelty of the concept as applied to oral health. Dentistry's interest in the dental home is driven primarily by the worsening epidemic of early childhood caries and the failure of system-wide approaches believed to work in older patients to lessen the problem. Only recently have health services researchers begun to look at evidence to support early intervention. A major obstacle in validating the dental home concept and early dental intervention and altering the antiquated view of when a child first needs to see a dentist is the lack of data, with few sources of nonemergent prevention available for study.

There are a few examples, with more emerging. Early work by Doykos (Doykos, 1967) in 1967 reported that introduction of dental care early resulted in less cost of care over time, suggesting a benefit to establishment of a dentist–patient relationship sooner rather than later. More recently, Savage et al. in a retrospective analysis of Medicaid data found that early involvement in oral health care led to less expenditures over time (Savage et al., 2004). In a structured community-based demonstration program that links very young children with the general dentists, the ABCD Program, Milgrom and Grembowski found that enrolled children had an increased use of dental services when compared to children who were not enrolled (Grembowski and Milgrom, 2000). Coulter and Brill found that in a private practice population, those children who were seen for the first time before 24 months had more preventive and fewer restorative visits than those seen later in childhood (Coulter and Brill, 2007). Lee and colleagues (Lee et al., 2007) were successful in encouraging physicians to refer very young children for dental care and found a lower rate of early childhood caries and in younger children a particularly notable lower rate of cavitated lesions.

Preventive services can be more successful with implementation of dental home concepts. Gagnon et al. achieved good compliance with fluoride supplements in mothers of 6- to 9-month-olds using a dental hygienist as a care coordinator (Gagnon et al., 2007). Luan et al. experienced more preventive visits and fewer restorative procedures with their preschool patients and suggest that services associated with a dental home such as preventive education, fluoride varnish application, and early restorative care can be beneficial (Luan et al., 2007).

In spite of limited data and the absence of randomized clinical trials, the dental home concept enjoys intuitive support, bolstered by small studies and indirect evidence at this point. Recent acceptance of the benefits of fluoride varnish and intensive patient counseling support a vehicle for provision of these services (Weinstein et al., 2004; Weintraub et al., 2006). The use of medical providers to offer these services continues to garner attention, but the medical literature strongly suggests that penetration of consistent, effective, and predictable oral health intervention by busy pediatricians will be limited. Of more critical importance is the fact that better surveillance of children from an early age by all types of health providers will undoubtedly result in identification of dental disease requiring the range of services available only in a dental home. When all is said and done, it is the refractory nature of early childhood caries in the face of the traditional preventive regimens that has focused efforts at establishment of an early dental home. At this writing, the dental home offers an empirical solution to a difficult problem.

CHARACTERIZING THE DENTAL HOME

The dental home is a relationship between a family and a dentist around the oral health care of a child and not a location as the term may imply. This distinction will become even more important as protected health information becomes more transportable over the next decade and more is known about the influence of cultural and social factors on oral disease. With the recognition that general dentists will be called upon more and more to provide the dental home for young children, certain characteristics not always present in an adult-oriented practice may need to be added or developed.

Accessibility has been used in health literature in a variety of ways. In its oldest sense, accessibility refers to barrier-free health facilities so that 16–18% of patients with some sort of disability can gain access to services with the same ease as someone without any physical or mental limitations. The concept has expanded to include removal of cultural and ethnic biases that have led to health care disparities in the past and currently prevent certain groups from seeking care. Evidence suggests that unless practices systematically eliminate biases throughout the care delivery system, patients will perceive a negative climate and be resistant to care (Kelly et al., 2005). In the dental home context, accessibility also refers to a geographical imperative to have comprehensive services available within a community, although in rural and certain urban areas, this ideal has proved difficult to achieve. The realization of the impact of finances on dental care seeking and compliance points to incorporation of case management, financial counseling, health care advocacy, and patient-focused or rational treatment planning. As health care evolves, accessibility in the form of a dental home will likewise take on new meanings.

Contemporary care assumes that the dental provider and office staffs are aware of contemporary science related to oral health and health care delivery. An example of this need for contemporary knowledge is the dynamic role of fluoride in dental caries prevention and management today as relates to children. In 2003, the Centers for Disease Control and Prevention introduced a risked-based model for caries prevention, a concept not yet fully appreciated by the practicing profession who may provide office fluoride treatments to children who are not at risk on a routine basis because of habit or reimbursement (Centers for Disease Control and Prevention, 2001). Very recently, the risk–benefit balance of fluoride supplementation has been challenged because of fear of fluorosis in permanent teeth due to mixing fluoridated water with formula (Bramson, 2007). The role of dentifrice in early childhood caries prevention is also under debate for similar fluorosis fears, potentially depriving at-risk children of its topical benefits. A recent maternal and child health–sponsored task force has revisited earlier recommendations on fluoride dentifrice use in high-risk children and will be recommending the use of a dentifrice for children under 2 years while being supervised (S. Levy, personal communication).

Another area of contemporary dentistry is the full use of auxiliary personnel in the dental home. Controversy swirls around the dental therapist concept, but many general practices do not even take advantage of the full range of preventive and therapeutic services by auxiliaries currently allowable under state law. As practices move to a dental home model, much of early intervention can be delegated to nondental staff; similarly minor restorative procedures needed by very young children may be performed by dental assistants trained as expanded-duties personnel and dental hygienists.

Comprehensive care is another hallmark of the dental home, which takes on new meaning because of the age of children involved and the need for recognition of diversity. Whether a typical general dental practice can fulfill this aspect of the dental home will remain to be shown as the concept evolves, but in the meantime, meeting the goal of comprehensive care may mean a linkage between general dentists and pediatric dentists within the community, each providing a contribution to the care of a child. Successful Head Start models employ a triad of oversight to the care of children, with a committed Head Start Program, an initial referral to a general dental practice dental home for basic services, and a backup pediatric dental practice for those children who have extensive needs, particularly those requiring sedation or general anesthesia (Casamassimo and Amini, 2005).

Family centeredness has assumed a broader context with the recognition of the effect of parenting on delivery of care in dentistry (Casamassimo et al., 2001) for children. Parental presence is both a challenge and a potential boon to oral health care and compliance with prevention at home. A key element of the dental home is a healthy, cooperative, supportive, and sharing relationship between dental provider and parent. Early dental intervention presumes full involvement of the parent and a dental home practice will need to determine the parameters of the parental role, both in and outside the office. The oral disease model proposed by Fisher-Owens et al. attributes a significant role to family, including the impact of such pragmatic issues as family size, functioning, social support, and parental health status (Fisher-Owens et al., 2007). It should be clear that a single parent with extensive personal unmet dental needs may be responsible for vertical transmission of cariogenic bacteria to a child. The same parent without a social network may be in greater need of education, motivation, and supervision to accomplish needed home care for a child. Finally, the competing life issues of that parent may place care seeking, payment for care, and attention to significant health changes in a young child at risk. The concept of family centeredness has taken on different dimensions than a generation ago.

Cultural effectiveness, often called cultural competency, is still another challenge in effecting a dental home in a traditional dental practice. Few professionals can claim the broad cultural and language skills needed to offer care to the full range of diverse patients needing it. However, culture effectiveness presumes that an office is welcoming to all types of families and can provide or obtain the services necessary to communicate and effect treatment. Cultural effectiveness may also mean that practices have appropriate resources available for language support and for referral.

MAKING A PRACTICE A DENTAL HOME

Table 7.2 provides a limited list of practice characteristics that correspond to the elements of the dental home directed at early dental intervention. The practice geared toward adults may need to refocus or broaden its approach to care to accommodate the very young child who because of developmental stages, third-party (parental) consent, parental oversight of home care, and an intensive early-life health supervision schedule, needs more focused attention.

A first step in creating the dental home is to develop a practice philosophy or set of goals that support the concepts of the definition. A practice might engage in a deliberative process in which current policies are challenged for appropriateness to the dental home for very young children. Areas of strength and weakness can be identified as a starting point for practice modification. Table 7.2 provides a partial checklist that can be used to facilitate the practice review. It is well established that general dentists do not routinely see children (Seale and Casamassimo, 2003), so facilitation of this process might be required by someone familiar with the needs of very young dental patients and their families. A next step is education of provider and staff in care of the very young child. Educational programs via the internet are available from a number of institutional sources. State

Table 7.2 Characteristics of the dental home and related practice.

Dental home characteristic	Practice applications
Accessibility	• Physical accessibility is insured • Welcoming office staff for all patients • Preappointment data collection is done to facilitate the first visit • Financial counseling and information are made available • Referral sources for financial need are available for families that need help • Familiarity of staff with public funding is present • Acceptance of Medicaid if possible
Family centered	• Policy on parental presence exists and is made clear to families prior to care • Preventive counseling keyed to lifestyle for families • Community location is conducive to access • Group practice policy allows provider choice • Appointment policies support varied needs of families as required for timing and duration and in cases of family visits, accommodation of multiple family members • Dental benefits for children, if different from those of adults are understood by staff • Written information is keyed to health literacy requirements • Parental oral health is considered and opportunities for improvement are available
Continuous care	• Same provider for child's lifetime if possible • Assistance with care transitions to other providers is insured if needed • Provision exists for access to practice 24 h a day, 7 days per week
Comprehensive care	• Prenatal, perinatal, and general health histories obtained • Anticipatory guidance is understood and practiced • Caries-risk assessment is understood and practiced • Primary prevention, secondary prevention, and all phases of treatment are provided • Practice has capability to secure sedation and general anesthesia services • For special needs children outside the scope of practice, referral and coordination of care is possible • Practice staff has requisite skills to work with very young children and those skills are updated on a regular basis • Dental issues are dealt with when children receive specialized home services like visiting nurse or physical/speech therapy • Continuing education plan exists to keep abreast of changes in dental science related to very young children

Table 7.2 (Continued)

Dental home characteristic	Practice applications
Coordinated care delivery	• Practice has network of nondental providers for referral for care of nondental problems • Established liaison with pediatric/family practitioners for medical issues is ongoing • Practice has the ability to work with medical providers in complex cases, or with schools, and other facilities • Protected health information is easily obtained and transferable if needed to other health professionals • Practice is aware of general health supervision guidelines for very young children including immunization schedules
Compassionate care	• Practice has policies on emergency care, pain management, and use of immobilization • Practice has grievance and parental feedback mechanisms • Practice has mechanism to identify and monitor individual patient's needs and requests
Cultural effectiveness	• Multilingual capability of staff • Telephone or other interpreter services • Multilingual health care information available • Practice participates in community-based health promotion activities • Practice has a role in community health activities such as health department or professional advisory boards of disability advocacy groups

and federal programs are available to help educate dental providers. A list of these through the internet is provided in Table 7.3.

Going beyond primarily dental aspects of early development to understand more global issues of child development may be helpful in dealing with general health issues that may have dental implications. This can be an entertaining exercise for young professionals who may have their own children. This can be done by a physician or a pediatric nurse practitioner in the community and focus on developmental stages and expectations of children from birth. The public relations benefit of establishing this type of learning environment should not be overlooked. In meeting the family-centered goal of a dental home, a well-educated staff who understands the demands and stages of early childhood can bond with parents and provide meaningful instruction and support.

A physical setting conducive to very young children and young families is another asset to a practice. Some pediatric dental practices have chosen novel ways to implement the dental home, including waiting

Table 7.3 Available learning tools for infant oral health.

Title/date/author	Description
First Dental Visit by Age One: A Guide to the New Recommendations 2004 Office of Oral Health, Arizona Department of Health Services	Contains information about anticipatory guidance for children ages 3 and younger, emphasizing the importance of establishing a dental home for children by age 1. Topics include the transmissible nature of dental caries, risk assessment for dental caries in children ages 3 and younger, the knee-to-knee position for oral screening, and indications for fluoride varnish application in children ages 3 and younger
http://www.azdhs.gov/cfhs/ooh/pdf/ce05.pdf	
Establishing the Dental Home: Using the American Academy of Pediatric Dentistry's Caries-Risk Assessment Tool (CAT) as a First Step 2007 American Academy of Pediatric Dentistry Foundation	Defines early childhood caries and provides information on dental caries process, use of the CAT, and dental home
http://www.aapd.org/foundation/pdfs/CAT.pdf	
Smiles for Ohio Fluoride Varnish Program for Primary Care Providers 2006 Bureau of Oral Health Services, Ohio Department of Health	Provides information about (1) how to assess the oral health of infants and young children at well-child examinations and (2) how to implement the Smiles for Ohio Fluoride Varnish Program to apply fluoride varnish to the teeth of high-risk children
http://www.mchoralhealth.org/materials/multiples/smilesforohio/	
Clinical Caries Risk Assessment 2003 Kids Get Care	Designed to help clinicians in King County, Washington, assesses children's oral health and habits as well as provides guidance to parents or other caregivers on preventive oral health practices
http://www.metrokc.gov/health/kgc/clinician-assessment.doc	
Oral Health Risk Assessment Timing and Establishment of the Dental Home 2003 American Academy of Pediatrics	Policy statement
http://www.aappolicy.aappublications.org/cgi/content/full/pediatrics; 111/5/1113	

Table 7.3 (Continued)

Title/date/author	Description
A Health Professional's Guide to Pediatric Oral Health Management 2003 National Maternal and Child Oral Health Resource Center	Includes information on performing oral screenings to identify infants and children at increased risk for oral health problems, offering referrals to oral health professionals, and providing parents with anticipatory guidance
http://www.mchoralhealth.org/PediatricOH/index.htm	
Dental Health Screening And Fluoride Varnish Application 2003 University of Minnesota	Provides training in oral health screening and fluoride varnish application for primary care health professionals; includes the following sections: etiology and prevention of dental caries, strategies for prevention, oral health screening, "lift the lip" examination (video clip), fluoride varnish application procedure (video clip), and the billing process
http://www.meded1.ahc.umn.edu/fluoridevarnish	
Integrating Preventive Oral Health Measures into Healthcare Practice: A Training Program for Healthcare Settings [Section 2] 2004 Oral Health Program, Wisconsin Department of Health and Family Services	Contains risk assessment checklists for identifying children at high risk for developing tooth decay, testing and presentation materials, and information on fluoride varnish application instructions and protocols
http://www.dhfs.state.wi.us/health/oral_Health/trainingresources.htm	
Oral Health Risk Assessment: Training for Pediatricians and Other Child Health Professionals 2006 American Academy of Pediatrics	Describes elements of oral health risk assessment and triage for young children; primary focus is early childhood caries in infants and children from birth through age 3
http://www.aap.org/commpeds/dochs/oralhealth/screening.cfm	
The Dental Home: It's Never too Early to Start 2007 American Academy of Pediatric Dentistry Foundation	Brochure
http://www.aapd.org/foundation/pdfs/DentalHomeFinal.pdf	

areas designed for parent–child interaction and treatment rooms more like physician offices than dental operatories because of the nature of infant oral health. A dental chair may be more a hindrance than an asset and the space required for a baby room is minimal and it can double as a consultation area. Decorations, restrooms, reading material, and office furniture are all considerations in making the practice family friendly. Another aspect of the dental home is conduciveness to special needs children and their families with more open space, decorations that are inclusive of all children, and instructional and promotional material written in first person style. Just making families aware of any professional and community relationships the dentist or other professional staff may have with special needs groups may cement a dental home relationship. Some practices have also used internet access to structure in-office and remote connections to culturally sensitive information or oral health information related to a particular disability. To have available web sites dealing with these issues at chairside or in consultation areas shows a family that the practice is sensitive to their unique issues.

Establishing relationships with other health professionals aids in comprehensive and coordinated care and also builds a practice. At a minimum, a dental home practice should have access to physicians and psychologists, as well as speech, physical, and occupational therapists within the community for referral. Access to these professionals is dynamic and over time, the interchange between the dental home practice and these health professionals will improve care and build the practice. An important element of these relationships is familiarity with the practice styles, philosophies, and treatment goals of the nondental health providers so that the dental home practice is comfortable with them and can build on their work with a child.

A reality of today's world is diversity and the access to care afforded patients from different cultural and ethnic backgrounds by improved employment and public programs. Dental practices need to pay attention to the requirements of a dental home that is sensitive to a wide range of patients, including those of majority background and varying socioeconomic abilities. A major challenge to dentists is the cultural imperative related to oral health present in ethnic, cultural, and socioeconomic groups. Understanding that the optimal treatment may be minimal treatment is a level of awareness that many dentists neither reach nor agree with in their practice philosophy. Learning the essential elements of a culture will help in designing preventive and care programs that are realistic and achievable. Staff development should incorporate education about the care seeking and dietary habits of various groups as well as very basic interactive "do's" and "dont's" that will determine how welcoming the dental home is.

Dentistry has looked at community involvement beyond the office walls as a practice building and marketing effort. In pediatric dentistry, the advocacy role of the dentist is primary, but this is not the case in all of dentistry. The dental home concept expands on that with two basic differences. The first is that the practitioner becomes more closely affiliated with the community, understanding its diversity and needs, and thus can better position the practice as a dental home. The second is that the dentist involved in advocacy and who understands the needs of the community will likely be more supportive of public health efforts to establish and operate alternate care programs for patients in entitlement programs, preventive programs to reach more children, and fullest use of health resources. The dental home practice is integrated with and not in conflict with the overall oral health care system.

The last novel concept of the dental home is that of care coordination. Dentistry has not needed to facilitate care of patients in the past, and in most practices in the United States, the concept of someone to oversee or coordinate care is foreign. The access crisis in oral health care delivery has exposed a need to help some groups of patients through the complexities of care. Minorities, the poor, and those with special health care needs illustrate patients whose pathway to oral health is complicated by regulation, medical problems, physical access and distance, and finances. The dental home practice incorporates a level of facilitation in delivering care, by either assisting the patient and family in overcoming obstacles or arranging for care in other venues if appropriate.

SUMMARY

The dental home is a new concept to the dental profession and is inextricably tied to early dental intervention and inclusion of diverse populations in dental care. For many practitioners and their staff, accommodation to a dental home concept will require training, changes in office policies, and perhaps even a different point of view on the public's right to health and health care. If the pattern of success established by implementation of the medical home concept extends to dentistry, the early childhood caries epidemic may be significantly reduced.

REFERENCES

American Academy of Pediatric Dentistry. 2008–2009 reference manual. *Pediatr Dent* 30 (suppl).

American Academy of Pediatrics. 2002. The medical home. *Pediatrics* 110:184–6.

Baker DW, Stevens CD, and Brook RH. 1994. Regular source of ambulatory care and medical care utilizations by patients presenting to a public hospital emergency department. *JAMA* 271:1909–12.

Bramson J. 2007. *A Letter Regarding the ADA's Interim Guidance on Fluoride Intake for Infants and Young Children*. American Dental Association. Available at http://www.ada.org/prof/resources/positions/statements/fluoride_infants.asp (accessed April 30, 2008).

Casamassimo PS and Amini H. 2005. *Development of a Strategic Plan to Increase the Number of Ohio Dentists Who See Head Start Patients: Report of Deliverables.* Columbus, OH: Ohio Department of Health.

Casamassimo PS, Wilson S, and Gross LC. 2001. Effects of changing U.S. parenting styles on dental practice: A study of diplomates of the American Board of Pediatric Dentistry. *Pediatr Dent* 23(1):46–50.

Centers for Disease Control and Prevention. 2001. Recommendations for using fluoride to prevent and control dental caries in the United States. *MMWR* 50(RR14):1–42.

Christakis DA, Wright JA, Koepsell TD, Emerson S, and Connell FA. 1999. Is greater continuity of care associated with less emergency department utilization. *Pediatrics* 103:738–42.

Coulter C and Brill W. 2007. *Benefits of Establishing a Dental Home: A Retrospective Chart Review.* San Antonio, TX: American Academy of Pediatric Dentistry 60th Annual Session.

Doykos J. 1967. Comparative cost and time analysis over a two-year period for children whose initial dental experience occurred between 4 and 8 years. *Harv Rev* 27(Winter):142–3.

Dye BA, Tan S, Smith V, Lewis BG, Barker LK, Thornton-Evans G, et al. 2007. Increase in caries among preschool children. Trends in oral health status: United States, 1988–1994 and 1999–2004. National Center for Health Statistics. *Vital Health Stat* 11:248.

Fisher-Owens SA, Gansky SA, Platt LJ, Weintraub J, Soobader M-J, Bramlett MD, and Newacheck PW. 2007. Influences on children's oral health: A conceptual model. *Pediatrics* 120:e510–e20.

Gagnon F, Catellier P, Artieu-Gauthier I, Simard-Tremblay E, Lepage-Saucier M, Paradis-Robert N, Michel J, and Lavalliere A. 2007. Compliance with fluoride supplements provided by a dental hygienist in homes of low-income parents of preschool children in Quebec. *J Public Health Dent* 67:60–63.

Grembowski D and Milgrom PM. 2000. Increasing access to dental care for Medicaid preschool children: The Access to Baby and Child Dentistry (ABCD) program. *Public Health Rep* 115:448–59.

Kelly SE, Binkley CJ, Neace WP, and Gale BS. 2005. Barriers to care-seeking for children's oral health among low-income caregivers. *Am J Public Health* 95:1345–51.

Lee G, Getzin A, Indurkhya A, Risko W, Chase I, Grove B, Webster R, and Ng MW. 2007. Changes in referrals and oral findings after implementation of an oral health program at the Children's Hospital Primary Care Clinic. San Antonio, TX : American Academy of Pediatric Dentistry 60th Annual Session.

Luan V, Rosenberg D, Tannen R, and Chu P. 2007. The impact of early intervention on nursing staff, parents and children. San Antonio, TX: American Academy of Pediatric Dentistry 60th Annual Session.

Nowak AJ and Casamassimo PS. 2002. The dental home: A primary care concept. *J Am Dent Assoc* 133:93–8.

Savage M, Lee J, Kotch J, and Vann W. 2004. Early preventive dental visits: Effect on subsequent utilization and costs. *Pediatrics* 114:418–23.

Seale NS and Casamassimo PS. 2003. Access to dental care for children in the United States: A survey of general practitioners. *J Am Dent Assoc* 134:1630–40.

St Peter RF, Newacheck PW, and Halfon N. 1992. Access to care for poor children: Separate and unequal? *J Am Med Assoc* 267:2760–64.

Weinstein P, Harrison R, and Benton T. 2004. Motivating parents to prevent caries in their young children. *J Am Dent Assoc* 135:731–8.

Weintraub JA, Ramos-Gomez F, and Jue S, Hoover CI, Featherstone JDB, and Gansky SA. 2006. Fluoride varnish efficacy in preventing early childhood caries. *J Dent Res* 85:172–6.

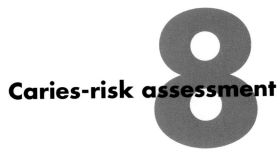

Caries-risk assessment

Rocio Quiñonez and James J. Crall

INTRODUCTION

Caries distribution and trends

Dental caries remains the most common threat to early childhood oral health. The percentage of U.S. children with clinically detectable decayed permanent teeth and the average number of decayed permanent teeth in children at different ages have been in decline for several decades

(USDHHS, 2000). However, comparisons of data from recent national surveys show that the prevalence of decayed (primary) teeth in 2- to 5-year-old U.S. children has increased from 24 to 28% in the past decade (Beltrán-Aguilar et al., 2005). Caries is a progressive disease such that, within a population, the percentage of children with decayed teeth (caries prevalence) tends to rise with increasing age. Thus, while the overall prevalence of caries in U.S. 2- to 5-year-olds is 28%, caries prevalence rates for children at the upper end of the preschool age range generally are reported to be 50% or higher (Dental Health Foundation, 2006).

Caries experience is not uniformly distributed within populations of children. In the United States, children who reside in poverty (<100% of the federal poverty level or FPL) or in low-income households (between 100 and 200% of the FPL) have rates of decayed teeth that are 3–5 times those of children who reside in more affluent segments of the population (Vargas et al., 1998; Mouradian et al., 2000). Race and ethnicity also are associated with higher prevalence of decayed teeth, with African American and Hispanic children having higher rates of decay (Vargas et al., 1998).

Increased emphasis on early interventions

A growing emphasis on early interventions has emerged as the cornerstone for strategies geared toward caries prevention, caries management, and optimal oral health in children. The transition from a paradigm focused primarily on treating the consequences of dental disease to an approach that emphasizes prevention and disease control as well as treatment elevates the importance of understanding the determinants of oral health and the factors that increase the risk of caries development in young children (Featherstone et al., 2003; Ismail, 2003; Stewart and Hale, 2003; Crall, 2007). Growing appreciation of dental caries as a complex, chronic, and infectious disease also has influenced this paradigm shift (Fejerskov, 2004; Crall, 2006), as has evidence suggesting that the traditional restorative approach is limited in terms of its ability to alter the underlying caries disease process. That is to say, restorative treatment generally has been shown to have only a minimal effect on bacterial loading and is not directly associated with individuals' oral self-care behaviors such as toothbrushing (Caufield et al., 1988; Featherstone, 2000).

Greater emphasis on risk assessment and earlier interventions is also motivated by workforce and delivery system considerations. Significant gaps currently exist between professional policies and delivery system performance concerning early oral health interventions. The vast majority of dentists are general dentists who provide the bulk of primary care dental services to children and adults (Crall, 2002). Despite policy statements by numerous dental and public health organizations recommending that children have their first dental visit by 1 year of age (AAP, 2003; AAPD, 2007a; ADA, 2007), results of a recent survey (Seale and Casamassimo,

2003) indicate that 54% of general dentists in the United States rarely or never perform infant oral examinations. A significantly higher percentage (roughly 75%) of general dentists report performing examinations on children between 1 and 3 years of age; however, only 46% do so often or very often. Pediatric dentists fill a substantial portion of this gap in services for young children, but with approximately 20 million U.S. preschoolers and relatively limited numbers of pediatric dentists, additional measures are necessary to achieve the goal of having infants' oral health and caries risk assessed starting by age 1. One such strategy involves training primary care medical providers, who frequently provide multiple well-child assessments during the first 2 years of a child's life, to perform caries-risk assessments along with counseling and referrals of high-risk children (AAP, 2003).

In summary, changing caries distributions, increased emphasis on caries prevention and early interventions in pediatric clinical practice, and the need to use scarce resources efficiently have brought about a greater interest in early risk assessment for caregivers and infants. Risk assessment can facilitate the process of early identification of children at elevated risk and assist in decision making to appropriately tailor interventions and the periodicity of services. Accordingly, the purpose of this chapter is to (a) define what constitutes caries-risk assessment, (b) provide an overview of important variables to consider when assessing children's risk for dental disease, (c) review current tools, and (d) assess policy implications of caries-risk assessment in clinical practice.

WHAT CONSTITUTES CARIES-RISK ASSESSMENT?

To best understand caries-risk assessment, a review of terminology is in order. Risk, in epidemiological terms, is the probability of an event (e.g., development of a carious lesion) occurring following an exposure (e.g., dietary intake) (Last, 2001). Similarly, a risk factor is defined as an:

> Environmental, behavioral, or biologic factor confirmed by temporal sequence, usually in longitudinal studies, which if present directly increases the probability of a disease occurring, and if absent or removed reduces the probability. Risk factors are part of the causal chain, or expose the host to the causal chain. Once disease occurs, removal of a risk factor may not result in a cure. (Beck, 1998)

The term "risk factor" is often used inconsistently or inappropriately in the literature—for example, in cases where the term "risk indicator" would be appropriate. Risk indicators can be risk factors, but lack the longitudinal studies or temporal aspect needed to confirm causality between an exposure and an event (Burt, 2001). Risk indicators are supported by cross-sectional study designs that allow only for correlation, not causality. Thus, risk assessment is the consideration of a set of dynamic risk indicators and/or factors that vary with a child's age and stage of development in order to gauge the likelihood of disease development within some future time frame.

Risk assessment has been used broadly in pediatric medicine in the context of conditions such as lead poisoning, infectious diseases, and childhood obesity (Granoff and Pollard, 2007; Toschke et al., 2005) (First Sign, http://www.firstsigns.org/screening/tools/index_tools.htm). In dentistry, risk-based frameworks have been used to develop radiation guidelines (AAPD, 2007b) and fluoride therapy recommendations (CDC, 2001; ADA, 2006). Specific to childhood caries, risk assessment has also been used to develop targeted approaches for reducing caries in young children (Jokela and Pienihäkkinen, 2003). Nested within the concept of population risk, however, is the notion of assessing an individual's risk for dental disease. Individual risk assessment can inform risk management and risk reduction strategies, decisions about periodicity of services, and motivation of caregivers and patients regarding their oral health (Reich et al., 1999; Zero et al., 2001; Berg, 2007). Some have argued that the assessment of risk at the level of individual teeth may also be of value in clinical decision making, as in the case of preventive measures such as sealant use in children (Rethman, 2000).

Although caries-risk assessment has been investigated for nearly three decades (Bader et al., 2005), limited work has been conducted in preschool-age children. A systematic literature review (Harris et al., 2004) on risk factors related to dental caries in children less than 6 years identified 106 risk factors significantly related to the prevalence or incidence of dental disease, but noted a shortage of high quality and longitudinal studies. Zero et al. (2001) conducted a systematic assessment of evidence in the literature to determine the predictive validity of currently available multivariate caries-risk assessment strategies. They determined that at the time of their review there existed only two longitudinal studies of good quality for caries-risk assessment in the primary dentition. The age of subjects for these two studies included 3–5 year-olds, thus precluding the infant years that are critical to fully implementing the concept of early risk assessment. Zero et al. (2001) also noted that in a number of instances, single risk indicators were as good as a combination of indicators in terms of predictive value. Among the strongest predictors reported were previous caries experience, followed by parental education, and socioeconomic status (Zero et al., 2001)—variables that while informative generally lie outside a clinician's sphere of influence.

Despite the shortcomings of current predictive models, the identification of caries-risk factors and indicators is generally considered to be a useful adjunct for assessing caries risk in populations and individuals. Therefore, the following section provides an overview of prominent risk factors and indicators related to caries development in children organized according to categories and a common conceptual model of the caries process.

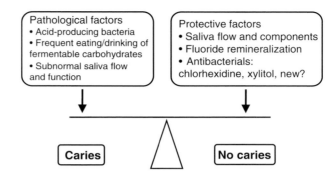

Figure 8.1   The caries balance.

RISK FACTORS AND INDICATORS FOR EARLY CHILDHOOD CARIES

The nature of the caries process has been described by Featherstone (1999, 2004a) in terms of a dynamic balance between protective and pathological factors (see Figure 8.1). This depiction illustrates the potential for states representing equilibrium or disequilibrium depending on the balance of factors that promote demineralization and remineralization of tooth structure. In this model, caries progression occurs when pathological factors dominate, and stasis or caries reversal occurs when protective factors prevail (Featherstone, 2004b). Although this model offers an excellent conceptual foundation for clinical considerations when performing caries-risk assessment in children and adults, its application is often limited to infectious disease concepts of agent, vector, and host (Keyes, 1960; Bokhout et al., 2000).

The nature of caries development encompasses broader considerations. Investigators and clinicians increasingly have come to recognize the important role that complex interactions involving environmental, social, and behavioral variables play in determining the balance between factors associated with caries risk and caries resistance or remission (Litt and Tinanoff, 1995; Ismail, 2003; Crall, 2006; Fisher-Owens et al., 2007). Accordingly, we incorporate this broader approach in our review of variables associated with caries risk in children.

Clinical

Dental history

As stated above, previous caries history is not well suited as a risk factor if the goal is to reach children prior to clinical manifestation of the disease. Nevertheless, young children who have experienced dental treatment in the form of restorations or extractions within the past year should be considered high risk. The exact nature of this history and the influence on a child's risk later in life is unclear. However, Skeie et al. (2006) found that, at age 5, the presence of two carious surfaces in primary second molars was a clinically useful predictor for being high risk at age 10. Equally compelling is evidence that 25–50% of children treated under general anesthesia require retreatment in the operating room within a 2-year period (Berkowitz et al., 1997; Almeida et al., 2000).

Another consideration related to a child's dental history concerns the presence of dental appliances. In very young children, these may include partial dentures to replace anterior teeth or space maintainers in posterior segments. Both pose additional oral hygiene challenges thereby increasing the child's risk profile. Although not documented in young children, reports indicate that the presence of fixed appliances in adolescents can pose a risk for caries development due to persistent high bacterial levels in spite of scrupulous oral hygiene instruction and overall reduction in the plaque index (Smiech-Slomkowska and Jablonsak-Zrobek, 2007).

Decalcified areas

White spot lesions (enamel caries) represent the beginning of the caries process and their presence indicates early clinical stages of the disease. Assessing whether white spot lesions are active or arrested at a single observation represents a significant diagnostic challenge. However, the presence of decalcifications in young children generally warrants an aggressive preventive approach to minimize caries progression. A study by Autio-Gold and Courts (2001) found that treating active incipient lesions with fluoride varnish doubled the percentage of lesions that remained stable (i.e., 81% of fluoride varnish-treated lesions did not progress to cavitation whereas less than 40% remained stable in the untreated group), confirming the role of fluoride varnish as a protective, non-surgical approach in preventing caries progression of incipient lesions.

Enamel defects

Enamel defects are defined as qualitative or quantitative disturbances in hard tissue matrices, resulting from insults during odontogenesis (Clarkson, 1989). Such defects may be the result of genetic, systemic, and/or environmental factors such as small gestational age, malnutrition, and infection (Seow, 1991; Slayton et al., 2001). Variations in defect location and types have been reported in the primary dentition, with hypoplasia and opacities most commonly cited (Montero et al., 2003).

Moreover, a strong association has been observed between enamel defects and caries development in low-income children and those born with very low birth weight (Lai et al., 1997; Quiñonez et al., 2001; Oliveira et al., 2006). In a Brazilian prospective study that examined children at multiple times prior to their third birthday, enamel defects, night breast-feeding, and poor oral hygiene practices were reported to be predictors of caries development at 18 and 24 months of age. The presence of enamel defects was the single best predictor of dental disease at 36 months of age (Oliveira et al., 2006; Chavez et al., 2007). With reports documenting prevalence rates for enamel defects in the primary dentition ranging from 6 to 80%, depending on race, ethnicity, socioeconomic status, and birth weight, enamel defects constitute a noteworthy risk factor for caries development (Slayton et al., 2001; Montero et al., 2003; Oliveira et al., 2006).

Bacteria

Mutans streptococci (MS) and lactobacilli have been implicated in the production of lactic acid, a prominent risk factor for tooth demineralization and ultimately cavitation (Loesche, 1986). Exciting research concerning the acquisition and transmissibility of these bacteria includes evidence of vertical (from mother or caretaker to child) and horizontal (from group members of similar age) transmission vectors, with vertical being the most prominent of the two, as demonstrated through genotypic markers (Caufield et al., 1988; Berkowitz, 2006).

The timing of bacterial acquisition has been termed the "window of infectivity." Initial studies suggested a period ranging from 19 to 31 months of age and highlighted the necessity of nonsquamous oral surfaces (e.g., teeth) for establishing cariogenic microbes in the oral cavity (Caufield et al., 1993). However, more recent literature points to an earlier window of infectivity, with furrows of the tongue as important ecological niches prior to tooth emergence (Tanner, 2002; Mohan et al., 1998). *Streptococcus mutans* and *Streptococcus sobrinus* have been detected as early as 3 months of age in approximately 30% of predentate infants, and in up to 80% of 24-month-old dentate children (Law et al., 2007). Children not infected during this earlier "window" may experience a second significant period of infectivity after permanent teeth emerge (Straetemans et al., 1998).

Bacterial acquisition and colonization of oral structures are complex processes with multiple potential determinants. For example, the acquisition of MS has been shown to be influenced by other indigenous bacterial species including *Streptococcus sanguinis* (Caufield et al., 2000). MS infectivity has also been associated with enamel hypoplasia (delayed), onset of toothbrushing after 12 months of age, lack of oral hygiene supervision, and visible plaque (Law and Seow, 2006). Early bacterial colonization has been linked to higher caries experience (Berkowitz, 2003). One study involving a cohort of over 700 children (Grindefjord et al., 1995) found that MS colonization in the first year of life was the best predictor of caries at 3.5 years of age. Roeters et al. (1995) reported on a cohort study demonstrating a significant relationship between levels of *Lactobacillus* in saliva and MS levels in saliva and plaque and the presence of caries in children at age 2.5 years and above. A systematic review assessing the validity of MS as a predictor of dental disease in preschool-age children (Thenisch et al., 2006) found a significant pooled risk ratio of 3.85 in studies using plaque tests and 2.11 in those using saliva testing. These investigators concluded that the presence of MS in plaque or saliva of young caries-free children is associated with a considerable increase in caries risk.

The possible protective effect of reducing maternal and child MS levels and delaying MS colonization pose exciting possibilities for clinical practice. Soderling et al. (2000) demonstrated that frequent use of xylitol gum by mothers during the period from 3 months to 2 years postdelivery resulted in a reduced maternal MS levels and caries reductions in their offspring. The xylitol-associated reduction in the probability of mother–child MS transmission persisted at ages 3 and 6 years (Soderling et al., 2001). Similarly, the use of polyol-containing chewing gum in a cohort of kindergarten children over a 6-month period showed a reduction in MS and plaque levels compared with controls (Makinen et al., 2005). The prospect of using sugar substitutes to reduce the incidence of caries in young children and their caregivers is an active area of research requiring further investigation to assess the long-term consequences of this strategy. Adoption of child-centered strategies necessitates the development of guidelines that address safety issues associated with chewing gum usage to minimize choking hazards in children (AAP, 2007).

Behavioral

Oral hygiene and diet

Providing anticipatory guidance concerning feeding practices and oral hygiene is grounded in classical work, implicating carbohydrates and bacteria as critical components in the caries process (Keyes, 1960). A recent systematic review of risk factors for dental disease by Harris et al. (2004) concluded that early colonization by MS was a key factor in caries development. Good oral hygiene practices (see sections below which emphasize the judicious use of fluoride toothpaste as part of oral hygiene routines in young children) and noncariogenic feeding practices were deemed to be protective for early childhood caries (ECC). Although typical counseling approaches have been shown to be largely ineffective in modifying oral health-related behaviors (Tinanoff, 1995), the use of techniques such as motivational interviewing to achieve positive knowledge and behavioral changes have demonstrated promising results (Weinstein et al., 2006; Harrison et al., 2007). These recent findings underscore the importance of understanding behavioral risk factors when designing interventions geared toward promoting oral health and disease prevention.

Within the context of childhood caries, general dietary considerations typically apply regardless of a child's age, with the exception of the infant and toddler years, a period that involves frequent feedings of breast milk and/or formula. Falling asleep while feeding has been shown to increase caries risk in children (Huntington et al., 2002; Hallett and O'Rourke, 2003). A systematic review of the relationship between breastfeeding and ECC indicated that breastfeeding beyond 1 year and at night once teeth were present may be associated with ECC (Valaitis et al., 2000). The moderate quality of the literature available precluded a more definitive statement regarding this association. More recent longitudinal studies involving a cohort of 600 Japanese children indicated that youngsters who were breast-fed beyond 18 months had higher levels of decayed and filled teeth compared to controls. Although human breast milk alone has a pH of 7.2 (Begg et al., 2002) and has been noted to lack an association with ECC, other literature considers it to have cariogenic potential by promoting enamel decalcification, particularly with the introduction of other sucrose-containing substrates at approximately the fifth month of life (Erickson and Mazhari, 1999; Iida et al., 2007).

As infants continue their development throughout the toddler stage and early childhood, dietary intake remains an important consideration for promoting a healthy "caries balance". With respect to liquid consumption beyond infancy, the American Academy of Pediatrics recommends a maximum of 4–6 ounces (the equivalent of half to three-quarters of a cup) of juice per day from ages 1 through 6 years. Common alternative sources of liquid include water, milk, and soda beverages. The high sugar content and low pH of sodas (e.g., 9.3 teaspoons of sugar, pH 3.12) do not make these good alternatives to juice from the standpoint of caries risk, and sports drinks may exhibit greater enamel dissolution potential than many sodas (Owens and Kitchens, 2007). Conversely, Levy et al. (2003) found milk consumption to be protective for caries development between 24 and 36 months of age. However, a cautionary note concerning total daily intake of milk is important. As children transition to cow's milk after 12 months of age, consuming greater than 24 ounces per day puts a child at risk for anemia, as their full stomach inhibits consumption of other food groups necessary to prevent iron deficiency (AAP, 2007). The frequent intake of large volumes of sugared beverages—regardless of the vehicle (i.e., bottle or sippy cup)—warrants counseling to discourage these feeding practices that elevate caries risk and adoption of practices that can help protect against ECC (Tinanoff and Palmer, 2000; Mariri et al., 2003). Similar principles apply when considering solid intake, with frequent ingestion of foods containing starches and sugars conveying increased risk for ECC (Mariri et al., 2003; Marshall et al., 2005).

A final note on the possible interaction with sugar ingestion and fluoride exposure seems in order. Burt and Pai (2001) have stated that sugar intake is a more powerful risk indicator among children who do not have adequate fluoride exposure, whereas sugar consumption with adequate fluoride exposure was deemed to have less cariogenic potential, the combination constituting a mild-to-moderate risk factor for dental disease. Their systematic review emphasized the importance of including topical fluoride (e.g., fluoride toothpaste) in oral hygiene caries prevention routines. Wendt et al. (1996) found that the probability of remaining caries free until 3 years of age in spite of the presence of dietary risk factors was highest if good oral hygiene practices, including the use of fluoride toothpaste beginning at 2 years of age, were employed. Similarly, in the Iowa Fluoride Study, Levy et al. (2003) demonstrated that fluoride toothpaste brushing in the fourth year of life was negatively associated with caries risk. Habibian et al. (2002) showed that children in a similar age cohort who started brushing their teeth or had their teeth brushed by 12 months of age were less likely to have detectable bacterial levels. With clinically visible plaque on teeth being a strong indicator for caries development in young children (Alaluusua and Malmivirta, 1994; Mattila et al., 1998), plaque removal via oral hygiene practices that combine judicious, supervised fluoride exposure (to minimize the risk of objectionable fluorosis) can exert protection against ECC.

General health

Systemic health status

A child's general health status is an important consideration in caries-risk assessment, as health conditions and treatments to address various diseases and medical conditions can influence the caries balance. For example, Ivancic et al. (2007) reported an average of 3.42 decayed and filled primary teeth (dft) in a cohort of disabled children (defined as those with conditions including cerebral palsy, Down syndrome, or autism) versus 1.43 dft in a control group. Children with gastric esophageal reflux also have been found to have a greater incidence of dental erosion and to be at higher risk for caries development (Linnett et al., 2002). Nearly one-half of infants with reflux have been reported to have an associated cow's milk allergy (Salvatore and Vandeplas, 2002), potentially compounding caries risk and warranting careful consideration of the medical history in these children.

The association between premature birth and enamel defects has prompted interest in the relationship between low birth weight and childhood caries (Lai et al., 1997). Although the evidence on this relation remains equivocal, Burt and Pai (2001) suggested that low birth weight should continue to be considered as a caries indicator, as it acts as a proxy for other social deprivation factors or altered immunological function, predisposing low-birth-weight babies to earlier colonization of cariogenic bacteria.

Systemic conditions can also contribute to reduced caries risk. For example, the persistent use of antibiotic medication in children with cystic fibrosis is hypothesized to convey caries protection (Fernald et al., 1990). Peterson et al. (1985) also found that altered urea metabolism in children with chronic renal failure contributed to enhanced buffering capacity in plaque and a more alkaline oral environment, thereby reducing caries risk.

Therapies and medications

Saliva plays an important role in the caries balance by providing minerals and proteins protective to the tooth surface, and by buffering acidity in the oral cavity (Featherstone, 2000). In this regard, therapies or medications that alter saliva quality and/or quantity are important considerations in caries-risk assessment. Use of radiation and chemotherapy in treating childhood cancers can alter the integrity of the rapidly dividing epithelial cells in salivary glands, often resulting in xerostomia or decreased salivary flow. A longitudinal study by Pajari et al. (2001) indicated that caries risk in children undergoing cancer treatment was highest if active caries was present at the time of cancer diagnosis. Such children were more likely to have positive findings for lactobacilli and candida over a 3-year period than those with a sound dentition at the time of cancer diagnosis.

The chronic use of liquid medications can pose another challenge to the caries balance. The use of high sucrose content to improve the palatability of liquid medications significantly elevates the cariogenic potential of such medications. Children on liquid oral medication therapies for more than 1 year have been shown to experience significantly more dental disease in the anterior primary dentition in comparison to their siblings (Maguire et al., 1996). Ersin et al. (2006) also found that among asthmatic children and adolescents, greater duration of asthma medication use was associated with lower salivary pH and elevated salivary levels of MS.

Patient education about ways to enhance oral clearance following medication intake has been promoted as a caries-risk reduction strategy (Feigal et al., 1981; Durward and Thou, 1997). Recommendations include taking medications in tablet form when possible, brushing with fluoride toothpaste or chewing sugarless gum after ingesting liquid medications, ingesting medications at mealtimes unless contraindicated, promoting sugar-free medication formulations, and avoiding ingestion of liquid medications just prior to bedtime.

Sociocultural and physical environment

Sociocultural

The emphasis on population health in recent decades underscores the need for an increased understanding of how social, cultural, and environmental factors influence caries risk in children (Public Health Agency of Canada, 2001). Indicators of socioeconomic status, such as poverty and caregiver educational levels, have been identified as major risk determinants for dental disease across the lifespan, with inverse correlations noted between the presence of dental caries in children and family's income level (Grindefjord et al., 1995; Vargas et al., 1998; Reisine and Psoter, 2001; Hallett and O'Rourke, 2003). With respect to oral health in early childhood, a 2007 report by the Centers for Disease Control and Prevention noted an increase in caries prevalence among U.S. preschool-age children during the preceding decade, with the greatest increase in untreated disease in the primary dentition occurring among children in households with incomes less than the federal poverty level (Dye et al., 2007).

Recent work has highlighted the importance of the interrelationships among various sociocultural factors. Larson et al. (2008) analyzed data from the 2003 National Survey of Children's Health and documented an 10-fold increase in the odds of parents reporting poorer oral health among their children in families with higher scores on an index of multiple social risks. Broad sociocultural indicators generally are helpful when considering population-based risk; however, addressing risk within specific groups (i.e., to further refine risk assessments among children within a specific group) is necessary in order to avoid oversimplifying the issue.

Mouradian et al. (2007) have noted the importance of family and community influences on caries risk. Early childhood is a time when caregivers are highly responsible for the well-being of their children. Accordingly, issues involving child–caregiver interactions, such as child temperament and family variables, have been examined as potential risk indicators for caries development. Although the literature on child temperament is equivocal, a number of authors point to an association between a "strong-tempered child" profile and inappropriate feeding practices or a shy child who responds strongly to novel experiences as being indicative of higher risk for ECC (Quiñonez et al., 2001; Jensen and Stjernqvist, 2002).

More specific to the role of family structure, single parents and those with more complex family compositions are found to be at higher caries risk (Crall et al., 1990; Mattila et al., 2000; Schroth and Cheba, 2007). Birth order and family size also have been investigated, with suggestions that caries risk may be higher in families with greater numbers of children (Primosch, 1982; Kinnby et al., 1995; Schroth and Cheba, 2007). In a 7-year prospective study, lack of family competence (with family competence being defined as improved child care knowledge, proper parental attitudes and child-rearing skills, and abilities suitable to the situation) emerged as a significant predictor for caries development (Mattila et al., 2005). Conversely, caregivers' appreciation for early teaching of healthy lifestyle choices and understanding the need for additional support when necessary were protective against ECC.

The dynamics within family systems are influenced by individuals' culture, ethnicity, and race. Although these factors may be confounded by issues of socioeconomic status and education, several investigations point to the need to understand the influence of these factors in oral health and disease progression. A study examining the effect of ethnic background on diet quality demonstrated that children of minority groups consume diets of lower quality than their non-Hispanic White counterparts (Hoerr et al., 2008). Similar findings have been documented among Hispanics and Asians, whose children are reported to have the highest rates of falling asleep while sipping milk or sweet substances (Shiboski et al., 2003). Among South Asian children ages 6–18 months, prechewing food practices by caregivers have also been shown to be associated with increased caries rates (Harrison et al., 2007). Persistent poor dietary behaviors such as those noted above have the potential to influence caries development and obesity patterns in children (Zive et al., 2002; Kranz et al., 2006).

Cultural beliefs, attitudes, and values are likely to influence caregivers' attitudes and beliefs about oral health behaviors. A study by Wong et al. (2005) found that Chinese mothers did not think it was important to preserve a child's primary dentition. Canadian aboriginal children's caregivers reported similar beliefs and failed to recognize the possible detrimental influence of poor oral health on systemic health (Schroth et al., 2007). The direct impact of these beliefs can have significant health effects as illustrated by Sohn et al. (2007) who, after accounting for insurance status and other risk indicators, demonstrated that caregivers who place higher value on their own oral health were more likely to have taken their children to visit a dentist. These findings point to the need for a greater appreciation of culture and behavioral influences that prevail among certain ethnic subgroups.

Physical environment

Physical environments represent an important dimension in caries-risk assessment. The presence of fluoride levels in drinking water is perhaps the clearest example. Fluoride has extensively documented effects on reducing demineralization and promoting remineralization in human enamel, and has been shown to be a cost-effective approach for reducing caries in children and adults (ten Cate and Featherstone, 1991; CDC, 2001; Do and Spencer, 2007). Although fluoride is protective for caries development, excessive fluoride ingestion is a risk factor for fluorosis, a condition that is most often mild in terms of its presentation and whose primary impact is esthetic in nature. Severe forms of fluorosis, which are relatively uncommon, can be a risk factor for caries development, however.

Neighborhood settings constitute an additional consideration when assessing a child's or family's environment. Tellez et al. (2006) assessed neighborhood characteristics and caries severity among African Americans living in low-income areas and found greater caries levels in areas with more grocery stores and lower caries levels in areas with more churches. The authors concluded that although socioeconomic status and individual risk factors are important considerations, neighborhood characteristics can also influence oral health and merit consideration when assessing caries risk in children.

RISK ASSESSMENT TOOLS

Diagnostic tools (e.g., various types of clinical examinations, radiographic tests, and microbiological assays) frequently are used by clinicians to identify individuals who have a particular disease or condition or to rule out the presence of a disease or condition. Risk assessment tools, on the other

Table 8.1 Representation of test findings and test characteristics.

	Positive test	Negative test
Caries present	True positive a	False negative b
Caries absent	False positive c	True negative d

Sensitivity = a/(a + c).
Specificity = d/(b + d).
Positive predictive value = a/(a + b).
Negative predictive value = d/(c + d).

hand, are used to help differentiate among individuals based on their risk, likelihood, or propensity for developing a specific condition or disease at some future time.

For children, risk assessment tools can help promote early identification of specific risk factors or indicators, allow for systematic evaluation and monitoring of risk over time, and serve as the basis for discussions with caregivers regarding children's conditions. Risk assessment tools have been used in pediatric medicine to identify individuals at risk for developmental and physical disorders, and behavioral or mental conditions, and have received considerable attention in the field of pediatric oral health care.

Parameters commonly used to assess the performance of diagnostic tools include characteristics such as sensitivity, specificity, and positive and negative predictive values (see Table 8.1). Assessment of clinical tools also necessarily involves consideration of epidemiological contexts (Berg, 2004; Sackett et al., 1991), with respect to the diagnosis of childhood caries:

- Sensitivity is the ability of a test or tool to determine the presence of caries in children who actually have the disease (i.e., the probability of a positive test result in an individual when caries is present or the proportion of positive test results in a group of individuals who have caries).
- Specificity is the ability of a test or tool to determine the absence of caries in children who do not have the disease (i.e., the probability of a negative test result in an individual when caries is not present or the proportion of negative test results in a group of individuals who do not have caries).
- Positive predictive value represents the likelihood that an individual with a positive test result actually has the disease in question (i.e., the probability that a child with a positive test result has caries) or the proportion of a group of individuals with positive test results that have caries or are considered caries active.

- Negative predictive value represents the likelihood that an individual who has a negative test result does not have the disease (i.e., the probability that a child with a negative test result does not have caries) or the proportion of a group of individuals with negative test results that do not have caries or are considered caries inactive.

These same characteristics can apply to risk assessment. However, in the case of risk assessment, the test or tool is used to identify factors that have been shown to be associated with the development of disease prior to the actual manifestation of the disease and/or to assess the probability that an individual will manifest a certain disease within some future time frame. Therefore, whereas evaluations of diagnostic tests or tools can involve concurrent comparisons of disease status and test results, evaluation of risk assessment tests or tools necessarily requires the passage of time following exposure to a risk factor to determine the accuracy of the risk assessment test or tool.

Overview of current caries-risk assessment tools (CAT) for children

The development of methods to identify caries-prone children has been of interest in the practice of dentistry for several decades. Complex epidemiological algorithms incorporating a multitude of risk factors have been formulated, but generally have been deemed inadequate, impractical, or unproven in terms of their ability to characterize an individual child's risk for developing caries. Investigations conducted heretofore generally have been limited by their study design or by the inherent characteristics of the tools being evaluated. Most risk assessment tools developed to date are better at predicting those who will not develop future disease rather than those who will. Although data concerning their performance are limited, the following section provides a brief overview of CAT used in pediatric clinical practice (See Table 8.2). With emerging evidence, additional tools continue to be developed and will require a close assessment of their validity and reliability for pediatric dental care.

American Academy of Pediatric Dentistry's caries-risk assessment tool

The American Academy of Pediatric Dentistry (AAPD) developed its CAT in 2002 based on clinical evidence and expert opinion. The structure of the initial version of the AAPD CAT included a number of risk factors organized into three general domains: clinical considerations, environmental considerations, and general health considerations (AAPD, 2002, 2007c). A more recent version of the AAPD CAT divides risk categories into child history (obtained via parental report), clinical evaluation, and supplemental professional assessment (Table 8.2). This tool is relatively broad in scope and is intended to be used from infancy through adolescence by dental and nondental health care providers. The AAPD CAT has undergone limited

Table 8.2 Comparison of various caries risk assessment tools.

	AAPD	CAMBRA (0–5 year)	Dundee CRM	Cariogram
Provider type	Intended for both dental and non-dental health care providers. One general form available.	Intended for dental and non-dental health care providers. Separate dental and medical forms tailored to each discipline.	Intended for dental providers.	Intended for dental providers.
Intended ages	Infancy through adolescence	Birth through 5 years (Ages 6 through adulthood available)	Preschool age children (Ages 6 through 16 yrs available)	Non-specific-childhood through adulthood
Risk Categories Total number of assessment items:	Low/Moderate/High Total N = 17 (100%)	Low/Moderate/High Total N = 21 (100%)	Low/Moderate/High Total N = 4 (100%)	Low/Moderate/High Total N = 10 (100%)
Distribution of questions by category:				
• Clinical/biological[a]	8 (47%)	9 (42%)	3 (75%)	7 (70%)
• Behavioral	2 (12%)	5 (24%)	0 (0%)	1 (10%)
• General health	2 (12%)	2 (10%)	0 (0%)	1 (10%)
• Sociocultural and physical environment	5 (29%)	5 (24%)	1 (25%)	1 (10%)
Weighting of factors according to their influence in the caries process	No	No	No	Yes
Management recommendations based on risk assessment derived from tool	No	Yes	Yes	Yes
Level of tool validation	Low	Low	Low	Moderate among 10- to 12-year-olds and the elderly. Low of young children
Language available	English	English	English	English and 12 additional languages
Computer based	No	No	No	Yes

[a] Clinical/biological category also includes the providers "clinical judgment," used in the Dundee CRM and cariogram tools.

Caries Risk Assessment Form for Age 0 to 5

Patient name:_____ I.D.#_____ Age _____ Date _____
Initial/base line exam date_____ Caries recall date_____ _____

Respond to each question in sections 1, 2, 3, and 4 with a check mark in the "Yes" or "No" column	Yes	No	Notes
1. Caries Risk Indicators — Parent Interview**			
(a) Mother or primary caregiver has had active dental decay in the past 12 months			
(b) Child has recent dental restorations (see 5b below)			
(c) Parent and/or caregiver has low SES (socioeconomic status) and/or low health literacy			
(d) Child has developmental problems			
(e) No dental home/episodic dental care			
2. Caries Risk Factors (Biological) — Parent Interview**			
(a) Child has frequent (greater than three times daily) between-meal snacks of sugars/cooked starch/sugared beverages			
(b) Child has saliva-reducing factors present, including:			
1. Medications (e.g., some for asthma or hyperactivity)			
2. Medical (cancer treatment) or genetic factors			
(c) Child continually uses bottle - contains fluids other than water			
(d) Child sleeps with a bottle or nurses on demand			
3. Protective Factors (Nonbiological) — Parent Interview			
(a) Mother/caregiver decay-free last three years			
(b) Child has a dental home and regular dental care			
4. Protective Factors (Biological) — Parent Interview			
(a) Child lives in a fluoridated community or takes fluoride supplements by slowly dissolving or as chewable tablets			
(b) Child's teeth are cleaned with fluoridated toothpaste (pea-size) daily			
(c) Mother/caregiver chews/sucks xylitol chewing gum/lozenges 2-4x daily			
5. Caries Risk Indicators/Factors — Clinical Examination of Child**			
(a) Obvious white spots, decalcifications, or obvious decay present on the child's teeth			
(b) Restorations placed in the last two years in/on child's teeth			
(c) Plaque is obvious on the child's teeth and/or gums bleed easily			
(d) Child has dental or orthodontic appliances present, fixed or removable: e.g., braces, space maintainers, obturators			
(e) Risk Factor: Visually inadequate saliva flow - dry mouth			

**If yes to any one of 1(a), 1(b), 5(a), or 5(b) or any two in categories 1, 2, 5, consider performing bacterial culture on mother or caregiver and child. Use this as a baseline to follow results of antibacterial intervention.	Parent/Caregiver Date:		Child Date:
(a) Mutans streptococci (Indicate bacterial level: high, medium, low)			
(b) Lactobacillus species (Indicate bacterial level: high, medium, low)			

Child's overall caries risk status: (CIRCLE) Extreme	Low	Moderate	High
Recommendations given: Yes _____ No _____ Date given _____		Date follow up: _____	

SELF-MANAGEMENT GOALS 1) _____ 2)_____

Practitioner signature_____ Date_____

Figure 8.2 CAMBRA assessment tool for 0–5-year-olds for dental provider use.

validity testing in clinical settings. A study by Nainar and Straffon (2006) showed high acceptance of the tool by dental students, with over 80% indicating that they were likely to use it in clinical practice, but raised concerns about the CAT's potential to "over-classify" children as being at increased risk for caries. An additional concern regarding the CAT's broad scope relates to its perceived complexity, lack of user-friendliness, especially for nondental providers (e.g., pediatricians or other primary care providers).

Caries management by risk assessment

Caries management by risk assessment (CAMBRA) was developed in 2002 and first introduced at a consensus conference dealing with caries management and risk assessment (Featherstone et al., 2003). CAMBRA provides separate caries-risk assessment forms for dental and medical professionals. The modified dental CAMBRA is illustrated in Figure 8.2 (Ramos-Gomez et al. 2007). Conceptually this tool is designed to identify risk and protective factors via a parent interview and clinical examination. Bacterial culturing is recommended for children who exhibit certain levels or combinations of risk factors. CAMBRA also seeks to serve as a tool for developing individualized treatment and preventive care recommendations based on caries-risk level and bacterial culture results.

Dundee caries-risk assessment model

The Scottish Intercollegiate Guidelines Network (SIGN) is focused on developing parameters to guide dental practice. In 1999, a cohort of over 1,000 children was followed from age 1 until they started school to identify risk indicators for caries development (Dental Health Services Research Unit, 2007). The Dundee caries-risk assessment model (DCRM) includes the following indicators that were deemed to be important for dental practice-based caries-risk assessment: (a) previous caries experience; (b) resident of a (socioeconomically) "deprived area"; (c) health care worker's opinion; and (d) oral MS counts (if feasible). The DCRM recommends that any child whose family lives in a deprived area should be considered as being at increased risk when delivering preventive programs (SIGN, 2005). A unique aspect of the DCRM is that each recommendation is accompanied by a "strength of the evidence" rating. The dental practice-based risk assessment approach and population-based guideline received "C" and "B" grades, respectively, indicating moderate levels of evidence for these recommendations.

Cariogram

The cariogram was developed in 1997 for use by dental providers. It is a computer-based tool aimed at illustrating the interaction of caries-related factors and the probability of developing new carious lesions. The cariogram uses a pie chart to show an individual's overall caries risk and the relative contributors to overall risk (Bratthall and Petersson, 2005). It relies primarily on assays of clinical specimens for the determination of caries risk, making it more complicated and potentially more costly to use given the need to obtain salivary secretion rates and MS and lactobacillus counts. One of the distinctive characteristics of this tool, however, is that it provides a "weighted" analysis of the various factors and indicators. Similar to the CAMBRA and DCRM approaches, it provides individualized strategies for the management of dental caries based on specific risk factors. Cariograms are easily accessible online and are available in 13 different languages (Bratthall et al., 2007). Although it has not been validated in young children, good data exist concerning its validity among 10- to 12-year-olds and the elderly (Hansel Petersson et al., 2002, 2003).

POTENTIAL USES, POLICY CONSIDERATIONS, AND NEED FOR DEVELOPMENT

Reliable, easy-to-use, low-cost CATs have the potential to promote more effective and more efficient approaches for addressing caries in children in a number of ways, including but not limited to the following:

- Differentiating children according to their relative caries risk
- Improving clinical decision making
- Individualized counseling and anticipatory guidance
- Clinical care strategies (guidelines) for groups having similar risk profiles
- Service delivery system performance and efficiency

Despite this widely recognized potential, the field of caries-risk assessment is relatively immature and requires additional investment in research and development geared toward cost-effective technological advances combined with field testing to determine which approaches demonstrate suitable validity, reliability, and utility.

For the most part, dental care for children consists of relatively frequent recurring episodes of diagnostic and preventive services supplemented, when necessary, by a considerable range of additional procedures to restore damaged teeth, alleviate pain and infection, and support the development of a functional dentition. Relative to other forms of health care, pediatric dental treatment services are provided with relatively high frequency, but are relatively low cost. Moreover, caries risk is subject to multiple changes throughout childhood. A major policy implication of this scenario for the central focus of this chapter is that methods used for caries-risk assessment must be relatively inexpensive and have a relatively high level of predictive accuracy in order to be cost-effective. For example, if microbiological assays are to be used as part of caries-risk assessment, the cost of the technology and analysis of results must have a favorable cost–benefit ratio in order to be recommended for inclusion in programs where cost-effectiveness is a paramount consideration. This financial imperative may necessitate the selective use of such technologies for subsets of children for whom preliminary assessments of other risk factors suggest elevated risk, rather than more universal applications of this technology. Cost-effectiveness may also be improved through workforce arrangements that look to use the most efficient combinations of personnel within systems of care (Jokela and Pienihäkkinen, 2003).

In conclusion, epidemiological trends and prevailing sociopolitical considerations underscore the need to develop more effective and more efficient methods for addressing childhood caries. Caries-risk assessment undoubtedly will be a core principle on which future changes in the delivery of pediatric oral health care are fashioned. Although approaches developed to date are encouraging, continued development is necessary to identify credible CATs and the most efficient approaches for using these tools as part of clinical or public health practice.

ACKNOWLEDGMENTS

The authors would like to thank Dr Carlos Quiñonez and Mr Mark Cummings for their assistance in developing this chapter.

REFERENCES

Alaluusua S and Malmivirta R. 1994. Early plaque accumulation—a sign for caries risk in young children. *Community Dent Oral Epidemiol* 22(5, Pt 1): 273–6.

Almeida AG, Roseman MM, Sheff M, Huntington N, and Hughes CV. 2000. Future caries susceptibility in children with early childhood caries following treatment under general anesthesia. *Pediatr Dent* 22(4):302–6.

American Academy of Pediatric Dentistry. 2002. Policy on use of a caries-risk assessment tool (CAT) in infants, children, and adolescents. *Pediatric Dent* 24(Suppl):15–17.

American Academy of Pediatric Dentistry. 2007a. Policy on the dental home. *Pediatr Dent* 29(7) Reference Manual 2007–2008. Available at http://www. aapd.org/media/Policies_Guidelines/P_DentalHome.pdf (accessed April 30, 2008).

American Academy of Pediatric Dentistry. 2007b. Guideline on prescribing dental radiographs for infants, children, adolescents, and persons with special health care needs. *Pediatr Dent* 28(Suppl):200–201. Reference Manual 2006–2007. Available at http://www.aapd.org/media/Policies_ Guidelines/E_Radiographs.pdf (accessed April 30, 2008).

American Academy of Pediatric Dentistry. 2007c. Policy on use of a caries-risk assessment tool (CAT) for infants, children, and adolescents. *Pediatr Dent* 29(7) Reference Manual 2007–2008. Available at http://aapd.org/media/ Policies_Guidelines/P_CariesRiskAssess.pdf (accessed April 30, 2008).

American Academy of Pediatrics (AAP). 2007. *Parents Corner Q&A: Chocking Prevention*. Available at http://www.aap.org/publiced/BR_Choking.htm (accessed April 30, 2008).

American Academy of Pediatrics Policy Statement. 2003. Oral health risk assessment timing and establishment of the dental home. *Pediatrics* 109(2):329. Available at http://aappolicy.aappublications.org/ (accessed April 30, 2008).

American Dental Association. 2007. *Current Policies. Statement on Early Child-hood Caries (2000:454)*, p 63. Available at http://www.ada.org/prof/resources/positions/doc_policies.pdf (accessed April 30, 2008).

American Dental Association, Council on Scientific Affairs. 2006. Professionally applied topical fluoride. *J Am Dent Assoc* 137:1151–9.

Autio-Gold JT and Courts F. 2001. Assessing the effect of fluoride varnish on early enamel carious lesions in the primary dentition. *J Am Dent Assoc* 132:1247–53.

Bader JD, Perrin NA, Maupome G, Rindal B, and Rush WA. 2005. Validation of a simple approach to caries risk assessment. *J Public Health Dent* 65(2):76–81.

Beck JD. 1998. Risk revisited. *Community Dent Oral Epidemiol* 26:220–25.

Begg EJ, Duffull SB, Hackett LP, and Ilett KF. 2002. Studying drugs in human milk: Time to unify the approach. *J Hum Lact* 18(4):323–32.

Beltrán-Aguilar ED, Barker LK, Canto MT, Dye BA, Gooch BF, Griffin SO, Hyman J, Jaramillo F, Kingman A, Nowjack-Raymer R, Selwitz RH, and Wu T. 2005. Surveillance for dental caries, dental sealants, tooth retention, edentulism, and enamel fluorosis—United States, 1988–1994 and 1999–2002. *MMWR* 54:1–44.

Berg J. 2007. Minimal intervention: Motivating parents through risk assessment. *Compend Contin Educ Dent* 28(3):162–4.

Berg JH. 2004. New technologies in pediatric dentistry: Dental caries detection and caries management by risk assessment. *Essence* 2(1):3–6.

Berkowitz RJ. 2006. Mutans streptococci: Acquisition and transmission. *Pediatr Dent* 28(2):106–9; discussion 192–8.

Berkowitz RJ. 2003. Causes, treatment and prevention of early childhood caries: A microbiologic perspective. *J Can Dent Assoc* 69(5):304–7.

Berkowitz RJ, Moss M, Billings RJ, and Weinstein P. 1997. Clinical outcomes for nursing caries using general anesthesia. *J Dent Child* 64(3):210–11, 28.

Bokhout B, Hopman F, Van Limbeek J, and Prahl-Andersen B. 2000. A "sufficient cause" model for dental caries. *J Epidemiol Biostatis* 5:203–8.

Bratthall D and Petersson GH. 2005. Cariogram—a miltifactorial risk assessment model for a multifactorial disease. *Community Dent Oral Epidemiol* 33:256–64.

Bratthall D, Petersson GH, and Stjernsward JR. 2007. *Cariogram: Information and Download page*. Available at http://www.db.od.mah.se/car/cariogram/cariograminfo.html (accessed April 30, 2008).

Burt BA. 2001. Definitions of risk. *J Dent Educ* 65(10):1007–8.

Burt B and Pai S. 2001. Does low birthweight increase the risk of caries? A systematic review. *J Dent Educ* 65(10):1024–7.

Caufield PW, Cutter GR, and Dasanayake AP. 1993. Initial acquisition of mutans streptococci by infants: Evidence for a discrete window of infectivity. *J Dent Res* 72(1):37–45.

Caufield PW, Dasanayake AP, Li Y, Pan Y, Hsu J, and Harding JM. 2000. Natural history of *Streptococcus sanguinis* in the oral cavity of infants: Evidence of a discrete window of infectivity. *Infect Immun* 68(7):4018–23.

Caufield PW, Ratanpridakul K, Allen DN, and Cutter GR. 1988. Plasmid-containing strains of *Streptococcus mutans* cluster within family and racial cohorts: Implication in natural transmission. *Infect Immun* 56:3216–20.

Centers for Disease Control and Prevention. 2001. *Recommendations for Using Fluoride to Prevent and Control Dental Caries in the United States*. Available at http://www.cdc.gov/mmwr/preview/mmwrhtml/rr5014a1.htm (accessed April 30, 2008).

Chavez AM, Rosenblatt A, and Oliveira OF. 2007. Enamel defects and its relation to life course events in primary dentition of Brazilian children: A longitudinal study. *Community Dent Health* 24(1):31–6.

Clarkson J. 1989. Review of terminology, classifications, and indices of developmental defects of enamel. *Adv Dent Res* 3(1):104–9.

Crall JJ. 2002. Children's oral health services: Organization and financing considerations. *Ambul Pediatr* 2(Suppl):148–53.

Crall JJ. 2006. Rethinking prevention. *Pediatr Dent* 28:96–101.

Crall JJ. 2007. Optimising oral health throughout childhood: The importance of caries risk assessment and strategic interventions. *Int Dent J* 57(Suppl 2): 221–6.

Crall JJ, Edelstein B, and Tinanoff N. 1990. Relationship of microbiological, social and environmental variables to caries status in young children. *Pediatr Dent* 12:233–6.

Dental Health Foundation. 2006. *Mommy, It Hurts to Chew: The California Smile Survey—An Oral Health Assessment of California's Kindergarten and 3rd Grade Children*. Available at http://www.kpbs.org/downloads/Kids/ CA_Oral_Health_Survey_2606.pdf (accessed April 30, 2008).

Dental Health Services Research Unit. 2007. *Targeted Caries Prevention for Pre-school Children*. Newsletter of the Chief Scientist Office. Available at http://www.sehd.scot.nhs.uk/cso/Publications/ReMat21/rm21-05.htm (accessed April 30, 2008).

Do LG and Spencer AJ. 2007. Risk-benefit balance in the use of fluoride among young children. *J Dent Res* 86(8):723–8.

Durward C and Thou T. 1997. Dental caries and sugar-containing liquid medicines for children in New Zealand. *NZ Dent J* 93(414):124–9.

Dye BA, Tan S, Smith V, Lewis BG, Barker LK, Thornton-Evans G, Eke PI, Beltran-Aguilar ED, Horowitz AM, and Li CH. 2007. Trends in oral health status: United States, 1988–1994 and 1999–2004. National Center for Health Statistics. *Vital Health Stat* 11(248):28–9.

Erickson PR and Mazhari E. 1999. Investigation of the role of human breast milk in caries development. *Pediatr Dent* 21(2):86–90.

Ersin NK, Gulen F, Eronat N, Cogulu D, Demir E, Tanac R, and Avdemir S. 2006. Oral and dental manifestations of young asthmatics related to medication, severity and duration of condition. *Pediatr Int* 48(6):549–54.

Featherstone JD. 1999. Prevention and reversal of dental caries: role of low level fluoride. *Community Dent and Oral Epidemiol* 27:31–40.

Featherstone JD. 2000. The science and practice of caries prevention. *J Am Dent Assoc* 131:887–99.

Featherstone JD. 2004a. The caries balance: Contributing factors and early detection. *J Calif Dent Assoc* 31(2):129–37.

Featherstone JD. 2004b. The continuum of dental caries. Evidence for a dynamic disease process. *J Dent Res* 83(Spec Issue C):C39–C42.

Featherstone JD, Adair SM, Anderson MH, Berkowitz RJ, Bird WF, Crall JJ, Den Besten PK, Donly KJ, Glassman P, Milgrom P, Roth JR, Snow R, and Stewart RE. 2003. Caries management by risk assessment: Consensus statement, April 2002. *J Calif Dent Assoc* 31(3):257–69.

Feigal RJ, Jensen ME, and Mensing CA. 1981. Dental caries potential of liquid medications. *Pediatrics* 68(3):416–9.

Fejerskov O. 2004. Changing paradigms in concepts on dental caries: Consequences for oral health care. *Caries Res* 38(3):182–91.

Fernald GW, Roberts MW, and Boat TF. 1990. Cystic fibrosis: A current review. *Pediatr Dent* 12(2):72–8.

Fisher-Owens SA, Gansky SA, Platt LJ, Weintraub JA, Soobader MJ, Bramlett MD, and Newacheck PW. 2007. Influences on children's oral health: A conceptual model. *Pediatrics* 120(3):e510–20.

Granoff DM and Pollard AJ. 2007. Reconsideration of the use of meningococcal polysaccharide vaccine. *Pediatr Infec Dis J* 26(8):716–22.

Grindefjord M, Dahllof G, Nilsson B, and Modeer T. 1995. Prediction of dental caries development in 1-year-old children. *Caries Res* 29(5):343–8.

Habibian M, Beighton D, Stevenson R, Lawson M, and Roberts G. 2002. Relationships between dietary behaviors, oral hygiene and mutans streptococci in dental plaque of a group of infants in southern England. *Arch Oral Biol* 47(6):491–8.

Hallett KB and O'Rourke PK. 2003. Social and behavioural determinants of early childhood caries. *Aust Dent J* 48(1):27–33.

Hansel Petersson G, Fure S, and Bratthall D. 2003. Evaluation of a computer based caries risk assessment program in an elderly group of individuals. *Acta Odontol Scand* 61:164–71.

Hansel Petersson G, Twetman S, and Bratthall D. 2002. Evaluation of a computer program for caries risk assessment in schoolchildren. *Caries Res* 36(5):327–40.

Harris R, Nicoll AD, Adair PM, and Pine CM. 2004. Risk factors for dental caries in young children: A systematic review of the literature. *Community Dent Health* 21(1, Suppl):71–85.

Harrison R, Benton T, Everson-Stewart S, and Weinstein P. 2007. Effect of motivational interviewing on rates of early childhood caries: A randomized trial. *Pediatr Dent* 29(1):16–22.

Hoerr SL, Tsuei E, Liu Y, Franklin FA, and Nicklas TA. 2008. Diet quality varies by race/ethnicity of Head Start mothers. *J Am Diet Assoc* 108(4):651–9.

Huntington NL, Kim IH, and Hughes CV. 2002. Caries-risk factors for Hispanic children affected by early childhood caries. *Pediatr Dent* 24(6):536–42.

Iida H, Auinger P, Billings RJ, and Weitzman M. 2007. Association between infant breastfeeding and early childhood caries in the United States. *Pediatrics* 120(4):e944–52.

Ismail AI. 2003. Determinants of health in children and the problem of early childhood caries. *Pediatr Dent* 25:328–33.

Ivancic JN, Majstorovic M, Bakarcic D, Katalinic A, and Szirovicza L. 2007. Dental caries I disabled children. *Coll Antropol* 31(1):321–4.

Jensen B and Stjernqvist K. 2002. Temperament and acceptance of dental treatment under sedation in preschool children. *Acta Odontol Scand* 60(4): 231–6.

Jokela J and Pienihäkkinen K. 2003. Economic evaluation of a risk-based caries prevention program in preschool children. *Acta Odontol Scand* 61(2):110–14.

Keyes P. 1960. The infectious and transmissible nature of experimental dental caries. *Arch Oral Biol* 1:304–20.

Kinnby CG, Lanke J, Linden AL, Widenheim J, and Granath L. 1995. Influence of social factors on sugary products behavior in 4-year-old children with regard to dental caries experience and information at child health centers. *Acta Odontol Scand* 53(2):105–11.

Kranz S, Smiciklas-Wright H, and Francis LA. 2006. Diet quality, added sugar, and dietary fiber intakes in American preschoolers. *Pediatr Dent* 28:164–71.

Lai PY, Seow WK, Tudehope DI, and Rogers Y. 1997. Enamel hypoplasia and dental caries in very-low birthweight children: A case-controlled, longitudinal study. *Pediatr Dent* 19(1):42–9.

Larson K, Russ SA, Crall JJ, and Halfon N. 2008. Influence of multiple social risks on children's health. *Pediatrics* 121:337–44.

Last JM (ed.). 2001. *A Dictionary of Epidemiology*, 4th edn. New York: Oxford University Press.

Law V and Seow WK. 2006. A longitudinal controlled study of factors associated with mutans streptococci infection and caries lesion initiation in children 21 to 72 months old. *Pediatr Dent* 28(1):58–65.

Law V, Seow WK, and Townsend G. 2007. Factors influencing oral colonization of mutans streptococci in young chidren. *Aust Dent J* 52(2):93–100.

Levy SM, Warren JJ, Broffitt B, Hillis SL, and Kanellis MJ. 2003. Fluoride, beverages and dental caries in the primary dentition. *Caries Res* 37(3):157–65.

Linnett V, Seow WK, Connor F, and Shepherd R. 2002. Oral health of children with gastro-esophageal reflux disease: A controlled study. *Aust Dent J* 47(2):156–62.

Litt MSR and Tinanoff N. 1995. Multidimensional causal model of dental caries development in low-income preschool children. *Pub Health* 110:607–17.

Loesche WJ. 1986. Role of *Streptococcus mutans* in human dental decay. *Microbiol Rev* 50(4):353–80.

Maguire A, Rugg-Gunn AJ, and Butler TJ. 1996. Dental health of children taking antimicrobial and non-antimicrobial liquid oral medication long-term. *Caries Res* 30(1):16–21.

Makinen KK, Saag M, Isotup KP, Olak J, Nommela R, Soderling E, and Makinen PL. 2005. Similarity of the effects of erythritol and xylitol on some risk factors of dental caries. *Caries Res* 39(3):207–15.

Mariri BP, Levy SM, Warrant JJ, Bergus GR, Marshall TA, and Broffitt B. 2003. Medically administered antibiotics, dietary habits, fluoride intake and dental caries experience in the primary dentition. *Community Dent Oral Epidemiol* 31(1):40–51.

Marshall TA, Broffitt B, Eichenberger-Gimore J, Warren JJ, Cunningham MA, and Levy SM. 2005. The roles of meal, snack, and daily total food and beverage exposures on caries experience in young children. *J Public Health Dent* 65(3):166–73.

Mattila M, Rautava P, Ojanlatva A, Paunio LH, Helenius H, and Sillanpaa M. 2005. Will the role of family influence dental caries among seven-year-old children? *Acta Odontol Scand* 63:73–84.

Mattila ML, Paunio P, Rautava P, Ojanlatva A, and Sillanpaa M. 1998. Changes in dental health and dental health habits from 3 to 5 years of age. *J Public Health Dent* 58(4):270–74.

Mattila ML, Rautava P, Sillanpaa M, and Paunio P. 2000. Caries in five-year-old children and associations with family-related factors. *J Dent Res* 79(3): 875–81.

Mohan A, Morse DE, O'Sullivan DM, and Tinanoff N. 1998. The relationship between bottle usage/content, age, and number of teeth with mutans streptococci colonization in 6–24 month-old children. *Community Dent Oral Epidemiol* 26(1):12–20.

Montero MJ, Douglass JM, and Mathieu GM. 2003. Prevalence of dental caries and enamel defects in Connecticut Head Start children. *Pediatr Dent* 25(3):235–9.

Mouradian WE, Huebner CE, Ramos-Gomez F, and Slavkin HC. 2007. Beyond access: The role of family and community in children's oral health. *J Dent Educ* 71(5):619–31.

Mouradian WE, Wehr E, and Crall JJ. 2000. Disparities in children's oral health and access to dental care. *J Am Med Assoc* 284(20):2625–31.

Nainar SH and Straffon LH. 2006. Predoctoral dental student evaluation of American Academy of Pediatric Dentistry's caries risk assessment tool. *J Dent Educ* 70(3):292–5.

Oliveira AF, Chaves AM, and Rosenblatt A. 2006. The influence of enamel defects on the development of early childhood caries in a population with low socioeconomic status: A longitudinal study. *Caries Res* 40(4):296–302.

Owens BM and Kitchens M. 2007. The erosive potential of soft drinks on enamel surface substrate: An in vitro scanning electron microscopy investigation. *J Contemp Dent Pract* 8(7):11–20.

Pajari U, Yliniemi R, and Mottonen M. 2001. The risk of dental caries in childhood cancer is not high if the teeth are caries-free at diagnosis. *Pediatr Hematol Oncol* 18(3)181–5.

Peterson S, Woodhead J, and Crall J. 1985. Caries resistance in children with chronic renal failure: Plaque pH, salivary pH, and salivary composition. *Pediatr Res* 19(8):796–9.

Primosch RF. 1982. Effect of family structure on the dental caries experience of children. *J Public Health Dent* 42(2):155–68.

Public Health Agency of Canada. 2001. Population and Public Health Branch. *The Population Health Template*. Available at http://www.phac-aspc.gc.ca/ph-sp/phdd/pdf/discussion_paper.pdf (accessed April 30, 2008).

Quinonez RB, Keels MA, Vann WF, Jr, McIver FT, Heller K, and Whitt JK. 2001. Early childhood caries: Analysis of psychosocial and biological factors in a high-risk population. *Caries Res* 35(5):376–83.

Ramos-Gomez FJ, Crall J, Gansky SA, Slayton RL, and Featherstone JD. 2007. Caries risk assessment appropriate for the age 1 visit (infants and toddlers). *J Calif Dent Assoc* 35(10):687–702.

Reich E, Lussi A, and Newbrun E. 1999. Caries-risk assessment: FDI Commission. *Int Dent J* 49:15–26.

Reisine ST and Psoter W. 2001. Socioeconomic status and selected behavioral determinants as risk factors for dental caries. *J Dent Educ* 65(10):1009–16.

Rethman J. 2000. Trends in preventive care: Caries risk assessment and indications for sealants. *J Am Dent Assoc* 131(Suppl):8S–12S.

Roeters FJ, Van Der Hoever JS, Burgerdijk RC, and Schaeken MJ. 1995. Lactobacilli, mutans streptococci and dental caries: A longitudinal study in 2-year-old children up to the age of 5 years. *Caries Res* 29(4):272–9.

Sackett DL, Haynes RB, Guyatt GH, and Tugwell P. 1991. *Clinical Epidemiology: A Basic Science for Clinical Medicine*, 2nd edn. Boston: Little Brown and Company, pp 82–90.

Salvatore S and Vandeplas Y. 2002. Gastroesaphageal reflux and cow milk allergy: Is there a link? *Pediatrics* 110:972–84.

Schroth RJ, Brothwell DJ, and Moffatt ME. 2007. Caregiver knowledge and attitudes of preschool oral health and early childhood caries. *Int J Circumpolar Health* 66(2):153–67.

Schroth RJ and Cheba V. 2007. Determining the prevalence and risk factors for early childhood caries in a community dental health clinic. *Pediatr Dent* 29(5):387–96.

Scottish Intercollegiate Guidelines Network (SIGN). 2005. *Prevention and Management of Dental Decay in the Pre-school Child: Quick Reference Guide*. Available at http://www.sign.ac.uk/pdf/qrg83.pdf (accessed April 30, 2008).

Seale NS and Casamassimo PS. 2003. Access to dental care for children in the United States: A survey of general practitioners. *J Am Dent Assoc* 134(12):1630–40.

Seow WK. 1991. Enamel hypoplasia in the primary dentition: A review. *ASDC J Dent Child* 58:441–52.

Shiboski CH, Gansky SA, Ramos-Gomez F, Ngo L, Isman R, and Pollick HF. 2003. The association of early childhood caries and race/ethnicity among California preschool children. *J Public Health Dent* 63(1):38–46.

Skeie MS, Raadal M, Strand GV, and Espelid I. 2006. The relationship between caries in the primary dentition at 5 years of age and permanent dentition at 10 years of age—a longitudinal study. *Int J Paedatr Dent* 16(3):152–60.

Slayton RL, Warren JJ, Kanellis MJ, Levy SM, and Islam M. 2001. Prevalence of enamel hypoplasia and isolated opacities in the primary dentition. *Pediatr Dent* 23(1):32–6.

Smiech-Slomkowska G and Jablonsak-Zrobek J. 2007. The effect of oral health education on dental plaque development and the level of caries-related *Streptococcus mutans* and *Lactobacillus* spp. *Eur J Orthod* 29(2):157–60.

Soderling E, Isokangas P, Pienihäkkinen K, and Tenovuo J. 2000. Influence of maternal xylitol consumption on acquisition of mutans streptococci by infants. *J Dent Res* 79(3):882–7.

Soderling E, Isokangas P, Pienihäkkinen K, Tenovuo J, and Alanen P. 2001. Influence of maternal xylitol consumption on mother-child transmission mutans streptococci: 6-year follow-up. *Caries Res* 35(3):173–7.

Sohn W, Ismail A, Amaya A, and Lepkowski J. 2007. Determinants of dental care visits among low-income African-American children. *J Am Dent Assoc* 138(3):309–18.

Stewart RE and Hale KJ. 2003. The paradigm shift in the etiology, prevention, and management of dental caries: Its effect on the practice of clinical dentistry. *J Calif Dent Assoc* 31(3):247–51.

Straetemans MM, van Loveren C, de Soet JJ, de Graaff J, and ten Cate JM. 1998. Colonization with mutans streptococci and lactobacilli and the caries experience of children after the age of five. *J Dent Res* 77(10):1851–5.

Tanner AC, Milgrom PM, Kent R, Jr, Mokeem SA, Page RC, Riedy CA, Weinstein P, and Bruss J. 2002. The microbiota of young children from tooth and tongue samples. *J Dent Res* 81:53–7.

Tellez M, Sohn W, Burt BA, and Ismail AI. 2006. Assessment of the relationship between neighborhood characteristics and dental caries severity among low-income African-Americans: A multilevel approach. *J Public Health Dent* 66(1):30–36.

ten Cate JM and Featherstone JD. 1991. Mechanistic aspects of the interactions between fluoride and dental enamel. *Crit Rev Oral Biol Med* 2(3):283–96.

Thenisch NL, Bachmann LM, Imfeld T, Leisebach Minder T, and Steurer J. 2006. Are mutans streptococci detected in preschool children a reliable predictive factor for dental caries risk? A systematic review. *Caries Res* 40(5):366–74.

Tinanoff N. 1995. Dental caries risk assessment and prevention. *Dent Clin North Am* 39(4):709–19.

Tinanoff N and Palmer CA. 2000. Dietary determinants of dental caries and dietary recommendations for preschool children. *J Public Health Dent* 60(3):197–206.

Toschke AM, Beyerlein A, and Kries R. 2005. Children at high risk for overweight: A classification and regression trees analysis approach. *Obes Res* 13(7):1270–74.

U.S. Department of Health and Human Services (DHHS). 2000. *Oral Health in America: A Report of the Surgeon General.* Rockville, MD: U.S. Department of Health and Human Services.

Valaitis R, Hesch R, Passarelli C, Sheehan D, and Sinton J. 2000. A systematic review of the relationship between breastfeeding and early childhood caries. *Can J Public Health* 91(6):411–7.

Vargas C, Crall J, and Schneider D. 1998. Sociodemographic distribution of pediatric dental caries: NHANES III, 1988–1994. *J Am Dent Assoc* 129:1229–38.

Weinstein P, Harrison R, and Benton T. 2006. Motivating mothers to prevent caries: Confirming the beneficial effect of counseling. *J Am Dent Assoc* 137(6):789–93.

Wendt LK, Hallonsten AL, Koch G, and Birkhed D. 1996. Analysis of caries-related factors infants and toddlers living in Sweden. *Acta odontol Scand* 54(2):131–7.

Wong D, Perez-Spiess S, and Julliard K. 2005. Attitudes of Chinese parents toward the oral health of their children with caries: A qualitative study. *Pediatr Dent* 27(6):505–12.

Zero D, Margherita F, and Lennon AM. 2001. Clinical applications and outcomes of using indicators of risk in caries management. *J Dent Educ* 65(10):1126–32.

Zive MM, Berry CC, Sallis JF, Grank GC, and Nader PR. 2002. Tracking dietary intake in white and Mexican American children from age 4 to 12. *J Am Diet Assoc* 102:683–9.

Family oral health education

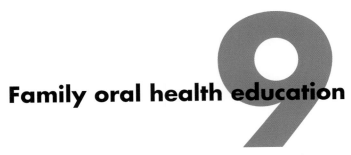

Tegwyn H. Brickhouse

INTRODUCTION

This chapter focuses on the family's role in the oral health status of the individual child and the impact caregivers may have in the prevention of early childhood caries (ECC). Caregivers play a vital role in filtering the interaction between the child and his or her environment through feeding habits, oral hygiene care, and other preventive practices/services they make available to their child. Predisposing, enabling, and reinforcing factors affect the caregiver's ability to instill healthy oral habits into their child's daily routines.

Oral health promotion and education framework for the prevention of ECC

Where a child lives contributes to an extremely complex environment that has an effect on the child's oral health and quality of life. There is no comprehensive model that exists for the promotion and education of oral health in early childhood, but there are existing frameworks that can be used. A theoretical framework adapted from Greene-Kreuter (1999) recognizes that the risk factors for ECC have many determinants and are caused by multiple factors. It also assumes that any strategies used to impact behavioral, environmental, and social change must be multidimensional (Hughes et al., 2002) (Figure 9.1).

The prevention and control of ECC and the promotion of oral health requires a complex set of strategies involving individual families, professional medical and dental services, public health activities, and health policy initiatives. Most evidence-based efforts to address ECC have focused on biologic processes or clinical care, not the constellation of factors that predispose a child to ECC. Family oral health education is a crucial and continuous component of a plan to prevent dental caries in early childhood. The characteristics of ECC and the availability of preventive methods support primary prevention as an important approach to address this pervasive pediatric health problem and its serious consequences (Figure 9.2).

Primary prevention involves (1) risk assessment to identify families at high risk for their children to develop ECC, (2) the timely delivery of appropriate educational material (anticipatory guidance) to families/caregivers/parents, and (3) families/caregivers/parents desire to receive,

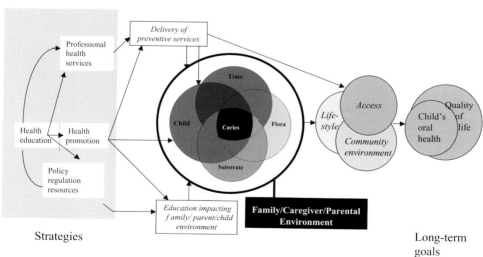

Figure 9.1   Framework for the prevention of ECC. (Modified from Hughes et al. 2002.)

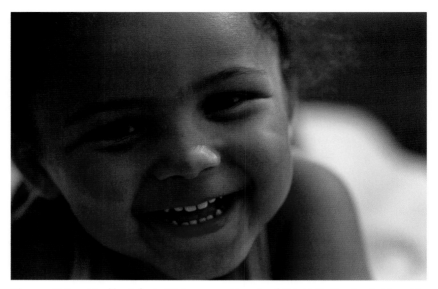

Figure 9.2   Healthy infant. (Picture compliments of Bright Smiles for Babies, Virginia Oral Health Partnership for Children, 2004.)

comprehend, and then implement preventive dental health measures. The oral health education needed to prevent ECC encompasses a wide variety of topics such as oral development, the transmission of oral bacteria, the dental disease process, oral hygiene, diet and feeding practices, and fluoride modalities. These areas of education are analogous and parallel to important preventive processes such as anticipatory guidance, risk assessment, and the establishment of a dental home (Nowak, 1995, 2002, 2007; AAP, 2003). Specific chapters have been devoted to these topics and provides a much more in-depth understanding of their impact on ECC.

This chapter focuses and expands on specific areas related to family oral health education such as oral health literacy, family/patient counseling, motivational interviewing (MI) versus traditional patient counseling, parental attitudes toward oral health, community-level education for families, and the effectiveness of oral health promotion and education.

ORAL HEALTH LITERACY

Oral health literacy is thought to be an important determinant of oral health that intersects with other factors (e.g., family attitudes and motivation) in numerous ways (Workgroup Report, 2005). Literacy is not the only pathway to improved oral health outcomes, but it is important that any preventive efforts aimed at impacting ECC should take this into account (USDHHS, 2003). A definition for oral health literacy is "the degree to

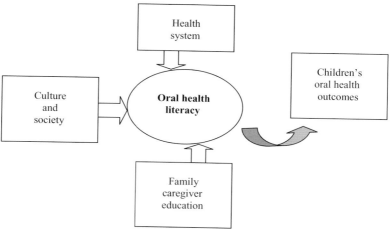

Figure 9.3   Oral health literacy framework. (Modified from NIDCR Workgroup Report on literacy, 2005.)

which individuals have the capacity to obtain, process, and understand basic oral health information and services needed to make appropriate health decisions" (ADA, 2006a; Office of Disease Prevention and Health Promotion, 2000). Figure 9.3 illustrates the relationship between oral health literacy, culture and society, the health system, and caregiver education in determining oral health outcomes.

The foundation of primary prevention is the delivery of educational information to the caregiver, yet this is just one part of the preventive process. The family must then be able to (1) visualize (e.g., read, watch, and listen), (2) comprehend the material given, and (3) implement the desired actions (e.g., behavior, toothbrushing, and feeding habits) as a part of the child's preventive health routine. Oral health literacy is a collection of skills that include not just the ability to function in the health care system but also to act upon the education being provided from that system or within the family's culture and community. Poor oral health literacy is associated with poorer perceptions of health, less utilization of services (particularly prevention related), and poorer understanding of verbal and written instructions for self-care (Jackson, 2006).

The American Academy of Pediatric Dentistry's Clinical Guideline on infant oral health calls for early risk assessment to identify parent–infant groups who are at higher risk for the development of ECC (AAPD, 2006a, b). For this reason, it is important to identify families with low oral health literacy skills as these children are most likely at risk for future decay and these parents are more likely to experience barriers to adequate education. Recent studies have identified screening tools that can be used effectively in a primary care setting to identify parents of children with low functional literacy skills (Bennett et al., 2003). Two health literacy instruments used in medicine have been modified for oral health and pilot tested with parents of children receiving oral health services (Lee et al., 2007). The dental literacy instruments appear to measure constructs that are different from the health literacy instruments. The Rapid Estimate of Adult Literacy in Dentistry (REALD) and the Test of Functional Health Literacy in Dentistry (TOFHLiD) have been demonstrated to be valid constructs and reliable measures of oral health literacy in addition to being correlated with the caregivers' perceived oral health quality of life and their child's oral health outcomes (Gong, 2007; Richman et al., 2007).

Once a family has been identified with literacy barriers, it is important to tailor preventive and educational interventions to the individual family for successful results. Suggestions regarding oral health communication for families consist of:

(1) communicating at a basic level, avoiding jargon terms;
(2) allowing the patient to explain his/her story without interruption;
(3) limiting new concepts to a maximum of three per visit;
(4) using pictures, graphics, and real devices for demonstration;
(5) asking questions using "how" or "why" to evaluate comprehension; and
(6) conveying material orally and using written material as backup (Figure 9.4).

Another effective strategy is to ask the parents to repeat the oral health information provided in their own words (Ebeling, 2003). Experts also

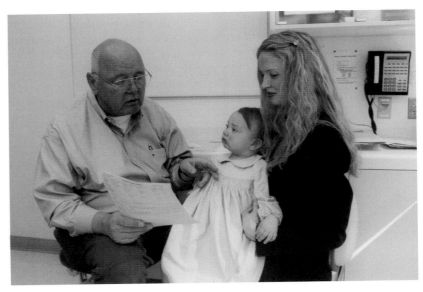

Figure 9.4   Caregiver education. (Picture compliments of Bright Smiles for Babies, Virginia Oral Health Partnership for Children, 2004.)

suggest finishing patient education appointments by providing written take-home materials such as pamphlets and brochures. Evidence suggests that pediatric dental patient education materials are difficult to read and above the recommended level for the general public using accepted readability measures (Amini et al., 2007). Parental health literacy skills have been shown to have an effect on their child's health (Berkman et al., 2004). The hypothesis is that higher parental educational levels will translate into increased likelihood of preventive dental care for their child. Oral health care providers are subsequently challenged with appropriately and effectively educating families with children at risk for ECC.

ORAL HEALTH EDUCATION AND PATIENT COUNSELING

Oral health education for families/caregivers/parents is a very broad concept that encompasses five major areas of prevention for ECC:

(1) Oral development
(2) Dental disease process
(3) Home care and oral hygiene training
(4) Diet and feeding habits
(5) Fluoride applications

The methods as to how family oral health education should be provided depend on the setting in which the education takes place. It may be a group setting in a community hospital, church, school, public health clinic, community aid program, or an office-based health care provider setting. Regardless, the educational program should be as tailored as possible to appropriately fit the audience and include basic information on oral development and the disease process, oral hygiene training, diet and nutrition, and fluoride interventions. Important aspects of educational programs are as follows:

(1) Visual and written information
(2) Demonstration of visual (knee-to-knee) examination and oral hygiene
(3) Counseling or motivation to instill preventive attitudes
(4) Evaluation of learning, hygiene procedures, acceptance, and needs of the family (Figure 9.5)

This chapter of family oral health education focuses on practical information for caregivers to utilize to impact the oral health of their children and prevent ECC in the prenatal period, infancy, and early childhood.

Prenatal education

Ideally, the oral health educational strategy for any family should begin with prenatal education. Medicine has long recognized the importance of prenatal counseling and medical care to expectant mothers. Maternal

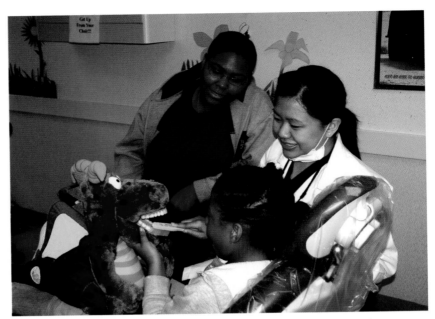

Figure 9.5   Parent counseling and motivation. (Picture compliments of Dr Tegwyn Brickhouse, 2008.)

oral health affects not only an infant's future oral health but also the infant's overall health. Periodontal disease has been linked to preterm labor (Jeffcoat et al., 2001). The outcomes of initial clinical trials suggest that periodontal therapy can decrease the risk of prematurity (Lopez et al., 2002; Jeffcoat et al., 2003). Pregnant women should be evaluated for cavities, poor oral hygiene, gingivitis, and loose teeth, as well as frequency of sugar consumption. Prenatal counseling should focus on referral to a dentist to treat existing caries and periodontal disease. Oral hygiene should be optimized with twice-daily toothbrushing using fluoride toothpaste and once-daily flossing. An over-the-counter, alcohol-free, 0.05% fluoride mouth rinse also may be recommended for women with active caries. Primary teeth begin to develop at approximately 6 weeks in utero. Adequate intake of calcium, phosphorus, and vitamins A, C, and D by mothers will help ensure the proper formation of infant's teeth.

Although often debated, there is no evidence that prenatal fluoride supplements prevent dental caries in the infants whose mothers took these supplements (Leverett et al., 1997).

Maternal oral health should also be stressed after the delivery of the infant because decreasing maternal *mutans streptococci* (MS) levels can reduce infant colonization and the child's subsequent caries risk (Kohler and Andreen, 1994). Several studies have determined that maternal levels of cariogenic bacteria are related to their child's subsequent bacterial acquisition and caries levels. It has been documented that the major source of caries-causing bacteria MS in children comes from the mother (Kohler et al., 1984; Kohler and Andreen, 1994; Caufield et al., 1993). It has also been suggested that mothers use xylitol chewing gum 4 times daily because this will decrease the transmission of MS and may subsequently reduce caries in their children (Isokangas et al., 2000). Mothers should be informed that in most cases, routine dental visits during pregnancy are not contraindicated.

Recent studies have documented that educational information related to children's oral health presented to expectant mothers resulted in improved oral health knowledge (Alsada et al., 2005; Kaste, 2007). The purpose of pre-natal education is to provide the family with information regarding their baby's dental development, the infectious nature of dental caries, diet and nutrition, oral hygiene, and recommended preventive measures such as fluoride, the timing of the first dental visit, and the importance of estab-lishing a dental home (AAP, 2003; AAPD, 2007).

Oral development

Family oral health education related to oral development should consist of dental and oral milestones such as eruption of the first tooth, eruption sequence and timing, teething, development of occlusion, and anatomical landmarks. Reasons for healthy teeth in early childhood are to provide a positive self-image, improved quality of life (i.e., not missing school due to tooth pain), and proper retention of the primary teeth to maintain space for the developing permanent dentition. Beginning in infancy, the first devel-opmental milestone discussed is the eruption of the first tooth somewhere between 6 and 8 months of age. The average age for eruption of the first primary tooth is 6 months. There is wide variability of tooth eruption and some children may be as old as 1 year before the first teeth appear. After the first tooth erupts, parents should understand the timing and sequence of tooth eruption and what teething might entail for their child. The primary incisors (centrals and laterals) typically begin to erupt between 6 and 12 months of age. The first molars erupt at about 1 year and the second molars at about 2 years. Most children have all 20 primary teeth erupted at 3 years of age. It is important to convey to parents that eruption patterns are pre-dictable but that variations are common and this should not be a source of anxiety. Parents should be advised that the earlier their child's teeth erupt, the more at risk the child is for early dental caries (Mohan et al., 1998). Figure 9.6 displays the primary dentition and timing of tooth eruption.

Although the first permanent teeth do not erupt until around 6 years of age, the enamel of these teeth is forming at birth. Parents should be aware that certain medications (e.g., tetracycline), if taken by the child or nursing mother during the first year of life, may cause discoloration of the devel-oping permanent teeth. Early childhood illnesses that result in high pro-longed fevers or poor nutrient absorption can disrupt the proper formation of the teeth as well.

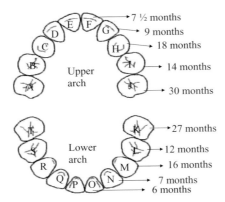

Figure 9.6   Guideline for the eruption timeline of the primary dentition. (Picture compliments of Access to Baby and Child Dentistry, Provider Training. Oral Health for Infant and Toddlers, University of Washington, 2007.)

Teething

Teething symptoms include fussiness, increased sucking behavior, and loose stools. Teething is a natural process and usually occurs with little or no problems, though some infants may exhibit a low-grade fever, diarrhea, gastrointestinal disturbances, increased salivation, and skin eruptions (Barlow et al., 2002). There is no evidence that teething causes fever and/or diarrhea. Temperatures higher than 38.1°C (100.6°F) are not associated with teething and should be evaluated for other causes (Macknin et al., 2000; Wake et al., 2000). If signs or symptoms persist for more than 24 h, parents should have the infant examined by their physician to rule out upper respiratory infection, ear infections, or other common childhood conditions.

Symptomatic relief of teething discomfort includes sucking on cold teething rings or washcloths. Palliative care for teething includes increased fluid consumption and nonaspirin analgesics. Parents should be aware of the symptoms of the teething process.

Teething symptoms
– Baby may become fussy, irritable, and sleepless
– Baby may have sore and tender gums when teeth begin to erupt
– Baby may have increased drooling and chewing behavior

Visual examination

With a visual examination the parent can be shown the oral anatomic landmarks such as the palate, alveolus, and frenulae attachments. They can be shown the difference between the incisor and molar teeth and the occlusal relationships that result in healthy occlusion. After the completion of the primary dentition (approximately 2 years of age), the purpose of the

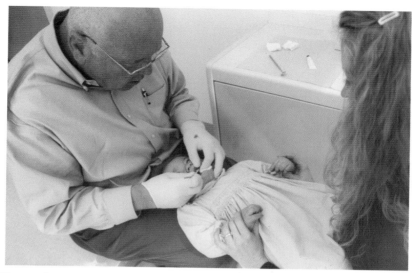

Figure 9.7   Knee-to-knee examination. (Picture compliments of Bright Smiles for Babies, Virginia Oral Health Partnership for Children, 2004.)

primary teeth as space maintainers for permanent teeth can be discussed. The development of permanent teeth and their position and timing can be discussed. The fact that maxillary permanent teeth develop facial/buccal to the primary teeth while mandibular permanent teeth develop, lingual to the primary teeth can be noted.

Positioning of the parent and child is an important aspect of a good visual examination. The parent must feel comfortable and be able to visualize the toothbrushing they provide their child. "Knee-to-knee" or "lift the lip" training for providers and parents is beneficial in providing for proper technique for both examining and brushing their child's teeth. Figures 9.7 and 9.8 show the ideal knee-to-knee position with a close-up of the lift the lip procedure for an infant examination and oral hygiene training.

Dental disease process

Early childhood caries is an infectious bacterial disease of teeth. Bacteria, predominately MS, metabolize monosaccharide and disaccharide sugars to produce acid that demineralizes teeth and causes cavities. The daily insults of bacteria and carbohydrate components of an infant's diet combine to build plaque accumulation that results in acid production. This environment encourages demineralization of the tooth enamel, which eventually results in cavitations of the teeth. ECC first presents with white spots or lines on the maxillary incisors and can progress to holes in both incisor and molar teeth. The interplay of these four etiologic factors (teeth, bacteria, carbohydrates, and time) controls the severity of the disease (see

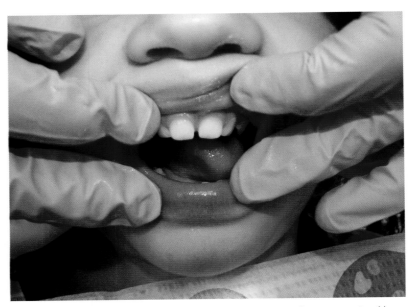

Figure 9.8   Lift the lip examination. (Picture compliments of Dr Tegwyn Brickhouse, 2008.)

Figure 9.1). Other factors such as the frequency of drinking/eating and salivary composition also contribute to caries levels in children.

The concept that dental caries is a transmissible and infectious disease is important knowledge for the family. There is a "window of infectivity" where MS, the bacteria which is responsible for dental caries, appears in a child's mouth (Caufield, 1997). The exact age at which MS colonization occurs in children is not known, but it usually does not happen until teeth erupt and often coincides with the eruption of the first primary molars. The earlier the colonization occurs, the greater the risk of caries (Kohler et al., 1988). Elevated maternal levels of MS, due to active or untreated caries and frequent sugar consumption, increase the risk of transmission (Kohler and Bratthall, 1978). MS typically originate in the mother. The bacteria found in the mouths of young children have been documented to be of the same genetic variance (fidelity) and virulence (clonality) as the caregiver's oral bacteria (Li and Caufield, 1995; Li et al., 2000).

The transmission of bacteria from mother to child can occur in any number of ways: kissing, sharing eating utensils, an infant putting his/her hand in the mother's mouth, and so on. It is impossible to completely stop the transmission, but reducing the bacterial count in the mother's mouth with preventive efforts such a restoring mother's active decay and chewing xylitol gum can delay and minimize this inoculation (Söderling et al., 2000, 2001). It is important that caregivers are aware of the impact their oral health has on their infant child. If they have untreated oral diseases, their children will be more at risk for dental disease.

Home care and oral hygiene training

Parents should be given guidance on how and when to start brushing their infant's teeth. The parents should be informed that it is their responsibility to carry out the oral hygiene practices for their children. Parents should begin cleaning an infant's gums with a moistened cloth or finger sponge before the teeth erupt. Positioning of the parent and child is an important component of oral hygiene. The parent should brush the child's teeth from behind the child while supporting the child's head. This position may have the parent sitting in a chair behind a standing child or sitting on the floor with the child's head between and arms under the parent's legs (Figure 9.9).

   Brushing should focus on removing plaque and debris. Important areas of the teeth to brush are the junction between the gingiva and teeth and pits and grooves of the molars. Toothbrushing should commence with the eruption of the first tooth. It has been shown that the earlier toothbrushing begins, the less likely children are to develop tooth decay (Creedon and O'Mullane, 2001). Children should participate in the brushing routine at an early age, but parents should supervise toothbrushing at all times and brush the child's teeth themselves at least once a day until the child is approximately 8 years of age. A common analogy used to determine when a child is capable of brushing their own teeth is when they are able to write in cursive letters.

   The use of fluoridated toothpaste by children is an extremely important practice to prevent ECC. The age at which brushing with fluoridated toothpaste should start has been debated; however, most children beginning at 2 years of age should start having their teeth brushed with a pea-sized amount of fluoridated toothpaste twice a day. Those children who are at high risk for ECC may need to start using fluoridated toothpaste before 2 years of age, at the advice of a dentist or physician. Parents should be aware that while some children's toothpastes have sweeter or milder flavors than their adult counterparts, they do contain fluoride. Most often they have the same 1,000 part per million (ppm) NaF that is present in adult toothpaste.

Chronological guidance for toothbrushing a child at risk for ECC

<1–2 years
   - Cleans teeth with cloth or soft toothbrush 1×/day
   - Smear of fluoridated toothpaste
2–6 years
   - Brush with pea-sized (or less) amount of fluoridated toothpaste 2×/day (Figure 9.10)
   - Caregiver performs

>6 years
- – Brush with fluoridated toothpaste 2×/day
- – Caregiver performs or supervises

A careful and complete toothbrushing before bedtime is recommended to remove the day's accumulation of plaque and debris in the child's mouth. This is often a difficult time when both the parent and the child

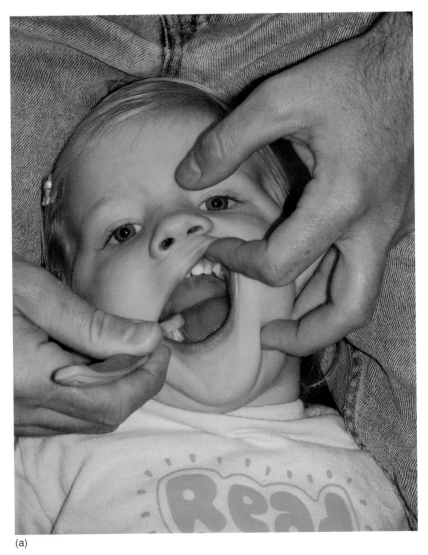

(a)

Figure 9.9   Positioning options for toothbrushing. (Pictures Compliments of Todd Brickhouse/Cara Brickhouse.)

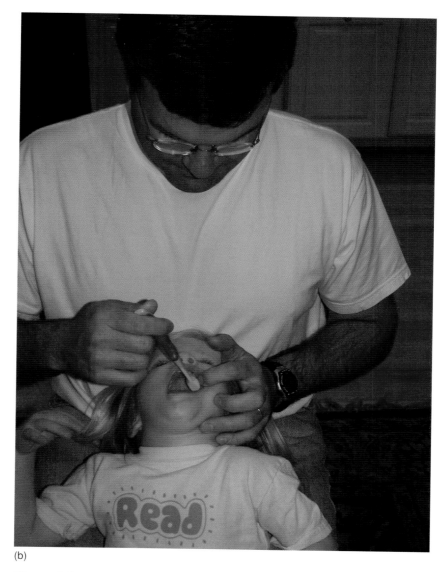

(b)

Figure 9.9   (Continued)

are tired. This is complicated by the fact that an infant is neither prepared nor expected to accept or understand the importance of brushing teeth. Just as taking a bath, toothbrushing should be incorporated
with games or music to create a positive experience. Over time, with per-
sistence by parents, toothbrushing can become a part of daily hygiene
routines.

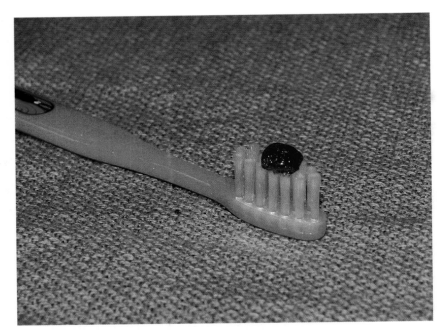

Figure 9.10   Pea-sized amount of toothpaste.

Diet and feeding habits

Initial counseling should focus on diet. Breast-feeding is the preferred source of infant nutrition. If the infant is bottle-fed, the mother should hold the infant when feeding, and the bottle should not be propped or placed in bed. Only formula or breast milk should be used in the bottle. ECC was historically attributed to inappropriate and prolonged bottle use, hence the older terms of "baby-bottle tooth decay" and "nursing caries." It is now understood that any dietary practice that allows frequent sugar consumption in the presence of MS may result in caries formation. Common contributing etiologic practices in children include propped bottles containing sweetened liquids, frequent consumption of sweetened liquids from infant- and toddler-size "sippy" cups, and frequent snacking. Beverages that are typically considered healthy such as infant formula or unsweetened fruit juices do contain carbohydrates that can produce dental caries if they are sipped frequently. Milk, juice, or other sweetened beverages should only be given at specific mealtimes. Small children should not be allowed to walk around drinking from a bottle or "sippy cup" throughout the day, unless it is filled with plain water. The caries risk generated by on demand breast-feeding is unclear. The buffering capacity of human milk is very poor. Therefore, human milk, formula, and bovine milk, and juice—all have the capacity to promote the development of dental caries when inappropriately provided to infants without daily oral hygiene care. For this reason, the parent should discontinue the use of the bottle by 12 months and should not allow their child to have constant access to a cup containing these liquids, especially during sleep times. Nap time or nighttime bottle of anything other then water should be discouraged.

The frequency of sugar consumption is the main dietary factor in the etiology of dental caries. A child's consumption of snacks or sugared beverages between meals increases the risk of dental caries (Tinanoff and Palmer, 2000). Bacteria metabolize sugars into acid and it takes 20–40 min for the acid to be neutralized or washed away by saliva. Therefore, the more frequent the snacking or drinks, the higher the potential for demineralization and greater the risk of cavities. Although MS can metabolize many different carbohydrates, they produce acids most efficiently from sugars, especially sucrose. Therefore, parents should limit the frequency and amount of sugary foods or beverages that their children consume.

As an infant child progresses to the toddler stage, the child has been introduced to a variety of foods and is being encouraged to self-feed. Parents should be aware of snack foods that are not only nutritious, but also safe for the teeth. Finger foods such as soft fruits, cereals without sugar coatings along with cheese, and salt-free crackers make healthy snacks for the teeth, while snacks with a high proportion of carbohydrates or sticky/adhesive foods should be avoided. Parents should be encouraged to develop a regular pattern of meals and set snack times should be developed, rather than "grazing." As the child grows, dietary advice should focus on limiting snacks and drinks between meals and limiting sweetened foods to mealtimes.

Fluoride

Community water fluoridation
Early in infancy, sources of systemic fluoride should be assessed. Community water fluoridation is one of the most effective tools in the prevention of dental decay and has been shown to reduce caries in young children by 40–50% (USPHS, 1979). Fluoride increases the resistance of the teeth to demineralization, promotes remineralization, and exerts bacteriostatic properties. Currently, 62% of the U.S. population has access to community water systems where water supplies are fluoridated to an optimal level of 1 ppm. Reductions in the severity of ECC from fluoridation now range from 13 to 68% (Locker et al., 1999). Homes with well water must be tested for fluoride content because levels vary even within neighborhoods from no fluoride to more than the optimal level of 1 ppm. Testing kits and services are widely available. Parents can receive direction from the dentist, physician, or local health department on how to utilize testing services.

Fluoride supplements
Fluoride supplements are an alternative source of dietary/systemic fluoride for children who do not have access to an optimally fluoridated water

system. This may occur if children either do not live in a community with an optimally fluoridated water system, have a private well, or live in a community with fluoridated water but they do not rely on this water for their primary source of fluid intake (i.e., drink and cook with bottled water). According to guidelines endorsed by the American Academy of Pediatric Dentistry, all children should receive appropriate systemic and topical fluoride beginning at 6 months of age (AAPD, 2007). If a child's home receives commercially fluoridated water, or the family's well water has more than 0.3 ppm of fluoride, no systemic supplementation should be given, even if alternative water sources are used at times (e.g., bottled water). Systemic supplementation is not recommended if the child is breast-feeding. If a child receives water from a nonfluoridated source or a well with less than 0.3 ppm of fluoride, supplementation should be considered starting at 6 months of age. Further recommendations based on age can be found in Chapter 4, Table 4.2. Recent recommendations place an emphasis on the importance of risk assessment by the health care provider to determine if the child is at high risk for dental caries. These recommendations call for fluoride supplements to be prescribed for children at high risk for dental caries and whose primary water source is not optimally fluoridated (CDC, 2001). Fluoride drops or chewable tablets should be specified because these increase oral (topical) levels of fluoride. Fluoride supplementation should not be given with formula or milk that may decrease absorption.

Professional fluoride applications

Professional applications of fluoride to children's teeth using gels or varnishes are safe and effective (Kanellis, 2000). Fluoride varnish is particularly appropriate for use in infants and young children because it can be painted on the teeth at any age. It reduces the occurrence of new caries lesions in primary teeth by 19–92% and is effective in halting the progression of already existing small lesions (Marinho et al., 2002; Marinho, 2006; Weintraub et al., 2006). Recent recommendations also stress that the use of topical fluoride treatments in the dental office be based on the child's risk of dental caries. These recommendations state that fluoride varnish is effective in prevention of caries in young children and that two or more applications a year are effective in preventing caries in high caries-risk populations. They also state that children at low risk for caries may not receive any additional benefit from professional topical fluoride applications. These recommendations point out that while fluoride gels and foams may be effective in preventing caries, this effectiveness requires a 4 min application. There is no evidence that a 1 min application provides any benefit. It is doubtful that infants or young children can tolerate a 4 min topical fluoride application. The recommendations state that fluoride varnish applications are proved to take less time, create less patient discomfort, and achieve greater patient acceptability than fluoride gel, especially in preschool-age children (ADA, 2006b). After a child receives a fluoride varnish application, it is important to let the parent know the child can drink something

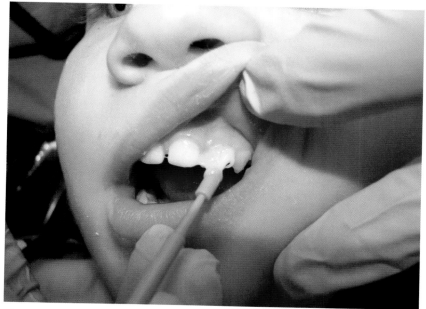

Figure 9.11   Fluoride varnish application. (Picture compliments of Dr Tegwyn Brickhouse, 2008.)

immediately and maintain a soft, nonabrasive diet for the remainder of the day. They should be advised not to brush their child's teeth that night but resume normal toothbrushing the next day (Figure 9.11).

Motivational interviewing (MI)

Strategies for providing education and direction to parents about their oral health are changing from the traditional persuasion approach of health education to individualized interventions such as anticipatory guidance and MI. Chapter 6 provides an in-depth understanding of anticipatory guidance, while motivational interviewing will be discussed here as a technique that may be used with parent counseling and guidance.

Motivational interviewing (MI) is defined as a brief counseling approach that focuses on the skills needed to motivate others and provides strategies to move patients from inaction to action (Britt et al., 2004). MI has been used successfully in a variety of health conditions such as drug addiction, diabetes, diet behaviors, and medication compliance. Evidence for the effectiveness of MI for both physiological and psychological conditions resulted in treatment effects ranging from 50 to 75% (Rubak et al., 2005).

MI has been used to counsel parents and mothers of infants and children at high risk for dental caries (Weinstein et al., 2004, 2006). Parents

Menu of Options for Infant Oral Health
Clean your baby's teeth as soon as they appear
Use a smear of fluoride toothpaste
Do not add anything sweet or sugary to bottle
Wean child from the bottle; focus on night-time
Hold baby when feeding
If baby wakens at night, give water
Limit sipping and snacking
Bring your baby to the dentist two times per year for fluoride varnish

Figure 9.12   Menu of options for infant oral health. (Figure from Weinstein et al. 2006. Copyright ©2006 American Dental Association. All rights reserved. Adapted 2008 with permission of the American Dental Association.)

receiving MI counseling in addition to traditional written and audiovisual education had infants with significantly lower levels of dental caries when compared to infants whose parents did not receive MI counseling. The goal of an MI counseling session is to establish rapport with the parents/ mothers and then provide and discuss a "menu of options" for infant oral health and caries preventive behavior (Weinstein, 2002). MI focuses on techniques such as open-ended questioning, affirmations, and the reinforcement of self-efficacy, reflective listening, and summarizing—all used in a directive manner (Harrison et al., 2007). Counselors encourage the parent to talk and are supportive listeners without judgment. They help the parent to identify the discrepancies between their current behavior and the goal of dental health for their child. Figure 9.12 displays a menu of dietary and nondietary options for caries prevention.

Parental attitudes of infant oral health

Parents and families often face difficult challenges on a daily basis, especially families at high risk for ECC. Some simply may not be aware of the risk factors and ramifications of living with and treating ECC. Often, parents do not understand the link between their child's oral health and overall health (Schroth et al., 2007). Education in the clinical setting often consists of direct persuasion or an advice giving approach by the health professional. This type of health education is ineffective. Parents play a critical role in their child's health, but little is known about their readiness to make behavior changes and how to impact the oral health care of their child. The parent's readiness for behavioral changes has four stages: (1) precontemplation, (2) contemplation, (3) preparation/action, and (4) maintenance (DiClemente, 1991). With ECC, parents may begin at the precontemplative stage where they are unaware or in denial of the condition or the risk of ECC. Next is the contemplative stage where they acknowledge the presence/risk of ECC but are ambivalent or may be considering the steps they want to take in addressing ECC. Next, the parent may take action by seeking treatment or preventive care or services. After taking action, the parents are then concerned about maintaining their child's oral health and avoiding recurrence. Several factors can influence a family's ability to make changes to its preventive oral health practices. These include cultural influences and often the parent's own dental anxiety or fear (Wong et al., 2005). Psychosocial factors that can influence parents' ability to engage in preventive health practices include poverty, stress, and depression. It has been documented that several maternal behavioral and psychosocial factors are associated with children's brushing practices at home and levels of ECC (Finlayson, 2005, 2007). Parents with low oral health self-efficacy have children with higher rates of dental caries (Reisine and Litt, 1993; Litt et al., 1995). These states of parental readiness and self-efficacy appear to be modifiable and are a point where interventions may cultivate oral health preventive habits and reductions in ECC.

Effectiveness of oral health promotion and education

Education of mothers and families has long been the strategy to promote healthy habits and to prevent ECC. These strategies have focused mainly on dietary habits, inappropriate use of the bottle, and oral hygiene (Bruerd and Jones, 1996; Seow et al., 2003). Systematic reviews of the literature have found that traditional oral health education/health promotion alone has a modest impact on the development of ECC (Ismail, 1998; Kay and Locker, 1998; Weinstein, 2006). Education should be promoted in high-risk families, but it should not be the only strategy for prevention. These children and families should be targeted with professional interventions such as oral screenings, risk assessment, effective counseling/anticipatory guidance (including MI), oral hygiene training, and effective preventive services such as the professional application of fluoride varnish.

A recent randomized controlled community trial found that home visits by dental health educators to mothers of infants at high risk for caries, during the first year of life, reduced disease in children by 83% (Kowash et al., 2000). This program was also found to be cost-effective when compared with other preventive programs (Kowash et al., 2006). At the community level, families at risk for having children with ECC should be identified early in programs such as WIC (Special Supplemental Food Program for Women, Infants, and Children), Early Head Start, or other similar settings.

REFERENCES

Alsada LH, Sigal MJ, Limeback H, Fiege J, and Kulkarni GV. 2005. Development and testing of an audio-visual aid for improving infant oral health through primary caregiver education. *J Can Dent Assoc* 71(4):241.

American Academy of Pediatric Dentistry. 2006a. Guideline on fluoride therapy. Pediatric dentistry reference manual 2006–2007. *Pediatr Dent* 28(7):29–30.

American Academy of Pediatric Dentistry. 2006b. Guideline on infant oral health care. Pediatric dentistry reference manual 2006–2007. *Pediatr Dent* 28(7):73–6.

American Academy of Pediatric Dentistry. 2007. Policy on the dental home. Pediatric dentistry reference manual 2007–2008. *Pediatr Dent* 29(7):22–3.

American Academy of Pediatrics. 2003. Oral health risk assessment timing and establishment of the dental home. *Pediatrics* 111(5, Pt 1):1113–6.

American Dental Association. 2006a. *ADA Resolution 13H-2006*. Available at http://www.ada.org/prof/resources/pubs/adanews/adanewsarticle.asp?articleid=2236 (accessed April 30, 2008).

American Dental Association. 2006b. *Evidence-Based Clinical Recommendations: Professionally Applied Topical Fluoride*. Available at http://www.ada.org/prof/resources/ebd/index.asp (accessed April 20, 2008).

Amini H, Casamassimo PS, Lin HL, and Hayes JR. 2007. Readability of the American Academy of Pediatric Dentistry patient education materials. *Pediatr Dent* 29(5):431–5.

Barlow BS, Kanellis MJ, and Slayton RL. 2002. Tooth eruption symptoms: A survey of parents and health professionals. *J Dent Child* 69(2):148–50.

Bennett IM, Robbins S, Al-Shamali N, and Haecker T. 2003. Screening for low literacy among adult caregivers of pediatric patients. *Fam Med* 35(8):585–90.

Berkman N, DeWalt D, Pignone MP, Sheridan SL, Lohr KN, Lux L, Sutton SF, Swinson T, and Bonito AJ. 2004. *Literacy and Health Outcomes*. Publication No.04-E007–2. Agency for Healthcare Research and Quality, Rockville, MD. Available at http://www.ahrq.gov/clinic/tp/littp.htm (accessed April 30, 2008).

Britt E, Hudson SM, and Blampied NM. 2004. Motivational interviewing in health settings: A review. *Patient Educ Couns* 53(2):147–55.

Bruerd B and Jones C. 1996. Preventing baby bottle tooth decay: Eight-year results. *Public Health Rep* 111:63–5.

Caufield PW. 1997. Dental caries—a transmissible and infectious disease revisited: A position paper. *Pediatr Dent* 19(8):491–8.

Caufield PW, Cutter GR, and Dasanayake AP. 1993. Initial acquisition of mutans streptococci by infants: Evidence for a discrete window of infectivity. *J Dent Res* 72(1):37–45.

Centers for Disease Control and Prevention. 2001. Recommendations for using fluoride to prevent and control dental caries in the United States. *MMWR Morb Mortal Wkly Rep* 50(RR–14):26.

Creedon MI and O'Mullane DM. 2001. Factors affecting caries levels amongst 5-year-old children in County Kerry, Ireland. *Community Dent Health* 18(2): 72–8.

DiClemente CC. 1991. Motivational interviewing and the stages of change. In: *Motivational Interviewing: Preparing People to Change Addictive Behavior*. New York: Guilford, pp 191–202.

Ebeling S. 2003. *Lessons and Tips for Addressing Health Literacy Issues in a Medical Setting*. Harvard School of Public Health: Health Literacy Website. Available at http://www.hsph.harvard.edu/healthliteracy/insights.html (accessed April 30, 2008).

Finlayson TL, Siefert K, Ismail AI, Delva J, and Sohn W. 2005. Reliability and validity of brief measures of oral health-related knowledge, fatalism, and self-efficacy in mothers of African American children. *Pediatr Dent* 27(5):422–28.

Finlayson TL, Siefert K, Ismail AI, and Sohn W. 2007. Maternal self-efficacy and 1-5-year-old children's brushing habits. *Community Dent and Oral Epidemiol* 35(4):272–81.

Gong D, Lee JY, Rozier RG, Pahel BT, Richman JA, and Vann WF. 2007. Development and testing of the test of functional health literacy in dentistry (TOFHLiD). *J Public Health Dent* 67(2):105–12.

Greene LW and Kreuter MW. 1999. *Health Promotion and Planning: An Educational and Ecological Approach*, 3rd edn. Mayfield: Mountain View.

Harrison R, Benton T, Everson-Stewart S, and Weinstein P. 2007. Effect of motivational interviewing on rates of early childhood caries: A randomized trial. *Pediatr Dent* 29(1):16–22.

Hughes TL, Dela Cruz GG, and Rozier RG. 2002. The prevention of oral diseases in early childhood. In: Gullota T and Bloom M (eds), *Encyclopedia of Primary Prevention and Health Promotion*, New York, NY: Springer Publishing Company, pp 756–67.

Ismail AI. 1998. Prevention of early childhood caries. *Community Dent and Oral Epidemiol* 26(Supp 1):49–61.

Isokangas P, Soderling E, Pienihakkinen K, and Alanen P. 2000. Occurrence of dental decay in children after maternal consumption of xylitol chewing gum, a follow-up from 0 to 5 years of age. *J Dent Res* 79:1885–9.

Jackson R. 2006. Parental health literacy and children's dental health: Implications for the future. *Pediatr Dent* 28(1):72–5.

Jeffcoat MK, Geurs NC, Reddy MS, Goldenburg RL, and Hauth JC. 2001. Current evidence regarding periodontal disease as a risk factor in preterm birth. *Ann Periodontol* 6(1):183–8.

Jeffcoat MK, Hauth JC, Geurs NC, Reddy MS, Cliver SP, Hodgkins PM, and Goldenberg RL. 2003. Periodontal disease and preterm birth: Results of a pilot intervention study. *J Periodontol* 74:1214–18.

Kanellis MJ. 2000. Caries risk assessment and prevention: Strategies for Head Start, Early Head Start, and WIC. *J Public Health Dent* 60(3):210–17, 218–20.

Kaste LM, Sreenivasan D, Koerber A, Punwani I, and Fadavi S. 2007. Pediatric oral health knowledge of African American and Hispanic of Mexican origin expectant mothers. *Pediatr Dent* 29(4):287–92.

Kay E and Locker D. 1998. A systematic review of the effectiveness of health promotion aimed at improving oral health. *Community Dent Health* 15:132–44.

Kohler B and Andreen I. 1994. Influence of caries-preventive measures in mothers on cariogenic bacteria and caries experience in their children. *Arch Oral Biol* 39(10):907–11.

Kohler B, Andreen I, and Jonsson B. 1984. Effect of caries preventive measures on *Streptococcus mutans* and lactobacilli in selected mothers. *Arch Oral Biol* 29(11):879–83.

Kohler B, Andreen I, and Jonsson B. 1988. The earlier the colonization by mutans streptococci, the higher the caries prevalence at 4 years of age. *Oral Microbiol Immunol* 3:14–17.

Kohler B and Bratthall D. 1978. Intrafamilial levels of *Streptococcus mutans* and some aspects of the bacterial transmission. *Scand J Dent Res* 86:35–42.

Kowash MB, Pinfield A, Smith J, and Curzon ME. 2000. Effectiveness on oral health of a long-term health education programme for mother with young children. *Br Dent J* 188(4):201–5.

Kowash MB, Toumba KJ, and Curzon ME. 2006. Cost-effectiveness of a long-term dental health education program for the prevention of early childhood caries. *Eur Arch Paediatr Dent* 7(3):130–35.

Lee JY, Rozier RG, Lee SD, Bender D, and Ruiz RE. 2007. Development of a word recognition instrument to test health literacy in dentistry: The REALD-30—a brief communication. *J Public Health Dent* 67(2):94–8.

Leverett DH, Adair SM, Vaughan BW, Proskin HM, and Moss ME. 1997. Randomized clinical trial of the effect of prenatal fluoride supplements in preventing dental caries. *Caries Res* 31(3):174–9.

Li Y and Caufield PW. 1995. The fidelity of initial acquisition of mutans streptococci by infants from their mothers. *J Dent Res* 74(2):681–5.

Li Y, Wang W, and Caufield PW. 2000. The fidelity of mutans streptococci transmission and caries status correlate with breast-feeding experience among Chinese families. *Caries Res* 34(2):123–32.

Litt MD, Reisine S, and Tinanoff N. 1995. Multidimensional causal model of dental caries development in low-income preschool children. *Public Health Rep* 110(5):607–17.

Locker D, Lawrence H, and Jokovic A. 1999. *Benefits and Risks for Water Fluoridation.* Report prepared for Ontario's public consultation on water fluoridation levels. Toronto: University of Toronto.

Lopez NJ, Smith PC, and Gutierrez J. 2002. Periodontal therapy may reduce the risk of preterm low birth weight in women with periodontal disease: A randomized controlled trial. *J Periodontol* 73:911–24.

Macknin ML, Piedmonte M, Jacobs J, and Skibinski C. 2000. Symptoms associated with infant teething: A prospective study. *Pediatrics* 105(4, Pt 1):747–52.

Marinho VC. 2006. Substantial caries-inhibiting effect of fluoride varnish suggested. *Evid Based Dent* 7(1):9–10.

Marinho VC, Higgins JP, Logan S, and Sheiham A. 2002. Fluoride varnishes for preventing dental caries in children and adolescents. Cochrane Database Syst Rev (3):CD002279.

Mohan A, Morse DE, O'Sullivan DM, and Tinanoff N. 1998. The relationship between bottle usage/content, age, and number of teeth with mutans streptococci colonization in 6–24-month-old children. *Community Dent Oral Epidemiol* 26(1):12–20.

Nowak AJ. 2007. Oral health policies and clinical guidelines. *Pediatr Dent* 29(2):138–9.

Nowak AJ and Casamassimo PS. 1995. Using anticipatory guidance to provide early dental intervention. *J Am Dent Assoc* 126(8):1156–63.

Nowak AJ and Casamassimo PS. 2002. The dental home: A primary care oral health concept. *J Am Dent Assoc* 133(1):93–8.

Office of Disease Prevention and Health Promotion. 2000. *Healthy People 2010*. Available at http://www.health.gov/healthypeople/Document/HTML/Volume2/21Oral.htm#_Toc489700403 (accessed December 15, 2007).

Reisine S and Litt MD. 1993. Social and psychological theories and their use for dental practice. *Int Dent J* 43(3, Suppl 1):279–87.

Richman JA, Lee JY, Rozier RG, Gong DA, Pahel BT, and Vann WF. 2007. Evaluation of a word recognition instrument to test health literacy in dentistry: The REALD-99. *J Public Health Dent* 67(2):99–104.

Rubak S, Sandbaek A, Lauritzen T, and Christensen B. 2005. Motivational interviewing: A systematic review and meta-analysis. *Br J Gen Pract* 55(513):305–12.

Schroth RJ, Brothwell DJ, and Moffatt MK. 2007. Caregiver knowledge and attitudes of preschool oral health and early childhood caries (ECC). *Int J Circumpolar Health* 66(2):153–67.

Seow KW, Cheng E, and Wan V. 2003. Effects of oral health education and toothbrushing on mutans streptococci infection in young children. *Pediatr Dent* 25(3):223–8.

Söderling E, Isokangas P, Pienihäkkinen K, and Tenovuo J. 2000. Influence of maternal xylitol consumption on acquisition of mutans streptococci by infants. *J Dent Res* 79(3):882–7.

Söderling E, Isokangas P, Pienihäkkinen K, Tenovuo J, and Alanen P. 2001. Influence of maternal xylitol consumption on mother-child transmission of mutans streptococci: 6-year follow-up. *Caries Res* 35(3):173–7.

Tinanoff N and Palmer CA. 2000. Dietary determinants of dental caries and dietary recommendations for preschool children. *J Public Health Dent* 60(3):197–206, 207–9.

University of Washington. 2007. *Access to Baby and Child Dentistry Provider Training. Oral Health for Infants and Toddlers*. ABCD Program. Available at http://www.abcd-dental.org (accessed April 30, 2008).

US Department of Health, Education, and Welfare. 1979. *Evaluatory Surveys of Long-Term Fluoridation Show Improved Dental Health*. Atlanta, GA: USPHS Publication No. 84-22647.

US Department of Health and Human Services. 2003. *A National Call to Action to Promote Oral Health*. Rockville, MD: USDHHS, PHS, CDC, NIH, NIDCR. NIH Publication No. 03-5303.

Virginia Oral Health Partnership for Children. 2004. *Bright Smiles for Babies*. Richmond, VA: Virginia Department of Public Health, Division of Dental Health.

Wake M, Hesketh K, and Lucas J. 2000. Teething and tooth eruption in infants: A cohort study. *Pediatrics* 106(6):1374–9.

Weinstein P. 2002. *Motivate Your Dental Patients: A Workbook*. Seattle, WA: University of Washington.

Weinstein P. 2006. Provider versus patient-centered approaches to health promotion with parents of young children: What works/does not work and why. *Pediatr Dent* 28(2):172–6.

Weinstein P, Harrison R, and Benton T. 2004. Motivating parents to prevent caries in their young children: One-year findings. *J Am Dent Assoc* 135(6):731–8.

Weinstein P, Harrison R, and Benton T. 2006. Motivating mothers to prevent caries: Confirming the beneficial effect of counseling. *J Am Dent Assoc* 137(6):789–93.

Weintraub JA, Ramos-Gomez F, and Jue B. 2006. Fluoride varnish efficacy in preventing early childhood caries. *J Dent Res* 85(2):172–6.

Wong D, Perez-Spiess S, and Julliard K. 2005. Attitudes of Chinese parents toward oral health of their children with caries: A qualitative study. *Pediatr Dent* 27(6):505–512.

Workgroup Report Sponsored by the National Institute of Dental and Craniofacial Research, National Institutes of Health, U.S. Public Health Service, Department of Health and Human Services. 2005. The invisible barrier: Literacy and its relationship with oral health. *J Public Health Dent* 65(3):174–82.

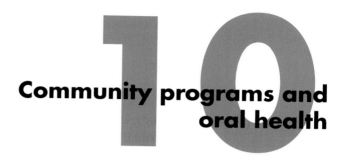

Community programs and oral health

Jessica Y. Lee

BACKGROUND AND OVERVIEW

Over the past 25 years the oral health of children in the United States has improved dramatically with the prevalence of permanent tooth caries declining precipitously. However, during this same time frame the prevalence of dental caries in primary teeth has remained the same nationally and increased among the most vulnerable children. Dental caries is now considered the most prevalent chronic childhood disease. Today, dental caries in preschool-age children is a major U.S. public health problem. This issue has come under scrutiny recently by policy makers, physicians, and researchers (Vargas et al., 1998).

The prevalence of early childhood caries and lack of access to dental care for young children was a major impetus for the Year 2000 Surgeon General's Conference, workshops and report being dedicated to children's oral health issues (US Department of Health and Human Services, 2000). In this report, the Surgeon General recommended that "partnerships be used to improve oral health of those who still suffer from oral disease." Because of the enormity of the crisis, the collective and complementary talents of community programs including public health agencies, federal programs, and social services organizations are vital in improving access to oral health care for young children. Many community programs, such as Women, Infants and Children's Supplemental Food Program (WIC) and Head Start (HS) were among those mentioned in the report that could participate in these partnerships. Community programs can improve the links between participants and the local dental community through referrals and networking (Jones et al., 2000).

The majority of studies (Cashion et al., 1999; Griffin et al., 2000) that have examined access to care or use of services focus primarily on individual characteristics such as health insurance, race, and income, but WIC, HS, and other programs like them can work on another level to improve access to dental care for young children. Andersen et al.'s (2001) revised access to care model includes more contextual factors, such as availability of providers (dentists and physicians) that play a role in access to care. The model also takes into consideration federal policies and programs. Because of the complex nature of access to dental care for young children a comprehensive model is needed. This modified Andersen model (Figure 10.1) is a conceptual framework for access to care that illustrates the manner through which community programs can act as enabling factors and translate into access to dental care. This model accounts for predisposing and enabling factors. Factors that may predispose persons toward or away from accessing oral health services include demographics (age, gender, and martial status) and social structure (education, ethnicity). Enabling characteristics refer to attributes specific to individuals such as income and insurance. Additionally, there are community-level enabling characteristics that include availability of providers and community programs.

A study conducted by Schuster et al. (1998) examined the influence of care coordinators, who visited families at home to assist with access to care, on access to well-baby checks. They tracked utilization of well-baby visits as a measure of realized access. Using a randomized design, they compared a sample of infants and children who received care coordination to those who did not. Their results indicated that care coordinators increased the number of well-baby visits by 21%. They also found that involvement in public programs (including WIC and HS) increased access to care. In many instances staff in community programs act as care coordinators. Identifying children from low-income families and those with oral health problems is important for both the overall health of the child and the cost associated with treating young children with severe dental caries. Community

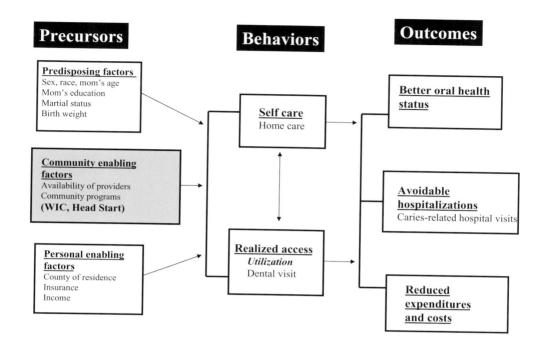

Modified from Andersen et al. (2001)

Figure 10.1   Conceptual model in the role of community programs.

program staff is well positioned to identify children at high risk for dental caries and make appropriate referrals for early management.

EARLY CHILDHOOD COMMUNITY PROGRAMS

The special supplemental food program for women, infants, and children

The WIC program is the nation's largest public health nutrition program and serves a large percentage of children and mothers with low income in the United States. In fiscal year 2004, the national WIC program served slightly less than 9 million participants (USDA, 2008). It was established by the Food and Nutrition Services of the Department of Agriculture (USDA) to target low-income women, infants, and children who are nutritionally at risk. The goal of the WIC program is to improve the health of its participants by providing nutritious foods, nutrition education, and medical and dental health referrals during pregnancy, the postpartum period, infancy, and early childhood. WIC nutritionists may be the only source of oral health and nutrition education accessible to some children (Faine and Oberg, 1995; North Carolina Food and Nutrition Services, 1999).

WIC and health outcomes

Many investigations have demonstrated associations between participation in WIC and positive health outcomes. These effects include reduced frequency of low-birth-weight deliveries (Edozien et al., 1976; Kotelchuck et al., 1984), reduced Medicaid costs for newborns (Schramm, 1985), reduced rates and costs of anemia in children (Kennedy and Gershoff, 1982), and increased nutrient intake in children (Rush et al., 1988). Often the beneficial effects of WIC participation are attributed to the direct nutrition-related benefits of the program rather than the effects of the health and welfare services coordination.

Few studies have addressed the effects of WIC on the utilization of health care services. One demonstrated that WIC participants used children's medical clinics more frequently than did nonparticipants (Kotch, 1989). Another suggested that children enrolled in WIC are more likely to have a "medical home" (Rush et al., 1988). For purposes of this study, a medical home was defined as having a regular source of care either in a private practice or in the local health department.

WIC and oral health

One approach that can prevent caries in the preschool population is an early oral health screening and referral, a model that WIC has tried to achieve. As an example, in North Carolina WIC (NC-WIC) clinics, oral health screenings are performed on a periodic basis for all enrolled children. This oral screening is one dimension of a standard physical assessment protocol used by all NC-WIC clinics to assess risk factors for children. To be recertified for WIC eligibility, children must have oral health screenings every 6 months until they are no longer eligible for WIC benefits at the age of 5.

WIC clinics rely on nurses and nutritionists to conduct the oral health screenings with a "lift the lip" examination. After the examination they make dental referrals for treatment if indicated. WIC nurses and nutritionists attend an annual training program update that includes an orientation to the recognition of healthy teeth and gums (North Carolina Food and Nutrition Services, 1999). When WIC nurses and nutritionists detect oral abnormalities, they make a dental referral. The referral can include informing the parents of the child's dental needs and providing resources to access dental care. The WIC screening manual has two oral health risk factors for infants and children. One addresses nursing or bottle caries (also referred to as early childhood caries or ECC) and inappropriate use of the bottle (B61) and the other addresses abscessed teeth (C61). The codes B61 and C61 are standard screening codes that are used by the WIC program to identify dental needs (North Carolina Food and Nutrition Services, 1999).

In addition to their referral options, WIC health care professionals have an education component that addresses oral hygiene and appropriate feeding behaviors. An Institute of Medicine (1990), evaluating the national WIC program, lists education on appropriate feeding behaviors as an area where WIC could have a significant impact.

Published, descriptive studies have examined WIC referrals for oral health care. McCunniff et al. (1998) examined dental referral rates by WIC clinics in Missouri, reporting that of the 1,850 participants seen during a 2-month period at a clinic site, 27% of children and 17% of infants were referred for services outside of the WIC clinic. Dental referrals comprised 10% of all referrals made for these infants and children. This study examined only the referral rates and not the outcomes. Sergeant et al. (1992) concluded from a survey of WIC employees in New York that dental referrals comprised the majority of all health care referrals made in an inner-city clinic. Shick et al. (2005) examined the effects of knowledge and confidence on dental referral practices among WIC nutritionists in North Carolina. They found that confidence in performing oral health risk assessments (OR = 2.12; 95% CI = 1.13, 3.96), confidence in making dental referrals (OR = 3.02; 95% CI = 1.45–6.29), and confidence in expected outcomes that parents would seek dental care when advised to do so (OR = 3.11; 95% CI = 1.62, 5.97) were associated with frequent dental referrals. The more confident WIC nutritionists feel about oral health, the more likely they are to make dental referrals. Screening and referral by WIC workers may benefit children by improving access to dental care as the WIC clinic is frequently the first point of contact with a health professional. Lee et al. (2004) examined how these dental referrals translated into realized access. They estimated the effects of WIC on dental services use by Medicaid children and found that children who participated in WIC had an increased probability of having a dental visit (OR = 1.46; 95% CI = 1.32, 1.56) compared to Medicaid-enrolled children who did not participate in WIC. Child WIC participation had a positive effect on the likelihood of using preventive and restorative services, and a negative effect on emergency services. In general, participation of children in the WIC program improved access to dental care services that should lead to improved oral health.

In summary, preschool-age children and their mothers are seen frequently in NC-WIC clinics, where nurses and nutritionists are trained to discuss oral health issues such as ECC. Moreover, NC-WIC nurses and nutritionists are required to screen for oral health abnormalities and refer as needed for dental follow-up. These screening and referrals lead to better access to dental care.

Early head start and head start

During the early 1960s the nation began to address the war on poverty and initiated preschool programs for children at socioeconomic disadvantage. Head Start is a program that focuses on assisting children from low-income families. Established in 1965, HS is the longest-running community child development program in the United States. The early goals of HS project included promoting social and behavioral competencies among children to ensure that they enter school with the same foundation as their non disadvantaged peers. It provides comprehensive education, health, and nutrition services to children and their families who are at or below the poverty level. Specifically, the services include (1) a comprehensive health services program that encompasses a broad range of medical, dental, nutrition, and mental health services; (2) preventive health services and ongoing early intervention; and (3) linkage to an ongoing health care system to ensure that these children receive comprehensive health care even after leaving the program. In 1990, Congress gave HS its largest budget increase. As of late 2005, more than 22 million preschool-age children have participated in HS. The US$ 6.8+ billion budget for 2005 provided services to more than 905,000 children, 57% of whom were 4 years old or older, and 43% were 3 years or younger (Office of Head Start, 2008).

Information about the prevalence of dental disease in HS children and the effects of this program on their oral health status suggests that by the time children from low-income families are enrolled in HS, the prevalence of dental caries is greater than the general population (Vargas et al., 1998). Studies of HS programs also suggest that access to dental care and thus use of dental services is limited, despite the federally mandated HS and Medicaid requirements for dental examinations and treatment.

Early Head Start (EHS) began in 1995 as an expansion of the longstanding HS program. It provides health and developmental services to low-income pregnant women and families with children from birth to 3 years of age. This new program has grown into a national initiative with more than 650 programs serving 70,000 children (Early Head Start, http://www.ehsnrc.org/AboutUs/ehs.htm). EHS has many performance standards that relate to oral health activities such as screening for dental disease, promoting access to dental care, and education for children and their families (Edelstein, 2000; ACF, 2006).

Hundreds of studies have been conducted on the impact of HS on physical, cognitive, and social development (Zigler et al., 1994). A systematic review by the Task Force on Community Preventive Services on the effectiveness of early childhood development programs in affecting health, however, found only one dental study that met the review criteria (Anderson et al., 2003). The Task Force concluded that insufficient evidence exists to determine the effectiveness of these programs on improving dental outcomes.

Two national studies are currently examining the impact of EHS and HS programs on child development, health status, and health services use, including dental visits. The Early Head Start Research and Evaluation project is a large-scale, random-assignment evaluation (Head Start Bureau, 2004). Reports from the Birth to Three Phase (1996–2001) of the evaluation found no effects of EHS on use of dental services. The second of these studies, the National Head Start Impact Study is a randomized controlled trial (RCT) of approximately 5,000 3- and 4-year-old children who were scheduled to be followed through 2006 (Head Start Bureau, 2005). After 1 year, use of dental services was 34–32% greater for 3- and 4-year-old children enrolled in HS, respectively, than those not enrolled. Both studies will provide important information on dental care use when they are completed. The Early Head Start Research and Evaluation project is scheduled to be completed in 2010 (http://www.acf.hhs.gov/programs/opre/ehs/ehs_resrch/ehs_overview.html) and the National Head Start Impact Study is scheduled to be completed in 2009 (http://www.acf.hhs.gov/programs/opre/hs/impact_study/).

Both HS and EHS must meet federally mandated "performance standards" that define the scope of services that programs must offer to enrolled families. The performance standards do not prescribe how these services must be carried out. Hence, each program is able to design services to meet the needs of those being served in their local communities (Office of Head Start, 2008).

The HS dental "performance standard" states that a child's oral health status must be determined by a dental professional within 90 days of entry into the program. If the children have treatment needs, they must be referred to a dentist for care. Currently, there are no EHS specific dental performance standards. Because EHS is a part of HS, they are expected to share the same performance standards.

A lack of information about EHS and its impact on the oral health of young children and their families emphasizes the need to examine all aspects of a problem about a population that has been documented to need care the most (Vargas et al., 1998). Partnerships that can increase utilization of dental services are needed as an additional means of enhancing health outcomes for these children.

Oral health care and the medicaid program

Federal mandates require the provision of dental services to Early and Periodic Screening, Diagnosis and Treatment (EPSDT) eligible Medicaid recipients. Despite the inclusion of this benefit in the Medicaid program, dental utilization among Medicaid children falls well below expectations. Several state-level studies found dental utilization rates among Medicaid recipients to range from 25 to 35% during the late 1980s (Lang and Weintraub, 1986). The dental utilization rate among North Carolina's (NC) Medicaid recipients from 1985 to 1992 was approximately 30%. Analysis of 7 years of claims data highlights the importance of race and duration of enrollment in determining the likelihood and extent of utilization of dental services among NC Medicaid recipients (Robinson, 1998). The recent national data documenting racial and socioeconomic disparities in children's dental caries come from the third National Health and Nutrition Examination Survey. Various publications have documented these disparities in the dental caries experience in terms of race, ethnicity, family income, and parental education (Vargas et al., 1998; U.S. General Accounting Office, 2000; U.S. Department of Health and Human Services, 2002). Two consistent findings from these analyses are relevant to this proposal: (1) disparities exist among racial and ethnic groups even within categories of income and; (2) gradients in disparities are more visible among preschool children than older children.

Access to private dental services can ensure availability of emergency dental treatment, preventive dental services, and restorative treatments to the vulnerable Medicaid population. Because untreated dental disease increases in severity over time and necessitates more extensive and costly treatment secondary to postponed care, adequate access to preventive and restorative dental services has great potential to decrease the overall costs associated with the Medicaid dental care benefit. The trajectory of dental disease and the high cost of treating chronically neglected dental disease highlight the need for analyses that explore Medicaid recipients' access to preventive and restorative dental services and justify the need for early referral by community-based programs. Children participating in the WIC program generally use more preventive and restorative services and less emergency services than nonparticipants (Lee et al., 2004).

Innovative medicaid dental access programs

Into the Mouth of Babes

Based on the successful pilot program, Smart Smiles initiative, North Carolina launched a statewide oral health program, training physicians to provide oral health services for children enrolled in the Medicaid program (Rozier at al., 2003). The medical intervention consisted of three primary components: (1) a risk assessment for dental disease, oral screening, and referral to a dentist; (2) application of fluoride varnish to the child's teeth; and (3) health education of the primary caregivers. All three must be done at a visit for the provider to be reimbursed. The program entitled "Into the Mouth of Babes" or IMB provided continuing medical education lectures and interactive sessions, practice guidelines for the patient interventions, case-based problems, practical strategies for implementation, a toolkit with resource materials, and follow-up training to the Medicaid providers.

In the first two years of the IMB program, 1,595 medical providers were trained. The number of providers billing for these services has steadily increased, and by the last quarter of 2002, the number of visits in which preventive dental services were provided in medical offices reached 10,875. A total of 38,056 preventive dental visits occurred in medical offices in 2002 (Rozier et al., 2003). The preliminary results from this program demonstrate that medical professionals can integrate preventive dental services into their practices. The program has increased access to preventive dental services for young Medicaid children whose access to dentists is restricted. Comprehensive assessments of this program are currently ongoing.

Access to Baby and Child Dentistry program

In 1994 a group of concerned dentists, dental educators, public health agencies, the state dental association, and State Medicaid representatives came together to address the problem of the severe lack of dental access by Washington State's high-risk preschool children. The proposed solution was the development of the Access to Baby and Child Dentistry (ABCD) program. ABCD focuses on preventive and restorative dental care for Medicaid-eligible children from birth to age 6, with emphasis on enrollment by age 1. It is based on the premise that starting dental visits early will yield positive behaviors by both parents and children, thereby helping to control the caries process and reduce the need for costly future restorative work. The first ABCD program opened for enrollment in Spokane, WA, in February 1995 as a collaborative effort between several partners in the public and private sectors. Its success has led other county dental societies and health districts in Washington to adopt the program, as well as prompted interest from other states (ABCD website, http://www.abcd-dental.org/).

The results of this program increased the number of dentists treating Medicaid-enrolled children. In the first 2 years of the program, 4,705 children were enrolled and approximately 51% visited a dentist. The ABCD program provides an avenue for dentists to treat children who otherwise would not receive care (Nagahama et al., 2002).

COMMUNITY PROGRAMS AND ACCESS TO DENTAL CARE

Research indicates that children who participated in WIC, HS, and other community programs are more likely to have had a dental visit, thus increasing their access to oral health care. Because inadequate access to dental care is common among children of families living in poverty and because ECC has become a childhood public health problem, community programs can serve as a vehicle to increase access to the oral health care system. Furthermore, children on Medicaid are a high-risk population who often need more frequent and extensive dental services than the general population. Evidence suggests that children participating in community programs may have a better connection to the health care system and this may allow their care to be more planned and less urgent. This is consistent with the fact that an important goal of these programs is to make appropriate referrals to health and social services.

Additionally, appropriate referrals may also lead to decreased costs of care. The estimated annual dental bill in the United States to restore children's dental caries exceeds US$ 2 billion, making it one if not the single most expensive uncontrolled disease of childhood. However, research documenting the total cost from this condition is limited. Cost estimates for individual children based on a review of dental records in an academic setting in 1992 ranged from US$ 170 to 2,212 per child and treatment costs increased greatly if care was provided in a hospital operating room under general anesthesia (Ramos-Gomez et al., 1996). In another study hospitalizations increased the cost as much as US$ 6,000 per patient (Weinstein, 1996).

There is no question that ECC plays a significant role in these expenditure data. Griffin et al. (2000) found the cost of dental treatment for children who had received care in a hospital operating room setting was far greater than for those who had not. These children consumed a disproportionate share of Medicaid dental resources with a reimbursement per hospitalized child that was 15 times greater than that of a nonhospitalized child (US$ 1,508 vs US$ 104). Findings demonstrate that enrollment in community programs may be effective in reducing dentally related costs for preschool children. Medicaid claims data can provide critical information about total resources spent for dental care provided to children from low-income families. To date, only the states of Iowa and Louisiana have reported on the portion of Medicaid dental reimbursements spent on young children (Griffin et al., 2000; Kanellis et al., 2000).

SUMMARY

Understanding the role of community-based programs and access to care should resonate with policy makers and providers. It is well documented that children on Medicaid have limited access to care and low utilization of dental services. There is evidence that Medicaid alone is insufficient to improve access and utilization of oral health care for high-risk preschool children. Community programs such as WIC and HS may be the first public programs to reach a population of high-risk low-income mothers and children under 5 years of age. Because of its first and early contact, these programs can serve as a vehicle for oral health anticipatory guidance and early access to dental care. For these reasons, the strategy for developing partnerships between WIC and HS/EHS (and other community-based programs) for the improvement of oral health is sound public health policy and has been shown to generate positive outcomes for preschool children enrolled in Medicaid. These partnerships should be expanded and strengthened in the future.

Inadequate access to dental care is common among children of families living in poverty. This has been documented by numerous national and state reports including the United States Office of the Inspector General (1996), the American Dental Association (http://www.ada.org), the U.S. General Accounting Office (2000), the U.S. Department of Health and Human Services (2000), and the North Carolina Institute of Medicine (1999). In the NC Institute of Medicine report on access to dental care, it was reported that less than 13% of the children ages 1–5 received any dental services. Findings indicate that participation in community programs increases this low participation. An explanation for such an increase is that the "enormity of the crisis, the collective and complementary talents of public health agencies, federal programs and social services organizations are vital in improving access to oral health care for young children" (U.S. Department of Health and Human Services, 2000). It has been documented that Medicaid alone is not enough to improve access to oral health care for young children, but when partnered with another public health program, access to oral care can be greatly improved. These programs offer a variety of food, nutrition and health education, and referral services. In 1988, WIC workers nationally were surveyed about the benefits of WIC. An overwhelming majority listed referral for health care and social services among the top benefits (Kotch, 1989). One of the goals of WIC and HS is to screen children for oral health risk criteria and then refer them into the health care system for care. Creation of partnerships to help facilitate this access can ensure timely and appropriate treatment.

Children on Medicaid are a relatively high-risk population, in need of more oral health care services than the general population (Cashion et al., 1999). During the time period of this study, children on Medicaid were in families with an income below 133% of the federal poverty level. The association of community program enrollment with higher use of services may mean that the oral health care needs of the children on Medicaid who participate in these programs are being better met. Studies have suggested that dental care is a serious unmet need among children in poverty.

In 2008, the American Academy of Pediatric Dentistry (AAPD) announced its partnership with the HS program. AAPD and HS are collaborating at the national, regional, state, and local level to develop a national network of dentists to link HS children with dental homes. A national network of pediatric dentists and general dentists will be created to provide quality dental homes for HS and EHS children; train teams of dentists and HS personnel in optimal oral health care practices; and assist HS programs in obtaining comprehensive services to meet the full range of HS children's oral health needs. This partnership will also provide parents, caregivers, and HS staff with the latest evidence-based information on how they can help prevent tooth decay and establish a foundation for a lifetime of oral health (AAPD Head Start Dental Home Initiative, http://www.aapd.org/headstart/). Partnering with community agencies like WIC and HS is one strategy to improve access to care and identify children at risk for dental caries early.

REFERENCES

Administration for Children and Families (ACF). 2006. *Oral Health-Revision.* ACF-PI-HS-06-03. Washington, DC: DHHS.

Andersen RM, Rice TH, and Kominski GF (eds). 2001. *Changing the US Health Care System,* 2nd edn. San Francisco: Jossy-Bass.

Anderson LM, Shinn C, Fullilove MT, Scrimshaw SC, Fielding JE, Normand J, Carande-Kulis VG, Task Force on Community Preventive Services. 2003. The effectiveness of early childhood development programs: A systematic review. *Ame J Prev Med* 24(3S):32–46.

Cashion SW, Vann WF, Rozier RG, Venezi RD, and McIver FT. 1999. Children's utilization of dental care in the NC Medicaid program. *Pediatr Dent* 21:1–7.

Edelstein BL. 2000. Access to dental care for Head Start enrollees. *J Public Health Dent* 60:221–9.

Edozien JC, Switzer B, and Bryan RB. 1976. *Medical Evaluation of the Special Supplemental Food Program for Women, Infants and Children.* Chapel Hill, NC: Department of Nutrition, University of North Carolina, School of Public Health.

Faine MP and Oberg D. 1995. Survey of dental nutrition knowledge of WIC nutritionists and public health dental hygienists. *J Am Diet Assoc* 95:190–94.

Griffin SO, Gooch BF, Beltran E, Sutherland JN, and Barsley R. 2000. Dental services, costs, and factors associated with hospitalization for Medicaid-eligible children, Louisiana, 1996–97. *J Public Health Dent* 60(1):21–7.

Head Start Bureau. 2004. Administration on Children, Youth and Families, U.S. Department of Health and Human Services. *Health and Disabilities Services in Early Head Start: Are Families Getting Needed Health Care Services? Office of Planning, Research, and Evaluation.* Available at http://www.acf.hhs.gov/programs/opre/ehs/ehs_resrch/index.html (accessed April 30, 2008).

Head Start Bureau. 2005. Administration on Children, Youth and Families, U.S. Department of Health and Human Services. *Head Start impact study: First year findings. Office of Planning, Research, and Evaluation.* Available at http://www.acf.hhs.gov/programs/opre/hs/impact_study/reports/first_yr_execsum/first_yr_execsum.pdf (accessed April 30, 2008).

Institute of Medicine. 1990. *An Evaluation of the WIC Program.* Washington, DC.

Jones C, Tinanoff N, Edelstein BL, Schneider DA, DeBerry-Sumner B, Kanda MB, Brocato RJ, Blum-Kemelor D, and Mitchell P. 2000. Creating partnerships for improving oral health of low-income children. *J Public Health Dent* 60:193–6.

Kanellis MJ, Damiano PC, and Momany ET. 2000. Medicaid costs associated with the hospitalization of young children for restorative dental treatment under general anesthesia. *J Public Health Dent* 60(1):28–32.

Kennedy ET and Gershoff S. 1982. The effect of WIC supplemental feeding on hemoglobin and hematocrit of prenatal patients. *J Am Diet Assoc* 80:227–30.

Kotch JB. 1989. Assessing the impact of WIC program on infants and children. In: *Final Report to the United States Department of Agriculture.* NC: Chapel Hill.

Kotelchuck M, Schwartz JB, Anderka M, and Finison KS. 1984. WIC participation and pregnancy outcomes: Massachusetts statewide evaluation project. *Am J Public Health* 74:1086–96.

Lang WP and Weintraub JA. 1986. Comparison of Medicaid and non-Medicaid dental providers. *J Public Health Dent* 46:207–11.

Lee JY, Rozier RG, Kotch JB, Norton ED, and Vann, Jr. WF. 2004. The effects of child WIC participation on use of oral health services. *Am J Public Health* 94:772–7.

McCunniff MD, Damiano PC, Kanellis MJ, and Levy SM. 1998. The impact of WIC dental screening and referral on utilization of dental services among low-income children. *Pediatr Dent* 20:(3):181–7.

Nagahama SI, Fuhriman SE, Moore CS, and Milgrom P. 2002. Evaluation of a dental society-based ABCD program in Washington state. *J Am Dent Assoc* 133(9):1251–7.

North Carolina Food and Nutrition Services. 1999. *The Supplemental Program for Women, Infants and Children Training Manual*. Raleigh, NC: North Carolina Food and Nutrition Services.

North Carolina Institute of Medicine. 1999. *Task Force Report on Dental Access*. Raleigh: North Carolina Institute of Medicine. Office of Head Start Web-site. Available at http://www.acf.hhs.gov/programs/hsb (accessed April 30, 2008).

Office of Head Start. 2008. *Head Start Program Fact Sheet*. Head Start Bureau. Available at http://www.acf.dhhs.gov/programs/hsb/research/2008.htm (accessed October 2008).

Ramos-Gomez FJ, Huang GF, Masouredis CM, and Braham RL. 1996. Preva-lence and treatment costs of infant caries in Northern California. *ASDC J Dent Child* 63(2):108–12.

Robinson V. 1998. *Dental Caries and Treatment Need in School Children Related to Medicaid Enrollment*. Unpublished doctoral dissertation. Chapel Hill, NC: University of North Carolina at Chapel Hill.

Rozier RG, Sutton BK, Bawden JW, Haupt K, Slade GD, and King RS. 2003. Prevention of early childhood caries in North Carolina medi-cal practices: Implications for research and practice. *J Dent Educ* 67(8): 876–85.

Rush D, Leighton J, Sloan NL, Alvir, JM, Horvitz, DG, Seaver WB, Garbowski GC, Johnson SS, Kulka, RA, Devore JW, Holt, M, Lynch JT, Virag TG, Wood-side MB, and Shanklin DS. 1988. The National WIC evaluation: Evaluation of the supplemental food program for women, infants and children. Study of infants and children. *Am J Clin Nutr* S2:389–92.

Schramm WF. 1985. WIC prenatal participation and its relationship to new-born Medicaid costs in Missouri: A cost benefit analysis. *Am J Public Health* 75:851–7.

Schuster MA, Wood DL, Duan N, Mazel RM, Sherbourne CD, and Halfon N. 1998. Utilization of well-child care services for African American infants in a low-income community: Results of a randomized, controlled case manage-ment/home visitation intervention. *Pediatrics* 101:999–1005.

Sergeant JD, Attar L, Meyers A, and Kocher E. 1992. Referrals of participants in an urban WIC program to health and welfare services. *Public Health Rep* 107:173–8.

Shick E, Lee JY, and Rozier RG. 2005. Determinants of dental referrals among NC WIC nutritionists. *J Public Health Dent* 65:221–7.

United States Office of the Inspector General. 1996. *Report on Children's Dental Services under Medicaid.* Report # OEI-09-93-00240. April 1996. Available at http://oig.hhs.gov/oei/reports/oei-09-93-00240.pdf (accessed October 2008).

U.S. Department of Health and Human Services. 2000. *Oral Health of America: A Report of the Surgeon General.* Rockville, MD: U.S. Department of Health and Human Services, National Institutes of Dental and Craniofacial Research, National Institutes of Health.

U.S. Department of Health and Human Services. 2002. *Healthy People 2010: Understanding and Improving Health,* 2nd edn. Washington, DC: United States Government Printing Office.

U.S. General Accounting Office. 2000. *Children's Dental Services under the Medicaid Program.* Washington, DC: United States Government Printing Office.

USDA Food, Nutrition and Consumer Services. 2008. *Nutrition Program Facts.* Available at http://www.fns.usda.gov (accessed April 30, 2008).

Vargas CM, Crall JJ, and Schneider DA. 1998. Sociodemographic distribution of pediatric caries: NHANES III, 1988–1994. *J Am Dent Assoc* 129:1229–38.

Weinstein P. 1996. Research recommendations: Pleas for enhanced research efforts to impact the epidemic of dental disease in infants. *J Public Health Dent* 56:55–60.

Zigler E, Piotrkowski CS, and Collins R. 1994. Health services in Head Start. *Annu Rev Public Health* 15:511–34.

11

The total health team: Working together to improve children's health

Wendy E. Mouradian and Russell Maier

BRINGING ORAL HEALTH INTO THE HEALTH TEAM

The primary goal of this chapter is to explore and outline how dental, medical, and other health professionals can work together effectively across their practices and in their communities to promote the oral health of children. This chapter will also provide dental professionals with a summary of some important issues related to children's overall health and development.

237

There is a growing awareness of the importance of oral health among nondental health professionals, due in part to the Surgeon General's Report on Oral Health (United States Department of Health and Human Services, 2000). This report highlighted the substantial national burden from oral diseases and the existence of oral health disparities in vulnerable populations such as children. Coincident with the release of the report, *The Face of the Child: Surgeon General's Conference on Children and Oral Health* further considered issues of relevance to pediatric oral health (National Institute of Dental and Craniofacial Research, 2000). Follow-up recommendations from the Surgeon General included supporting community collaborations and revamping health professional education to include oral health—two policies of special relevance for children's oral health (United States Department of Health and Human Services, 2007).

Within the dental profession itself, children's oral health has also been the focus of intensified efforts, including partnerships with other professionals caring for children. The American Dental Association now oversees "Give Kids a Smile Day," (American Dental Association, 2008) and supports the policy of a 1-year oral health examination for all infants. The American Academy of Pediatric Dentistry (AAPD) and the American Academy of Pediatrics (AAP) have collaborated on policy statements to assist child health professionals in identifying children at risk for oral disease by age 1 (Hale, 2003; Hale et al., 2008). The American Academy of Family Physicians (AAFP) has highlighted the physician's role in children's oral health (Douglass et al., 2004), while the Society of Teachers of Family Medicine (Stearns, 2004; Douglass et al., 2008), the American Academy of Pediatrics (American Academy of Pediatrics, 2008), and others (National Maternal and Child Oral Health Resource Center, 2006) have released training materials for medical professionals.

Now these insights and policies must be translated into effective, working systems of care at the level of community practitioners. The majority of children receive their oral health care from general dentists, making it critical that dental educators provide all dental students with the knowledge, attitudes, and skills needed to deliver this care effectively to infants and young children and their families. As the many chapters illustrate, early childhood oral health education emphasizes prevention and health promotion; the skills needed to examine infants and young children; the use of risk assessment tools and both medicinal and surgical approaches; and the capacity to work sensitively and respectfully with families of many different cultural and ethnic backgrounds.

A core competency for general dentists is also the ability to collaborate with other health professionals to support children's oral and overall health. Since most children are cared for by private dental and medical practitioners, this discussion will be oriented to the private health sector. However, the points addressed are very applicable to public health settings.

CREATING A COORDINATED APPROACH TO CHILDREN'S HEALTH

The best care for children includes a coordinated approach to health care. While they should take the leadership role for children's oral health, dental professionals also need an understanding of children's overall health and development, and the role of primary medical providers in caring for children. Conversely, medical professionals should play the principal role for systemic health issues, but they also must possess enough oral health knowledge to promote oral health as part of regular medical care and understand the role of dental professionals. Dentists and physicians must also communicate well with each other. They are the role models for other members of the health team—dental hygienists and dental assistants, nurses and nurse practitioners, physician's assistants and other medical professionals, who must also work together across professions to create seamless team care. Dental professionals in training today have the unique opportunity to make this "total health team" a reality by setting a new standard of dental–medical collaboration. Similarly medical professionals in training can also model this collaboration. Such partnerships will also ensure a steady flow of referrals between medical and dental professionals to better serve the needs of children and their families. Such an integrated approach makes sense for many reasons:

First, children at high-risk for oral health disparities will benefit from a team approach to health care. Children at higher risk for oral diseases include those from families disadvantaged by poverty, minority or ethnic status, recent immigration, educational, linguistic, or cultural factors or the existence of special health care needs. Medical–dental professional partnerships that ensure coordinated care over the long term will make it easier for families who may not understand our health care system, who may be fearful of dental visits, or may be experiencing other difficulties accessing care. Since multiple biological, sociocultural, and environmental factors contribute to children's health disparities, a team of medical, dental, social service, and other health professionals is often needed to support these families.

A team approach will also get children to dentists early when prevention opportunities are maximal. Since any entry into this health care system can lead to a dental referral, coordinated care will facilitate prevention of oral disease and health promotion as well as early identification of dental disease. The resultant reduction in the burden of oral diseases will lower overall costs, benefiting both families and society. Perhaps most importantly, such an approach will impart early the values of good oral health to children and the steps needed to maintain their own oral health.

Finally, the emerging science makes it clear that oral health is an integral part of children's overall health. Oral diseases and disorders can affect children's growth and development, while medical conditions and interventions can influence children's oral health and dental treatment options. This is true for all children, but especially for children with special health care needs (CSHCN), about 10–15% of children, who experience complex or chronic diseases, developmental disabilities, or other serious medical conditions. Dental and medical professionals need each other to understand the oral–systemic interactions for these children (see Box 11.1).

Health system issues also complicate access to care for this population. For example, some families have their financial resources depleted by health care costs. For other families, medically necessary oral health care may not be covered and require time-consuming authorizations and advocacy for needed services. Indeed, dental care is the largest unmet health care need for this group of children (Newacheck and Kim, 2005). The complexity of their care highlights the need for a coordinated team approach to their care—as recommended by an earlier Surgeon General's report (Office of Maternal and Child Health, 1987). Children with craniofacial conditions need especially close collaboration and coordination between medical and dental professionals (see Box 11.2).

To create the new health care teams, the traditional separation of dentistry from medicine and the rest of the health care system will have to be challenged. Most dental and medical education, especially at the predoctoral level, takes place separately. While there may have been an early

---

Box 11.1   Caring for children with special needs.

Children with special health care needs (CSHCN) are defined as those who "have or are at risk for chronic physical, developmental, behavioral or emotional conditions, and who also require health and related services of a type or amount beyond that required by children generally" (McPherson et al., 1998). Examples of such medical conditions include asthma, cleft lip and palate, and developmental disabilities. Factors that increase risk of disease in CSHCN include, enamel hypoplasia, use of medications that cause xerostomia or contain sugar, or prolonged bottle-feeding. Other factors can impact delivery of dental care, such as behavioral issues or positioning problems. Most CSHCN can be cared for in the community by general or pediatric dentists. Oral health care can typically proceed normally once the practitioner has a basic understanding of the medical issues. Discussing the child's medical history with the family and communicating with the child's primary care physician will make for optimal clinical care. In addition, there are excellent educational resources to orient community dentists to the care of CSHCN (Isman, 2000; Mouradian, 2001b; American Academy of Pediatric Dentistry, 2004; Maternal and Child Health Bureau, 2006; National Institute of Dental and Craniofacial Research, 2007; Nowak and Cassamassimo, 2007). A smaller portion of CSHCN needs dental care provided in hospitals or specialty centers.

Box 11.2 *Craniofacial teams: An example of medical and dental integration.*

A child born with cleft lip and palate or other craniofacial condition can experience feeding and nutritional problems, middle ear problems, hearing loss and/or speech difficulties, dentofacial and orthodontic anomalies, and psychosocial or developmental problems. The best care for such children is an interdisciplinary craniofacial team of medical, dental, and other specialists working together. One of the best examples of medical–dental collaboration that exists, craniofacial teams demonstrate the effectiveness of coordinated, interdisciplinary care. Craniofacial teams do not provide primary care, but work with community dentists, orthodontists, primary care physicians, and other providers to coordinate optimal care for these children and families. Craniofacial teams are most often located at children's hospitals, within universities, or in association with regional health department activities. Standards of care for children with cleft lip and palate and other craniofacial conditions, and for craniofacial teams, have been established and guide approaches to care for these children nationwide.

For clinical guidelines see *Cleft Lip and Palate: Critical Elements of Care*, 4th edn (Children's Hospital and Regional Medical Center in conjunction with the Washington State Department of Health, 2006).

For team standards see *The American Cleft Palate-Craniofacial Association, the Cleft and Craniofacial Teams* at http://www.acpa-cpf.org/teamcare/ccteam.htm.

An example of a craniofacial team: http://craniofacial.seattlechildrens.org/

rationale for this schema due to the technical nature of much of dental education (Formicola, 2002), the isolation of dentistry has effectively excluded oral health from the training of physicians and the formulation of public policy, and even affected the oral health research agenda to some extent. Only in the past decade or so have researchers begun to explore the full range of oral–systemic interactions, for example, or sought more effective methods for caries detection. Indeed, it is possible to draw a line from the isolation of dentistry to oral health disparities (Mouradian, 2002). If physicians do not learn about oral health, they cannot counsel families about caries in young children, screen patients for oral cancer, or anticipate the impact of medications on oral health. If dentists do not learn enough about general health and development, they will not be able to care for infants or children with special needs or recognize developmental or systemic problems that require attention. These impacts will be experienced more by patients who are disadvantaged by socioeconomic status, educational level, or for other reasons.

The division between dentistry and medicine also blurs the enormous overlap in the biomedical and social sciences shared by the two professions. Both professions appreciate the need for both medical and surgical therapies, the importance of risk assessment and health promotion, and the need for behavior change strategies that are family centered and effective. These shared training goals make the overlap between the two professions more apparent, and present opportunities for educational collaboration (Formicola et al., 2008). Medicine and dentistry, and indeed all the health professions, are adopting a more holistic, interdisciplinary approach to the skills needed to provide health care in today's changing environment. All health professionals need broad competencies including good communication skills, cultural competency, a strong sense of professionalism and ability to work in teams, critical thinking, and the ability to practice evidence-based care, enact quality improvement steps, and engage in lifelong learning, among others (Greiner and Knebel, 2003; American Dental Education Association, 2006). (For more discussion of cross-cutting competencies, see the Institute of Medicine Report, *Health Professions Education: A Bridge to Quality* at http://www.nap.edu/books/0309087236/html/ and the American Dental Education Association, *Commission on Change and Innovation in Dental Education* at http://www.adea.org/cci/CallforComments09292006.pdf.)

For most medical and dental professionals, the move from isolation to collaboration will not happen without deliberate effort. Yet such collaborations are part of effective models of community care for children. A discussion of how to implement successful community networks is included below (see section "Dentists and Physicians in Practice: Establishing Collaborative Networks.").

UNDERSTANDING CHILD DEVELOPMENT AND CHILDREN'S UNIQUE NEEDS

In order for dental professionals to evaluate and treat infants and young children, they need to understand children's unique characteristics and needs (Wehr and Jameson, 1994; Mouradian, 2001a). Child health and development are important for general (as well as pediatric) dentists because they provide the majority of oral health care for children.

Children are constantly changing. Children are in the most rapid time of change of their life cycle—tripling their body in less than 2 years, acquiring physical, verbal, and cognitive skills in rapid succession. Their early development and later school learning may not proceed optimally if impeded by disease. For example, infants and toddlers with chronic pain of dental disease may not gain weight normally (Acs et al., 1999; Sheiham, 2006). Later they may not be able to concentrate on educational tasks. School absences due to dental disease disadvantage children. Rates of absenteeism for dental problems are especially high among poor and minority children, who, arguably, have the most to benefit from school opportunities (United States General Accounting Office, 2000). These developmental changes also require that health professionals act differently with children of different developmental (not just chronological) ages. This tailoring of style to age impacts the health provider's communication style and handling of the oral examination, approaches to behavior and disease management, choice of medical and surgical therapies, and use of medications and dosing regimens. The "experience ladder" discussed in Chapter 6 is an example of a developmental approach to children's dental care. For a listing of some common developmental milestones see Table 11.1.

Children are at the beginning of the lifespan when prevention opportunities are maximal. Since they are in the beginning of their lives, children have the chance to develop good, lifelong oral health habits. During these early years children are learning many things related to oral health— whether their mouth hurts, how other children view them when they smile, whether dental visits are associated with pain, whether parents fear dental visits, and whether oral health habits are practiced in their homes. They are also learning habits of eating and nutrition that will impact their oral and overall health for years to come. Early childhood in particular is a time when modest preventive efforts can alter potential outcomes for years to come. Consider, for example, the advantages of preventing early transmission of cariogenic bacteria from a primary caregiver, or of applying fluoride varnishes to prevent caries or arrest their progression. Attention to well-balanced diets and reduced intake of refined carbohydrates could also have benefits for other health outcomes such as rates of childhood obesity and type 2 diabetes. The dental science of prevention is well developed; indeed, most dental disease is preventable—a fact underscored by the low rates of dental disease among socioeconomically "advantaged" children. Many adolescents who have benefited from advances in dental science have never experienced tooth decay.

A comprehensive approach to health promotion and disease prevention for children, including oral health, is provided through *Bright Futures.* "*Bright Futures* is a national health promotion initiative dedicated to the principle that every child deserves to be healthy and that optimal health involves a trusting relationship between the health professional, the child, the family, and the community as partners in health practice" (Bright Futures, 2008). There are guidelines for parents and providers on *What to Expect and When to Seek Help* for every age (Bright Futures, Developmental Tools for Family Providers, 2008). Bright Futures guidelines are available in specific subject areas as well including oral health, nutrition, and mental health. Components of oral health promotion relating to injury prevention, oral hygiene, prevention of malocclusion, caries, and periodontal disease are summarized in the handy oral health pocket guide, available online (Casamassimo and Holt, 2004).

Children's developmental vulnerability and the impact of early experiences make the use of minimally invasive techniques particularly attractive. When it has not been possible to prevent caries with good oral hygiene or the use of fluorides, alternative restorative technique (as highlighted in Chapter 3) may provide an acceptable alternative to traditional interventions. This technique may be utilized under the appropriate circumstances to remove infected material in an easily tolerated procedure that avoids

Table 11.1 Some common developmental milestones.

What a child can do

By the end of 7 months
- Responds to own name
- Babbles chains of consonants
- Enjoys social play (e.g., "peek-a-boo")
- Sits with, then without, support of hands
- Tracks objects with both eyes

By the end of 12 months
- Is shy or anxious with strangers
- Says "dada" and "mama"
- Uses simple gestures (shakes head for "no")
- Uses pincer grasp (thumb and index finger)
- Pulls to stand, may take a few steps

By the end of 18 months
- Follows one-step command with gesture (dbpeds)
- Imitates housework (dbpeds)
- Points to body parts (dbpeds)
- Speaks 15 or more words
- Can walk

By the end of 24 months
- Uses two- to four-word sentences
- Follows simple instructions
- Walks alone
- Points to object or picture when named
- Begins to show defiant behavior

By the end of 3 years
- Uses four- to five-word sentences
- Runs easily
- Turns book pages one at a time
- Imitates adults and playmates
- Plays make-believe with animals and toys (e.g., "feed" a teddy bear)

By the end of 4 years
- Goes upstairs and downstairs without support
- Speaks in five- to six-word sentences
- Follows three-step commands
- Dresses, undresses
- Cooperates with other children

By the end of 5 years
- Counts to 10 or more objects
- Correctly names at least four colors
- Prints some letters
- Wants to please friends
- Able to tell fantasy from reality

Table 11.1 *(Continued)*

In dental context

By the end of 7 months, many infants can
• Lie on their caretaker's lap facing him or her with legs straddled around the waist while the dentist examines teeth and mouth (knee-to-knee position: dentist and caretaker in chairs facing)

By the end of 12 months, many children can
• Open their mouth in imitation
• Allow their teeth to be brushed by caretaker
• Allow the dentist to check teeth and gums (knee-to-knee position)

By the end of 18 months, many children will
• Allow the dentist to check their teeth and gums (knee-to-knee position)
• Imitate toothbrushing
• Allow their teeth to be brushed by caretaker

By the end of 3 years, many children will
• Sit independently in a dental chair
• Allow the dentist to check their teeth and gums
• Brush their own teeth (with supervision)
• Allow their teeth to be brushed by caretaker

By the end of 4 years, many children will
• Sit independently in a dental chair
• Allow the dentist to check teeth and gums
• Allow dentist to place instruments in their mouth
• Cooperate with simple instructions, spit
• Brush their own teeth (with supervision)

By the end of 5 years, most children will
• Sit independently in a dental chair
• Allow the dentist to check teeth and gums
• Allow dentist to place instruments in their mouth
• Cooperate and follow simple instructions, spit
• Brush their own teeth (with supervision)

Adapted from *Your Baby and Young Child: Birth to Age 5*, Steven Shelov, Robert E. Hannermann, ©1991, 1993, 1998, 2004 by AAP (Bantam) except those indicated "dbpeds," from Developmental milestones, Cynthia Dedrick, Ph.D., University of South Florida, http://www.dbpeds.org/milestones.html.

pain and helps children (and parents) maintain a positive outlook toward future dental care.

Children are dependent on others. Children are dependent on adults for home health care and access to health services. They are also dependent on adults to provide caring, nurturing, and healthful environments. This seemingly obvious fact has several important implications for dental and medical professionals. First, it means that health providers must work effectively with parents to benefit children. The health professional must develop a trusting, supportive, and respectful relationship with parents in order to bring the best care to their child patients. Rapport is easily established with many families, but with families from different educational, social, or cultural backgrounds or with negative dental experiences of their own, this may be challenging. Understanding families in order to promote healthy habits for their children is an important goal. When families have many health behaviors that must be changed, special behavioral strategies—such as "motivational interviewing"—can be utilized that empower families to make step-by-step changes successfully (see Chapter 9). Alienating a family by simply reiterating its shortcomings is rarely helpful, while identifying barriers to change and positive initial steps can encourage good oral health practices. Knowing how to work with families from different backgrounds is particularly important for today's dental graduates, who will practice in a complex and changing society.

Because of shifting demographics, more of today's children are at risk for dental disease. As we become increasingly diverse, a larger number of children are from minority backgrounds—a third of the whole population and almost half of children under age 5 are from minority backgrounds (Cohn and Bahrampour, 2006; United States Census Bureau, 2006). Rates of child poverty are also high: about 40% of children grow up in low-income homes (Douglas-Hall and Chau, 2008)—defined as <200% of the federal poverty level. In 2008, the federal poverty level was $ 21,200 for a family of four (income guidelines as published in the Federal Register Vol 73, No. 15, January 23, 2008). Families need at least 200% of the federal poverty level to meet the basic necessities of children (Douglas-Hall and Chau, 2008). Despite advances in the science of caries prevention, the latest data reveal that among young children caries rates are actually increasing (Beltrán-Aguilar et al., 2005). Clearly not all children have had an opportunity to benefit from advances in dental science, and today's changing demographics may aggravate this inequity.

Children's vulnerability creates a moral imperative for health professionals to act in their best interests. All health professionals have an obligation to be proactive on behalf of children—especially those who are disadvantaged. Children are not responsible for their poor health outcomes and do not choose their social circumstances. Health professionals have an obligation to reach out whenever possible to help families provide care for their children. This may involve reminder cards, phone calls, and communication with others involved—such as medical, social, or school personnel. On the other hand, dental and other health professionals are *not* required to fulfill parents' requests for treatments that seem unreasonable, or are not in the children's best interests or may harm them. The health professional's primary legal and moral obligation is to the child, not the parent, even as the parent is intimately involved in the care of and decision making for the child (Mouradian, 1999). It is important to engage the child in the decision-making process as age and abilities permit and gain their "assent," along with "informed, parental permission" (not *consent*) (Bartholome, 1989) (see Table 11.2).

Children's health can be promoted through joint advocacy. Many dental and medical professionals join hands at the community level to support water fluoridation, ban soda machines from schools, or support other efforts that will benefit children. Others participate in community-based programs providing access to care for underserved children and families. Still others work together as advocates for important policy-level changes

Table 11.2 Making decisions for children.

Obtaining assent from a child	Guidelines for providers

1. Provide information
  • Nature of the condition in child's terms
  • Treatments/tests proposed
  • Child's understanding of above
2. Assess decisional capacity
  • Depends on developmental (not just chronological) age
	1. Apply best interest's standard
	  • Assess potential harms, benefits, and make recommendations for child's care
	
	2. Assess parental decision making
	  • Is decisional capacity adequate?
	  • Do parents consider best interests of child?
	  • Are decisions within a range of acceptable choices?
	  • Are there unusual beliefs with potential harm to child?
	  • Report abuse, neglect, or incompetence
	  • Refer for social services, or other resources for help if needed
	  • Strive for a partnership and shared decision making
	  • Seek consultation if needed for conflict resolution

3. Consider voluntariness
  • Assess for undue pressure on child
4. Obtain child's assent if possible
  • Provider solicits assent of child
  • Respects dissent when possible
  • Explains when child's wishes must be overruled
5. Obtain informed, parental permission
	3. Obtain informed, parental permission
	
	4. Obtain assent from child as age and abilities allow

Adapted from Mouradian (1999). See also AAP Committee on Bioethics (American Academy of Pediatrics, 1995) and Bartholome (Bartholome, 1989).

at county, state, or national levels. Because health disparities are multifactorial, the most effective efforts will be those that amplify dental professional efforts by creating systemic solutions to complex problems (Mouradian, 2006). Examples include the Access to Baby and Child Dentistry (ABCD) program in Washington State and the Into the Mouths of Babes (IMB) program in North Carolina (see Boxes 11.3 and 11.4) (Rozier et al., 2003). Both programs were cited as "best practices" by the American Academy of Pediatric Dentistry in 2003. Still other dental professionals are involved in the education and training of their medical colleagues in oral health issues. Many resources exist to assist dentists in sharing this information with nonoral health professionals (Stearns, 2004; National Maternal and Child Oral Health Resource Center, 2006; American Academy of Pediatrics, 2008).

While there are clear moral imperatives for child advocacy based on children's vulnerability and importance to society, access to dental care for all children is actually considered a "right" by the American Academy of Pediatric Dentistry, "All infants, children, and adolescents are entitled to oral health care that meets the treatment and ethical standards set by our specialty." This framing provides dental professional caring for children with the strongest possible mandate for advocacy and action.

Because of children's vulnerability and their importance to the future society, their health is everyone's responsibility. For this reason, child maltreatment, when it occurs, is also everyone's responsibility especially for professionals working with children. Although relatively rare, some children are seriously neglected or abused. When child abuse/neglect is suspected, health professionals are legally mandated to report these findings

---

Box 11.3   The ABCD program—an award winning model.

The ABCD program was started in 1994 as a partnership between the University of Washington School of Dentistry, the state dental association, state Medicaid agency, local health departments, and the Washington Dental Service Foundation. In the ABCD model pediatric dentists help train general dentists to provide care for young Medicaid-eligible children. In turn Medicaid provides a slightly enhanced reimbursement rate for dentists and a hotline number for billing questions. The health department assists with case management (e.g., transportation and reminder calls) to help ensure children get to their appointments. Washington Dental Service Foundation provided grant dollars to launch the ABCD program, which has now expanded from one county to more than half of the state's 35 counties. The ABCD program emphasizes prevention and the establishment of a dental home for young children, and addresses some common barriers to access to care that families may experience. The program has won awards and citations from a number of entities over the years. In a later innovation, ABCD"E" (Expanded), ABCD dentists train physicians and their staff to provide oral health risk assessment, fluoride varnishes, and health education. For more information about ABCD program, see http://www.abcd-dental.org/

Box 11.4   Into the Mouths of Babes: Taking physician prevention seriously.

In an effort to address high rates of dental disease in young children in North Carolina (NC), six key entities jointed forces to develop an innovative model of care. Primary care physicians and their office staff receive training to provide oral health risk assessment and screening examination, application of fluoride varnish, parent education, and referral for establishment of a dental home. Targeting children at age 3 and under, the package is reimbursed under a special Medicaid program that has now expanded from a pilot project to include all Medicaid providers. The six partners included the NC Academy of Family Physicians, the NC Pediatric Society, the NC Division of Medical Assistance, the NC Oral Health Section, the University of North Carolina (UNC) School of Dentistry, and the UNC School of Public Health. Initial grant funding was provided by the Centers for Disease Control, the Center for Medicare and Medicaid Services, and the Health Resources and Services Administration. Research and evaluation components were supported by the National Institute of Dental and Craniofacial Research at the National Institutes of Health. Studies have demonstrated that with IMB training (a 1.5 h American Medical Association approved Continuing Medical Education session), physicians are able to screen children with caries with a high degree of accuracy (Pierce, 2002). Physicians and staff also receive information on filing Medicaid claims, an oral health toolkit and starter supplies.
    For more information on IMB, see http://www.ncafp.com/imb/tools.html

---

to the appropriate authorities. It is important that dental professionals are able to identify the signs and symptoms of children maltreatment and understand reporting requirements (see Box 11.5).

MAKING THE MOST OF PRIMARY HEALTH CARE: COORDINATED DENTAL AND MEDICAL HOMES

In a well-working system of primary care, dental professionals provide expertise in children's oral health and access to a dental home (American Academy of Pediatric Dentistry, 2006), an ongoing source of comprehensive dental care that is continuous, coordinated, family centered, and culturally appropriate (see Chapter 7). A dental home includes provisions for appropriate afterhours and weekend care. Dental professionals can also promote children's overall health by taking a careful medical history and acting on general health or developmental issues. This is particularly important in the case of children in whom complaints must often be inferred. Through careful evaluation of oral health, medical, and family history, the dental professional may discover medical problems, missed immunizations, signs of abuse or neglect, or developmental or social issues that need to be addressed. The presence of established relationships within the medical community will facilitate the necessary communication and referrals.

Box 11.5 The dental professional's role in identifying child abuse and neglect.

The majority—65–75%—of child abuse injuries occur in the mouth, face, or head. Dental professionals are in a position to detect such findings, yet as a group have been much less likely to report suspected abuse/neglect. In 1992, concerned dentists in Missouri formed the PANDA (Prevent Abuse and Neglect through Dental Awareness) coalition to call attention to this problem. Since then most states in the United States and a number of foreign countries have emulated the Missouri model. PANDA educational programs include information on the history of family violence in our society, clinical examples of confirmed child abuse and neglect, and discussions of legal and liability issues involved in reporting child maltreatment. Federal law[a] mandates that dentists, physicians, nurses, and others working with children report suspected child abuse or neglect to the appropriate agency, usually Child Protective Services or other child welfare agencies. For more information see the following:

(1) One of the many state PANDA web sites at http://www.modental.org/forthedentist/PreventAbuse.aspx
(2) American Academy of Pediatric Dentistry Guidelines on oral and dental aspects of child abuse and neglect at http://www.aapd.org/media/Policies_Guidelines/G_Childabuse.pdf
(3) Child abuse reporting, state-by-state contact information at http://www.childwelfare.gov/pubs/reslist/rl_dsp.cfm?rs_id=5&rate_chno=11-11172
(4) Spencer DE (2004) *Child Abuse: Dentists' Recognition and Involvement* at http://www.cdafoundation.org/who_we_are/publications/cda_journal_april_2004/

[a]Child Abuse Prevention and Treatment Act (CAPTA), federal legislation covering reporting and handling of child maltreatment cases, web site: http://www.childwelfare.gov/pubs/factsheets/about.cfm (accessed November 30, 2008).

Medical professionals should provide access to the parallel medical home, an ongoing source of comprehensive, coordinated, family-centered, and culturally appropriate medical care (American Academy of Pediatrics, Ad Hoc Task Force on Definition of the Medical Home, 1992; Center for Medical Home Improvement, 2006). They should also possess enough oral health knowledge to promote children's oral health and act on emergent dental needs when necessary. Oral health promotion will be optimal when dentists and physicians have enough overlapping knowledge to reinforce important health messages for families and complement each other's areas of expertise. All dental and medical professionals caring for children need general knowledge in the following areas, although the depth of information will depend on whether the practitioner is a dental or medical provider (see Table 11.3).

Table 11.3 Important pediatric health issues for both dental and medical professionals.

- *Risk factors for oral disease*: past history of dental caries, low socioeconomic status, minority background, history of oral disease in family members or primary caregiver, presence of a special health care need (see Chapter 8)
- *Maternal oral health*: transmission of cariogenic organisms, maternal oral health practices, past dental experiences, last dental visit; regular source of medical care; pregnancy conditions that may affect fetal health or risk for premature delivery
- *Nutrition and feeding*: practices that promote oral and overall health, for example, appropriate use of bottles/sippy cups, healthy snacks, avoiding frequent or high intake of soda/juices, and cariogenic carbohydrates
- *Fluorides*: preventive role in caries process, general mechanisms of action, sources of fluoride (water, supplements, appropriate use of fluoride varnishes, etc)
- *Oral hygiene practices/habits*: cleaning gums and teeth after feedings (including breast-feeding), use of soft toothbrush and small amount of toothpaste, adequate adult supervision, management of finger sucking, other oral habits
- *Normal growth and development*: Growth grids, table of dental development, and common speech and language milestones are available at the American Academy of Pediatric Dentistry web site at http://www.aapd.org/media/policies.asp and immunization guidance is available at the American Academy of Pediatrics web site at http://www.cispimmunize.org/IZSchedule_Childhood.pdf
- *Common oral pathology and diseases and conditions with oral manifestations*: for example, oral candidiasis, Coxsackie B (hand-foot-and-mouth disease), herpes type 2, HIV, and other sexually transmitted diseases, craniofacial/other congenital conditions affecting oral cavity, other major medical conditions. For photos see these atlases at http://www.uiowa.edu/~oprm/AtlasWIN/AtlasFrame.html
- *Common systemic conditions that can impact delivery of oral health care*: for example, bleeding diatheses, immune conditions, cardiac conditions, developmental disabilities, and major medical conditions (Nowak and Casamassimo, 2007)
- *Medications and therapies that impact oral health*: for example, medications that cause xerostomia or mucositis, special dietary or feeding regimens, radiotherapy (Nowak and Casamassimo, 2007; The ADA/PDR guide to dental therapeutics, 4th edn. *Drugs Used in Medicine*: Chapters 14–18. Chicago: American Dental Association, 2008)
- *Common oral injuries and emergencies*: recognition and emergent management
- *Family history*: major health conditions, dental problems, teenage mother
- *Social history*: recent immigration/move, family makeup, caregivers, day care

Table 11.4 Community resources for children and families.

- *Medicaid—State Children's Health Insurance Program (SCHIP)*: jointly financed by state and federal agencies, SCHIP provides health and dental coverage for children in low-income families up to age 19. For more information see http://www.cms.hhs.gov/home/schip.asp or state Medicaid agency.
- *Women, Infants and Children's program (WIC)*: provides nutritional support services for pregnant women, mothers, and young infants. For more information see http://www.fns.usda.gov/wic/Contacts/tollfreenumbers.htm or listings by state http://www.fns.usda.gov/wic/Contacts/statealpha.HTM
- *Head Start/Early Head Start (HS/EHS)*: promotes school readiness by enhancing the children's social and cognitive development through educational, health, nutritional, social, and other services. For more information see http://www.acf.hhs.gov/programs/ohs/about/index.html# mission; to locate a center see http://www.eclkc.ohs.acf.hhs.gov/hslc/ HeadStartOffices
- *Child-Find*: a component of Individuals with Disabilities Education Act (IDEA) that requires states to identify, locate, and evaluate all children with developmental disabilities, aged birth to 21, who are in need of early intervention or special education services. For more information see http://www.childfindidea.org/overview.htm or specific state programs.
- *Special Education programs*: available through the public school system typically provide services by age 3 as mandated by IDEA http://www.idea.ed.gov/
- *Community health centers*: often provide medical, dental, mental health, and other social services and prescriptions, all with sliding scales. To locate federally funded community health centers by county/state see http://www.ask.hrsa.gov/pc/

Both medical and dental professionals should also know about resources in their community available to promote the healthy development of families. There are many resources for children, and if they are not getting services, it is often because families have not had assistance in determining which services they qualify for and how to access them (see Table 11.4).

AGE AND FREQUENCY OF DENTAL VISITS: ASSESSING RISK AND PRIORITIZING REFERRALS

The recommended age for the first dental visit or oral health assessment is at or before age 1, with follow-up dependent on the results of the assessment (American Academy of Pediatric Dentistry, Clinical Affairs Committee, 2004). Since the first teeth are erupting by 4–6 months, colonization with cariogenic bacteria, in the presence of fermentable carbohydrates, can result in early oral disease. Although every child can benefit from the oral health care provided by a dental home, there will be communities, often in rural or other underserved areas, in which shortage of dentists precludes this arrangement. Under such circumstances it is critical that dental resources prioritize high-risk children—those with identified dental disease or at high risk for developing it (Jones and Tomar, 2005). It is also important that other available health professionals promote oral health effectively. Regular medical visits begin at birth, with frequent preventive visits in the first 2 years of life, usually 10 or more (American Academy of Pediatrics, Committee on Practice and Ambulatory Medicine, 2008), providing medical professionals with the opportunity to prevent disease or identify it early when treatments are simpler and fewer teeth are affected. In rural or underserved communities, children's oral health can also be promoted by other community-based programs, for example, Head Start/Early Head Start or school oral health screening or sealant programs. Water fluoridation, when available, can help decrease baseline caries rates. However, due to the multifactorial nature of caries, children can still experience high rates of disease in communities with water fluoridation.

TRAINING FOR COLLABORATION: DENTAL AND MEDICAL STUDENT PROGRAMS

While some dentists and physicians communicate regularly and coordinate care, such collaboration is not as common as it needs to be. To promote greater cooperation, dentists and physicians must begin to change the way they think about each other: from parallel professions each addressing a portion of overall health, to colleagues whose areas of health concern and interventions are interrelated.

The best way to facilitate medical–dental collaboration is to begin early by bringing medical and dental trainees together whenever possible and emphasizing areas of overlap. This could occur during dental and medical school through required courses or electives, or in shared community-based experiences in underserved communities. Many medical and dental schools have common basic science course requirements (e.g., gross anatomy, histology, microbiology), where joint learning and collaboration could be encouraged. Both dental and medical students need curricula that include important oral health topics within basic and clinical courses. An ideal approach is a spiral curriculum in which the desired content is presented to students across the years to reinforce important concepts (Stearns, 2004; Mouradian et al., 2005). It would also be possible to create overlapping courses in patient history taking and examination, communication skills, professionalism and ethics, cultural competency, evidence-based care, and public health, for example. Clinical rotations could include experiences in medicine for dental students/residents and in pediatric dentistry or family dentistry for medical students/residents.

Regardless of the setting, collaboration can be encouraged through faculty role modeling and by using students or residents in a mentoring role across their respective disciplines. For example, at the University of Washington, third- and fourth-year dental students provide oral examinations and talk to parents in the pediatric clinic, along with medical students and pediatric medical residents. In the University of Washington oral health elective for medical students, dental students and pediatric dentistry residents have acted as mentors for medical students learning the oral health examination and how to apply fluoride varnishes (Mouradian et al., 2006). The topic of overlapping curricula for dental and medical students has recently been the subject of a national panel report organized by the American Dental Education Association and American Association of Medical Colleges. This report provides learning objectives and resources for dental and medical schools seeking to make such changes (Formicola et al., 2008).

Student-led efforts can have a unique impact at the national level as well. Recently the American Medical Student Association launched its Achieving Diversity in Dentistry and Medicine project funded by the Health Services and Resource Administration, sponsoring annual week-long joint leadership conferences for medical and dental students on critical emerging issues, developing curricula in cultural competency to be piloted at medical and dental schools, and hosting other activities (American Medical Student Association, 2008).

DENTISTS AND PHYSICIANS IN PRACTICE: ESTABLISHING COLLABORATIVE NETWORKS

Even without early joint training experiences, dentists and physicians can still establish close collaborative networks at the community level. There are many ways to do this—calling on nearby medical colleagues when new to a community, joining the hospital medical staff (necessary for dentists providing comprehensive oral health care for children anyway), presenting at grand rounds on oral diseases, and calling the local dental or medical society for referrals. Calling or sending letters or reports on children who have been referred by a medical provider or when there is an important health concern is an especially valuable approach. Many physicians are unaccustomed to receiving follow-up from their patients' dentists, so this contact can be an especially effective way to build a relationship. Often the only dentist the medical provider knows is his/her own personal dentist. Dentists and physicians should get in the habit of expecting feedback from each other in the same way they typically expect calls or letters from specialists in their respective disciplines. Not only will this serve to establish a network for referrals in both directions, it will often provide additional oral health information for the medical office, reinforcing important health messages or calling attention to risk factors that may require monitoring as part of regular medical care. Dental professionals can also develop relationships by joining in community advocacy efforts for children, or by inviting physicians to support oral health policies. It will also be important for dentists and physicians to set a collaborative tone with their office staffs—who will be the ones fielding telephone, referral requests, etc.

Referrals between health professionals can be fraught with difficulty when there is misunderstanding or lack of clarity in roles. More integrated training during medical and dental school will help to decrease barriers between dentists and physicians. Although some national organizations see "turf" issues with shared care, at a local level medical and dental providers see the community they are serving. In most instances the community is better served by collaborative relationships. Medical providers are not interested in providing dental care, but they are committed to preventing disease and helping their patients access needed dental care. Conversely, dental professionals are not interested in providing medical care, but are interested in promoting overall health and seeing high-risk children early before rampant caries develop. By developing some overlapping expertise, both professions can promote children's health by timely identification of health issues that need attention. In fact, health professionals with more knowledge in a particular area are usually more, not less, likely to refer, because of their heightened awareness of the health implications.

Expected norms for referral usually include noting the reason for the consultation, including the question to be answered or the problem to be addressed, along with an appropriate abbreviated history (see Table 11.5). Most physicians desire direct verbal or written feedback from the specialist providing the consultation, and probably most dentists do as well. A personal phone call will often accelerate referral to a dental or medical office with a waiting list. Frequent communication is especially important when dealing with CSHCN, who often have complex health issues. Failure to do so may result in less optimal health outcomes for these children.

One barrier to effective collaboration is the resistance of some dentists to accept patients on Medicaid for both financial and nonfinancial reasons

Table 11.5 Ten commandments for an effective consultation.

1. The consultant should determine the question that is being asked
2. Establish the urgency of the consultation
3. Gather primary data
4. Communicate as briefly as appropriate
5. Make specific recommendations
6. Provide contingency plans
7. Understand his or her own role in the process
8. Offer educational information
9. Communicate recommendations directly to the requesting physician (dentist)
10. Provide appropriate follow-up

Adapted from Goldman et al. (1983). See also Salerno et al. (2007).

(Milgrom and Riedy, 1988). In the case of children, Medicaid services are typically better funded than adult services, making participation in Medicaid feasible for most dentists. In fact, pediatric dentists as a group and general dentists in underserved areas all have a higher than average rates of participation in Medicaid. Many feel a moral obligation, or just compassion for children needing care, and thus include disadvantaged children in their practice. Primary care physicians also share these values, which can help reinforce referral networks built on commitment to the needs of all children in a community. The ABCD(E) partnerships and the IMB model in North Carolina provide strong evidence for how effective collaboration can change policies, rates of access to care, and ultimately oral health outcomes for children (Boxes 11.3 and 11.4).

Not everyone who reaches out across the medical–dental divide will initially meet with success. Some old habits are hard to change, but it is clear that today's graduates in dentistry and in medicine have more awareness of each other's areas than previously. New educational curricula, changing policies in professional organizations, board examinations, and other credential standards are also moving this agenda forward. While business as usual may seem easier, it is clearly not better for children's health outcomes, and it may not really mean better business. Improved communication and collaboration between dental and medical practices will be better for business, better for patients, and better for overall satisfaction with the health care professionals provide.

SUMMARY

Infants and children are among our most vulnerable patients, and of special importance to our collective future. Today's children are increasingly diverse, often from low-income families, and experiencing rising rates of caries. To care for these children effectively requires an understanding of their overall health and development, the health conditions that uniquely affect them, and the sociocultural factors that contribute to their health behaviors and health outcomes. Determining the best approaches to care requires working collaboratively with their families and other professionals in their lives to understand their needs and preferences, as well as applying current dental and medical science and treatment modalities.

High-risk children need dual management—that is, dental and medical homes that coordinate care effectively. Providing optimal care for children will require overcoming the historic distance between dentistry and medicine. Rather than worrying about contested areas ("scope-of-practice" battles), dentists and physicians need to focus on the best interests of the child, family, and community. When dentists and physicians of the future collaborate to improve children's oral and overall health, patient's health will improve, family's satisfaction increase, and referral networks grow (see Table 11.6).

Table 11.6 Dental professionals of the future.

- Understand overall health issues and importance of sociocultural factors
- Care for a diverse population
- Understand public and private systems of care
- Use medicinal *and* surgical approaches to disease
- Engage in lifelong learning as knowledgeable consumers of science and technology
- Participate in community health efforts as the oral health expert
- Are part of the health team ensuring oral health is part of overall health
- Communicate and share responsibility with medical providers

Many policy changes are underway that indicate that the trend toward greater integration of medicine and dentistry will continue. The American Academy of Pediatrics recently placed oral health among its top five priorities in 2006, and in October, 2008, highlighted oral health as a centerpiece at its national meeting; the AAP is also leading an effort to update the Surgeon General's Report on Oral Health in the area of children's oral health. The American Academy of Pediatrics and American Academy of Family Physicians have incorporated oral health into their board examinations and residency requirements, respectively. Nationally, curricula on medical–dental approaches to oral health care have been developed and implemented. The stage is set for the recognition of the importance of oral health and its inclusion in overall health considerations. The future of oral health for children has the potential to be much better. That is certainly worth smiling about.

REFERENCES

Acs G, Shulman R, Ng MW, and Chussid S. 1999. The effect of dental rehabilitation on the body weight of children with early childhood caries. *Pediatr Dent* 21:109–13.

American Academy of Pediatric Dentistry. 2004. *Policy and Guidelines: Guidelines on Management of Persons with Special Health Care Needs*. Available at http://www.aapd.org/media/Policies_Guidelines/G_SHCN.pdf (accessed November 30, 2008).

American Academy of Pediatric Dentistry. 2006. *Definition of Dental Home*. Available at http://www.aapd.org/media/Policies_Guidelines/D_DentalHome.pdf (accessed November 30, 2008).

American Academy of Pediatric Dentistry, Clinical Affairs Committee—Infant Oral Health Subcommittee. 2004. *Guideline on Infant Oral Health Care*. Available at http://www.aapd.org/media/Policies_Guidelines/G_InfantOralHealthCare.pdf (accessed November 30, 2008).

American Academy of Pediatrics. 1995. Committee on bioethics. Informed consent, parental permission, and assent in pediatric practice. *Pediatrics* 95(2):314–7.

American Academy of Pediatrics. 2008. *Oral Health Risk Assessment Training for Pediatricians and Other Child Health Professionals.* Available at http://www. aap.org/commpeds/dochs/oralhealth/screening.cfm (accessed November 30, 2008).

American Academy of Pediatrics, Ad Hoc Task Force on Definition of the Medical Home. 1992. The medical home. *Pediatrics* 20:744.

American Academy of Pediatrics, Committee on Practice and Ambulatory Medicine. 2008. *Recommendations for Preventive Pediatric Health Care (RE9535).* Available at http://www.aappolicy.aappublications.org/cgi/reprint/pediatrics;105/3/645.pdf (accessed November 30, 2008).

American Dental Association. 2008. *Give Kids a Smile Day.* Available at http://www.ada.org/prof/events/featured/gkas/index.asp (accessed November 30, 2008).

American Dental Education Association. 2006. *Commission on Change and Innovation in Dental Education, Competencies for the New General Dentist.* Available at http://www.adea.org/about_adea/governance/Pages/CompetencesfortheNewGeneralDentist.aspx (accessed November 30, 2008).

American Medical Student Association. 2008. *Achieving Diversity in Dentistry and Medicine (ADDM).* Available at http://www.amsa.org/addm/index.cfm (accessed November 30, 2008).

Bartholome WG. 1989. A new understanding of consent in pediatric practice: Consent, parental permission, and child assent. *Pediatr Ann* 18(4): 262–5.

Beltrán-Aguilar ED, Barker LK, Canto MT, Dye BA, Gooch BF, Griffin SO, Hyman J, Jaramillo F, Kingman A, Nowjack-Raymer R, Selwitz RH, and Wu T. 2005. Surveillance for dental caries, dental sealants, tooth retention, edentulism, and enamel fluorosis—United States, 1988–1994 and 1999—2002. *MMWR Surveill Summ* 54(03):1–44.

Bright Futures. 2008. *Bright Futures at Georgetown University.* Available at http://www.brightfutures.org/ (accessed November 30, 2008).

Bright Futures, Developmental Tools for Families and Providers. 2008. *Bright Futures What to Expect and When to Seek Help.* Available at http://www.brightfutures.org/tools/index.html# tools (accessed November 30, 2008).

Casamassimo P and Holt K (eds). 2004. *Bright Futures in Practice: Oral Health—Pocket Guide.* Washington, DC: National Maternal and Child Oral Health Resource Center.

Center for Medical Home Improvement. 2006. *Medical Home Measurements.* Available at http://www.medicalhomeimprovement.org/outcomes.htm (accessed November 30, 2008).

Cohn DV and Bahrampour T. 2006. *Of U.S. Children Under 5, Nearly Half Are Minorities.* Available at http://www.washingtonpost.com/wp-dyn/content/article/2006/05/09/AR2006050901841.html (accessed November 30, 2008).

Douglas-Hall A and Chau M. 2008. *Basic Facts about Low-Income Children: Birth to Age 18.* Columbia University, National Center for Childhood Poverty. Available at http://www.nccp.org/publications/pub_762.html (accessed November 30, 2008).

Douglass A, Gonsalves W, Maier R, Silk H, Tysinger JW, and Wrightson AS. 2008. *Smiles for Life: A National Oral Health Curriculum for Family Medicine.* Available at http://www.stfm.org/oralhealth (accessed November 30, 2008).

Douglass JM, Douglass AB, and Silk HJ. 2004. A practical guide to infant oral health. *Am Fam Physician* 70(11)2113–20. Available at http://www.aafp.org/afp/20041201/2113.html (accessed November 30, 2008).

Formicola A. 2002. Dentistry and medicine, then and now. *J Am Coll Dent* 69(2):30–34.

Formicola A, Valachovic RW, Chmar JE, Mouradian W, Bertolami CN, Tedesco L, Aschenbrener C, Crandall SJ, Epstein RM, da Fonseca M, Haden NK, Ruffin A, Sciubba JJ, Silverton S, and Strauss R. 2008. Curriculum and clinical training in oral health for physicians and dentists: Report of Panel 2 of the Macy Study. *J Dent Educ* 72(2 Suppl):73–85.

Goldman L, Lee T, and Rudd P. 1983. Ten commandments for effective consultations. *Arch Intern Med* 143:1753–5.

Greiner AN and Knebel E (eds). 2003. *Health Professions Education: A Bridge to Quality.* Washington, DC: Institute of Medicine of the National Academies of Science, National Academies Press.

Hale K. 2003. Oral health risk assessment timing and the establishment of a dental home. *Pediatrics* 111(5):1113–15.

Hale K, Keels MA, Thomas HF, Davis MJ, Czerepak CS, and Weiss PA. 2008. Preventive oral health intervention for pediatricians. *Pediatrics* 122:1387–94. Available at http://pediatrics.aappublications.org/cgi/content/abstract/peds.2008-2577v1 (accessed November 30, 2008).

Isman B, Newton R, Bujold C, and Baer MT. 2000. *Planning Guide for Dental Professionals Serving Children with Special Needs.* University of Southern California Affiliated Program. Los Angeles, CA: Children's Hospital. Available at http://www.mchoralhealth.org/PDFs/OHguide.pdf (accessed November 30, 2008).

Jones K and Tomar SL. 2005. Estimated impact of competing policy recommendations for age of first dental visit. *Pediatrics* 115:906–14.

Maternal and Child Health Bureau. 2006. *Special Care: An Oral Health Professional's Guide to Serving Young Children with Special Health Care Needs.* Available at http://www.mchoralhealth.org/Special/mod1_0.htm (accessed November 30, 2008).

McPherson MH, Arango P, Fox H, Lauver C, McManus M, Newacheck PW, Perrin JM, Shonkoff JP, and Strickland B. 1998. A new definition of children with special health care needs. *Pediatrics* 102:137–40.

Milgrom P and Riedy C. 1988. Survey of Medicaid dental services in Washington State: Preparation for a marketing program. *J Am Dent Assoc* 129:753–63.

Mouradian W. 1999. Making decisions for children. *Angle Orthod* 69(4):300–305.

Mouradian W. 2001a. The face of a child: Children's oral health and dental education. *J Dent Educ* 65(9):821–31.

Mouradian W (ed.). 2001b. *Promoting Oral Health of Children with Neurodevelopmental Disabilities and Other Health Care Needs.* Conference Proceedings. Children's Hospital: Seattle, May 4–5. Available at http://www.mchoralhealth.org/PDFs/LEND2001.pdf (accessed November 30, 2008).

Mouradian W. 2002. Commentary on M Michael Cohen: Disparities, diversity and dental education. *J Dent Educ* 66(3):374–9.

Mouradian W. 2006. Band aid solutions to the dental access crisis: Conceptually flawed—a response to Dr. David Smith. *J Dent Educ* 70(11):1174–9.

Mouradian W, Reeves A, Kim S, Evans R, Schaad D, Marshall S, and Slayton R. 2005. An oral health curriculum for medical students at the University of Washington. *Acad Med* 80(5):434–42.

Mouradian W, Reeves A, Kim S, Lewis C, Keerbs A, Slayton R, Gupta D, Oskouian R, Schaad, D, Kalet T, and Marshall S. 2006. A New oral health elective for medical students at the University of Washington. *Teach Learn Med* 18:336–47.

National Institute of Dental and Craniofacial Research. 2000. *Surgeon General's Conference on Children and Oral Health,* June 12–13, 2000, Washington, DC. Available at http://www.nidcr.nih.gov/DataStatistics/SurgeonGeneral/Conference/ConferenceChildrenOralHealth/ (accessed November 30, 2008).

National Institute of Dental and Craniofacial Research. 2007. *Oral Conditions in Children with Special Needs: A Guide for Healthcare Providers.* Available at http://www.nidcr.nih.gov/HealthInformation/DiseasesAndConditions/ChildrensOralHealth/SpecialNeeds.htm (accessed November 30, 2008).

National Maternal and Child Oral Health Resource Center. 2006. *A Health Professional's Guide to Pediatric Oral Health Management.* Available at http://www.mchoralhealth.org/PediatricOH/index.htm (accessed November 30, 2008).

Newacheck PW and Kim SE. 2005. A national profile of health care utilization and expenditure for children with special health care needs. *Arch Pediatr Adolesc Med* 159:10–17.

Nowak AJ and Cassamassimo P (eds). 2007. *The Handbook: Pediatric Dentistry,* 3rd edn. Chicago: American Academy of Pediatric Dentistry.

Office of Maternal and Child Health, U.S. Dept of Health and Human Services. 1987. *Surgeon General's Report: Children with Special Health Care Needs.* Rockville, MD.

Pierce KM. 2002. Accuracy of pediatric primary care providers' screening and referral for early childhood caries. *Pediatrics* 109(5):E82.

Rozier RG, Sutton BK, Bawden JW, Haupt K, Slade GD, and King RS. 2003. Prevention of early childhood caries in North Carolina medical practices: Implications for research and practice. *J Dent Educ* 67:876–85.

Salerno SM, Hurst FP, Halvorson S, and Mercado DL. 2007. Principles of effective consultation: An update for the 21st-century consultant. *Arch Intern Med* 167:271–5.

Sheiham A. 2006. Dental caries affects body growth, weight and quality of life in pre-school children. *Br Dent J* 201(10):625–6.

Stearns J. 2004. *Society of Teachers of Family Medicine, Curriculum Resources, Special Topics: Oral Heath.* Available at http://www.fammed.musc.edu/fmc/data/pdf/Oral_Health.pdf (accessed November 30, 2008).

United States Department of Health and Human Services. 2007. *National Call to Action to Promote Oral Health.* Available at http://www.surgeongeneral.gov/topics/oralhealth/nationalcalltoaction.htm (accessed November 30, 2008).

United States Department of Health and Human Services, National Institute of Dental and Craniofacial Research, National Institutes of Health. 2000. *Oral Health in America: A Report of the Surgeon General-Executive Summary.* Rockville, MD. Available at http://www.nidcr.nih.gov/DataStatistics/SurgeonGeneral/sgr/ (accessed November 30, 2008).

United States General Accounting Office. 2000. *Oral Health: Dental Disease Is a Chronic Problem among Low-Income Populations.* Washington, DC: GAO/HEHS-00-72.

US Census Bureau. 2006. *Nation's Population One-Third Minority.* Available at http://www.census.gov/Press-Release/www/releases/archives/population/006808.html (accessed November 30, 2008).

Wehr E and Jameson EJ. 1994. Beyond health benefits: The importance of a pediatric standard in private insurance contracts to ensuring health care access for children. *Future Child* 4:115–33.

12

Building an infant- and toddler-friendly practice

David K. Curtis

Building an infant- and toddler-friendly practice can be a rewarding and profitable endeavor for both generalists and specialists. This chapter covers the fundamentals of incorporating infants and toddlers into the busy practice without undue additional requirements or challenges.

The rationale for incorporating babies into the dental practice begins with an understanding of the gradual but dramatic change in the public's perceptions and expectations, why these changes are occurring, and why practice patterns have shifted and will continue to shift as a result. From a historical perspective, we are in a different cultural place now with respect to infant oral health compared to two decades ago. In Chapter 6, Casamassimo and Nowak discuss the implementation of anticipatory guidance as a rational approach to clinical decision making. However, until recent years the prospect of identifying environmental, cultural, behavioral, and perhaps even genetic factors that would put some children at risk for oral disease has been more of an academic discussion than a driver of clinical practice.

As recently as 1990, the age 1 dental visit was nothing more than a conceptual ideal shared by a relatively small group of visionaries. The young parent of 1990 would have considered age 4 or 5 to be appropriate for the first dental visit. Most pediatricians would have shared this view, and the typical dentist would have considered an appropriate entry age to be whenever a child could cooperate for a set of bitewings and a rubber cup prophylaxis. This mindset was fortified by the prevailing view in the 1970s and the early 1980s that dental caries would continue to decline and would not be a significant health issue for children in the next century. During those years, oral health was not considered essential to a child's overall well-being, and dental caries was not considered to be a major health issue for children.

As amazing as it may seem, the problem of dental caries did not go away. The myths that the caries vaccine was just a matter of time and that caries was about to be eradicated were pure fallacy. To the contrary, caries exploded to assume epidemic proportions. Equally remarkable, a general awareness of the early childhood caries problem was not widely known until the Surgeon General's report *Oral Health in America* was published in 2000.

During that same 20-year period a major educational campaign was waged by the American Academy of Pediatric Dentistry to mitigate the cultural paradigm that rampant tooth decay could simply be a normal part of childhood. This campaign was directed toward the entire medical/dental community, the public health community, and most importantly to the general public. The results of these efforts are the growing acceptance of the validity and efficacy of the age 1 examination, and the adoption of early intervention policies by the American Dental Association, the American Academy of Pediatrics, and the American Academy of Public Health Dentistry. The resultant new paradigm has as its centerpiece the recognition of dental caries as an infectious transmissible disease and the necessity to shift both preventative and treatment strategies toward a medical approach. The principles of the medical approach to caries management are simply to reorient management from treatment of cavities (end stage) to management of caries (infection)—that is to treat the cause rather than just the manifestation of the disease.

Under the old model, caries was considered inevitable, with surgical intervention of the effects of disease the standard of care. The new model supports early examination, risk assessment, anticipatory guidance, and appropriate intervention. Under the new paradigm the first dental visit at age 3 can no longer be supported as the standard of care.

It is remarkable to note the increased parental awareness with regard to the importance of their children's oral health as well as noticeable changes in their attitudes and expectations of the dental community. In the 1970s and 1980s the only babies in dental practices were the ones who presented with catastrophic oral disease. Even then the child would often not be presented to the dentist until the condition of the child began to affect other family members (i.e., loss of sleep). Until the 1990s the idea of babies visiting the dentist as a normal part of well-baby care seemed unusual if not strange to most parents. Many of today's parents, however, understand the importance of their children's oral health and seek out dentists who are willing to see babies and are skilled at treating them. This phenomenon is largely attributable to the health media. Most baby/parent publications give considerable attention to oral health as it relates to hygiene practices and nutrition, etc. Visiting the dentist is also frequently discussed in such articles.

Children's oral health is also a frequent subject on early morning news shows both locally and in the national markets.

We have observed a gradual but dramatic swing from a time when the public was being sold on the importance of baby teeth to the present day when large segments of American society place great value in oral health. In fact, it is not unusual in some communities for the demand to outstrip the supply—that is health-conscious parents having difficulty finding a dentist willing to see their babies.

It is clear that for some communities, barriers remain in place that impede parental understanding of the importance of good oral health and thus the importance of early visits. Much effort will continue to be required to bridge the gap for those communities. However, for many families very little marketing is required for them to enroll their babies in a dental home. For many families it is "build it and they will come."

It is important to recognize that dentists who regularly see preschoolers and school-age children in their practices have an entire market of babies sitting in their reception rooms. Mothers who have their babies with them during their own or other family members' dental visits present the perfect opportunity to broach the topic of infant oral health and to establish the dental home for these babies. Mothers are usually very receptive to early enrollment and are invariably impressed with the practitioner who is comfortable and skilled at physically handling their infants or toddlers. These occasions present opportune moments to establish a bond between the practitioner and the family (usually the mother) or to deepen an existing relationship. Families who enroll their babies are also likely to keep their older children in the practice longer than they might otherwise. Establishing such a strong bond with the family is the underpinning for the concept of enrollment.

The idea of enrollment implies that it is not just about having parents make an appointment for their child at a certain age. It affords us the opportunity to build the kind of relationship necessary for us to be effective, trusted advisors because we must have families enroll their children in our practices with the same emotional commitment that they would enroll them in a particular day care, preschool, Sunday school class, etc. It is important to understand that a single encounter with the families is not enough to change the way they think about teeth and health. A single encounter will not cause a change in behavior. In fact, research has demonstrated that no amount of information will lead a family to change behavior such as oral hygiene and dietary practices, until the families (primarily the mother) come to the realization that their own actions are at odds with their desired outcomes. This critical level of self-efficacy can only be achieved through motivational interviewing, whereby the parents are led through a series of discussions that result in the parents reaching their own conclusions regarding home practices (ADA Council on Scientific Affairs, 2006). Having the opportunity to establish a trusted relationship with the families over an extended period of time increases the likelihood of helping them to reach milestones of self-efficacy with measurable positive outcomes for their children. This is the basis for dental home.

THE INITIAL CONTACT

In order for families to enjoy the benefits of a positive dental experience, it is incumbent for the practice to create an internal culture that is focused on managing the experience and is capable of doing so. This is especially true for families enrolling their babies and it begins with the initial contact.

The initial phone call for an infant appointment is usually initiated by the mother, and there is always a compelling reason that leads the mother to do so. Perhaps her pediatrician has advised her that her baby is at high risk for oral disease and she is encouraged to see the dentist. In other instances it may be an allied community health professional, such as a school nurse, who prompts the mother to initiate the first visit. Some families will start their babies earlier than older siblings were started based on the dental history of those older siblings, and for others it is simply a deliberate effort based on their level of understanding and health awareness.

Regardless of what constellation of events leads a mother to initiate contact, it is imperative for the staff member to understand that each mother comes to that point from a unique perspective based on the total context of her experience and present situation. Often, parents will not know what to expect on the first visit, and their expectations will be based on their own experiences. The very idea may be disconcerting or even frightening. This is to be expected. Without question, parents' attitudes regarding oral health and dentistry are influenced by their own experiences, often beginning during childhood.

Any experienced practitioner can relate a story in which a patient's very first comments after introduction convey his dread of dental visits. On further investigation these feelings are often traced to childhood experiences, and often just the smell of the dental office is sufficient to elicit a negative emotional response. It is impossible for parents to make purely objective decisions without being powerfully affected by their own experiences and attitudes.

In other instances it may not be the mother's personal experience with dentistry but the influences of other family members. Family dynamics play a large role in the decisions that most mothers ultimately make, and cultural attitudes expressed through grandparents, spouses, and even close friends are significant. A mother may be conflicted by the advice given by her pediatrician to get her children to the dentist versus the admonition of other family members who might view dentistry for children a waste of money or even worse—as assault.

A mother who calls with a child who is suffering with advanced dental disease comes to the initial visit with a sense of guilt, and how that experience is managed relative to her feelings of guilt will dictate the ultimate outcome of the experience. Other parents will be in total denial that their child's situation is a result of parental practices, and they will adopt a defensive mindset at the suggestion that they might be even remotely responsible for their child's illness.

The well-trained staff member understands the multiplicity of attitudes, experiences, education, and cultural diversity that she faces during the initial telephone conversation. It is important to navigate that first conversation in such a manner that is neither insensitive nor condescending but rather provides the information the parent needs to make an informed decision and, more importantly, to address the mother's primary concerns in such a way that relieves fears and anxieties. The staff member must field a host of questions and concerns. Here are a few common examples:

(1) "My pediatrician has recommended that I take my baby to the dentist. Why is it necessary to take a 2-year-old to the dentist, and what do you do to a 2-year-old anyway?"

(2) "I've heard that I should take my 18-month-old in for her first visit. She really doesn't like it when I try to brush her teeth, and I don't push the issue too hard because I don't want to cause any psychological harm. What if she doesn't want to open for the doctor? I'm afraid she might cry."

(3) "I sort of get the creeps when I go to the dentist, especially when I lie down in the dental chair. Will my baby have to lie down in the dental chair, and can I be with her to relieve her fears?"

Competently responding to such questions and concerns requires thorough training. Real-time role playing for any conceivable situation or scenario is a very effective training tool. In each scenario the salient points that should be communicated pertinent to the situation must be memorized and rehearsed. In most lines of communication the staff person is encouraged to use her own words and unique style of speech to communicate the messages. With regard to the initial phone call from a parent who is making an appointment for a baby or toddler, the line of communication is more tightly scripted and memorized to ensure the correct use of key phrases and buzzwords and the absolute avoidance of others.

An important skill for staff to develop is the avoidance of straight-up answers to a mother's concerns or questions, unless that is indeed the most appropriate response. This can be a challenging behavior change for people who are accustomed to giving direct answers to questions rather than delving into the nature of the questions. For example, the mother asks, "Is this procedure going to hurt my child?" If the staff person answers "no," the question has been answered, but the underlying concern has not been sufficiently addressed. The question offers an opportunity to communicate, and advantage of the moment should be taken. What the mother may be communicating with the simple question "Is it going to hurt?" is "I'm worried that you might hurt my child; I need to know how much it's going to hurt so that I can prepare my child appropriately, and I need you to offer me some reassurance that everything is going to be all right." Adequate training and role playing ensure the staff's ability to respond in a fashion that inspires trust and confidence.

Another important skill for phone managers to master is the creation of a positive image of the upcoming experience. For many mothers the preconceived image is that of the dentist placing their infants in a dental chair and proceeding with a routine that is consistent with their own experiences as a dental patient. The initial phone call is the perfect opportunity to build a new image, and this can be accomplished by walking the mother through the first appointment and by using positive imagery.

Example of telephone dialogue is as follows:

> STAFF: Thank you for calling the children's dental center. This is Kelly; how may I help you?
> CALLER: Yes, I'd like to make an appointment for my child, but I have a few questions first.

This first statement alerts Kelly as to the direction the conversation might be headed. The fact that the mother has questions before she even offers her name is a verbal clue of some worry or anxiety. Her questions could very well concern her insurance or if the office is a Medicaid provider, etc., but probably not. Rather than proceed directly to the mother's questions, the response should be as follows:

> KELLY: Yes, I'll be happy to assist you. I'm sorry but I didn't get your name.
> CALLER: Mrs Williams.
> KELLY: Thank you, Mrs Williams. May I ask the child's name please?

It is important for Kelly to repeat the mother's name and the child's name as many times as possible for the remainder of the conversation. Calling a person by name conveys to her that the staff member to whom she is speaking values her, and this is the very first and most important step in establishing a relationship built on trust:

> MRS WILLIAMS: Yes, his name is Trey.
>
> KELLY: Wonderful, Mrs Williams. We look forward to meeting you and Trey. May I ask how old Trey is?

Note that Kelly does not ask the age of "the child" since she now knows the child's name. Note also that Kelly does not ask for the child's birthday. That type of demographic and technical information should come later in the conversation. For the moment Kelly need know only the child's name and roughly how old he is:

> MRS WILLIAMS: Yes, he's eighteen months old.
>
> KELLY: Terrific! Mrs Williams, it's wonderful that you have chosen to get Trey started early with his dental visits, and we're pleased that you have chosen us for Trey's dental home. I promise you that you and Trey are going to have an enjoyable experience when you visit us. Mrs Williams, you mentioned that you have a few questions for me. Are there any special concerns that you have regarding Trey that you would like for us to address?

Invariably there will be at least one clinical issue with which the mother is concerned. These include teething pain, tooth eruption patterns, difficulty brushing, perceived pathology, previous problems with older siblings, and medical conditions. However, the most common concern is the simple need to know what the first visit will entail:

> MRS WILLIAMS: How is Dr Jones going to get Trey to lie still in the dental chair? I mean I can hardly open his mouth to look at his teeth much less get them brushed very well. I had such a horrible experience with my older son, and I just don't want Trey to have a bad experience.

What this mother is communicating is that she knows the importance of getting Trey enrolled early. She clearly understands that part, but she does not have the reassurance that everything is going to be all right or that the dentist and his staff are adequately prepared to deal with her toddler. At this point Kelly's most important job is to empathize with Mrs Williams and to demonstrate that her concerns are being heard. Kelly can demonstrate this by rephrasing with a positive inflection, the concerns that Mrs Williams has just voiced:

> KELLY: Mrs Williams, I can tell from your questions that you really want Trey to have a positive experience.
>
> MRS WILLIAMS: Yes, I really do!
>
> KELLY: Mrs Williams, let me just offer a word of reassurance. Our goal is to offer all our children a positive dental experience, and we are very good at doing so. When you and Trey arrive at our office, you will immediately notice that it doesn't have the look or feel

of a typical clinical environment. Trey will think of it as one of the most fun places he has ever been. Once you have been checked in, you will be given a tour of the clinic, and then you will be invited to make yourself comfortable in one of our consultation rooms. Dr Jones will visit with you there and address any concerns that you have about Trey. He will also examine Trey while Trey is sitting or lying in your lap, and Dr Jones will also demonstrate proper cleaning and brushing.

MRS WILLIAMS: You mean that Dr Jones is not going to put Trey into the dental chair?

KELLY: No, Mrs Williams. Trey will not be asked to lie in the dental chair.

MRS WILLIAMS: You mean that Trey won't have his teeth cleaned with the dental tools and everything?

KELLY: Mrs Williams, a professional cleaning is certainly something that will be appropriate for Trey as he gets a little older, but for now what is important is for Dr Jones to have the opportunity to get to know you and Trey, to get you started doing the right things for Trey's oral health, and for you to know that you have a place to come for all of your children's dental needs. Mrs. Williams, I guarantee that you're going to enjoy the experience. Now may I take a few moments to get some additional information from you please?

At this point the caller should be feeling less anxious and perhaps even enjoying the conversation. This is a good time to begin receiving demographic information such as addresses, birth dates, and insurance information, and to invite the mother to visit the office web site. She should be advised to expect a packet of information from the office in a day or two. This packet will include a welcome letter, an office brochure explaining insurance and financial policies, and health history forms for each enrolled child. The mother is encouraged to have the appropriate forms completed prior to arrival or to fax or e-mail the forms in advance of the first appointment. For the mother to attempt to complete the various forms in the reception area while also attending to small children or babies is stressful, and having these items taken care of prior to the appointment ensures a smooth and timely transition from the reception area to the clinic. In addition to relieving the mother's stress, attending to the first appointment in a timely manner adds to the culture of professionalism and gives parents a sense of confidence in the practice.

After the demographic information is obtained, a friendly sign-off is important:

KELLY: Mrs Williams, I have really enjoyed talking with you this morning, and we look forward to meeting you and Trey on the seventeenth.

The initial conversation sets the stage for the upcoming encounter. The mother should now feel more relaxed with a positive image of the ensuing experience. In a few short minutes the phone handler can lay the foundation for the beginning of a solid, trusting relationship with the family.

SCHEDULING THE INFANT/TODDLER EXAMINATION

The most important aspect of scheduling the infant/toddler examination is to make the parent and child wait as short a time as possible. It is imperative that the patient be appointed within 2 weeks of the initial phone call. Once the parent has decided to schedule the initial examination, she is mentally prepared to take the next step in her child's dental experience. Delays may provide an opportunity for any apprehension or anxiety regarding the appointment to intensify. Likewise, scheduling the infant/toddler at a time the clinician can attend to him promptly is essential. As clinicians with a wide variety of practice styles and scheduling templates, it vital that we set aside certain predetermined times when we are confident that we will be able to see these patients punctually. This time may be at the beginning of the day or just after lunch when the office should be "running on schedule." Another favorite time for these appointments is during "re-care" visits or other preestablished short appointments during which there are frequent breaks in the schedule that will allow the clinician to be prompt. Ultimately, one should avoid appointing infants and toddlers during procedures that either take longer to complete or are unpredictable in nature, such as heavy restorative dentistry or conscious sedation cases.

Some may feel that when dealing with an infant or toddler it is best to schedule after nap time in order to prevent trying to examine an unhappy or cranky child. Others believe it is best to schedule a young child just before nap time in order to try to catch a somewhat sleepy child. It is prudent to ask the parent during the initial telephone interview what time of day she feels would be the best for her child and then try to accommodate her if at all possible. Therefore, if the appointment does not go well, the parent will not feel that she was forced into a time that was not optimal for her child. The best scheduling of these visits is often a balance between the best time for the clinician and his schedule and the best time for the parent's and patient's schedules.

THE PHYSICAL ENVIRONMENT

The physical plan often may contain the limiting factors that affect the ability to smoothly incorporate babies and toddlers into everyday activities. The entryway/foyer should be large enough for parents with strollers and baby carriers to be clear of traffic at the check-in area. The greeter should be in the open rather than behind a glass window, with a countertop low enough for clear visibility of young children. Segmented lobbies are helpful in segregating babies, toddlers, and preschoolers from school-age children

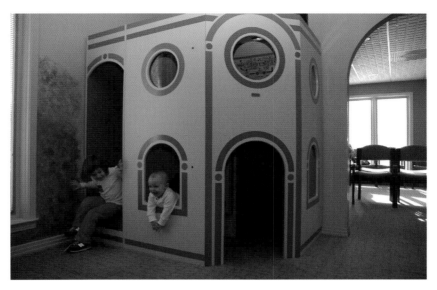

Figure 12.1   Reception area for toddlers and preschoolers.

and teenagers, with age-appropriate games, toys, and movies in each area (Figures 12.1–12.3). Segmented lobby areas create a feeling of coziness without being crowded and help to decrease overall background noise.

If possible, it is ideal to have spaces away from the clinical area for visits with parents. The dental operatory is the least desirable area in which to

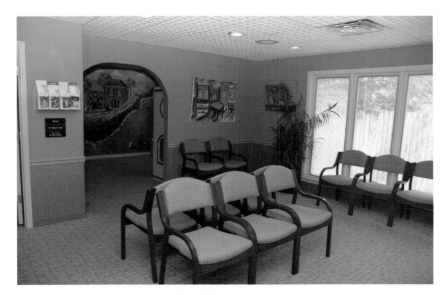

Figure 12.2   Reception area for adults.

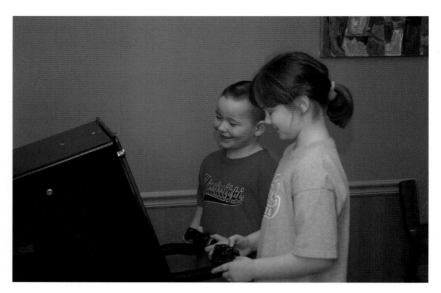

Figure 12.3   Reception area for school-aged children.

have a relaxed conversation with mothers about their babies. Despite our best efforts to design friendly dental cubicles, the truth remains that the normal sights, sounds, and smells of dentistry can elicit anxiety in the parents, and we must do whatever is possible to counter that affect. It is, therefore, best to be as far away from the dental operatory as possible when dealing with babies. This can be accomplished by appointing small consultation areas or rooms specifically for babies and small children (Figure 12.4). These cozy areas are very nonclinical in their appearance and feel, with carpeted floors and comfortable seating. There are interactive materials such as wall-mounted games or floor activities for toddlers (Figures 12.5 and 12.6) and a rounded-edge countertop for educational materials, a computer terminal, and the preset examination tray. These rooms can be enclosed for purposes of privacy, but with glass walls and doors for a more open relaxed effect. Semiprivate open consultation areas are equally useful (Figure 12.7). These consultation rooms or areas should be positioned away from the view or sound of high-speed handpieces or high-volume suctions. If these rooms are designed and appointed thoughtfully, the child should be completely unaware that he is in a clinical environment.

Every effort should be expended to mitigate the smell of dentistry. Fortunately, this is no longer difficult to accomplish. First, it is imperative to eliminate the presence and use of eugenol or formocresol, which are largely responsible for the typical and well-recognized dental office smell. Neither of these items is necessary because there is a host of modern

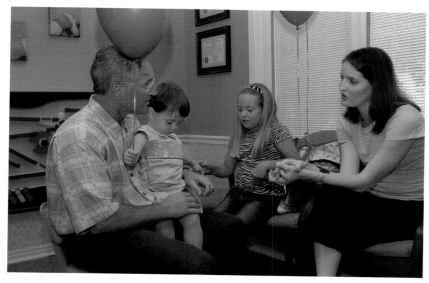

Figure 12.4   Consultation area designed for children.

suitable alternatives available. The additional use of ozone generators and HEPA filtration air purifiers can totally eliminate the additional odors common to dentistry such as cutting tooth structure and autoclave smells. Finally, the use of candles, essential oil vaporizers, or scent diffusers is helpful in producing a spa-like or home-like atmosphere.

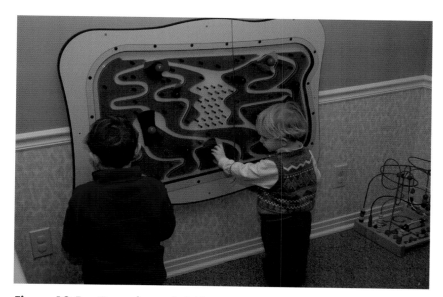

Figure 12.5   Games for small children in consultation room.

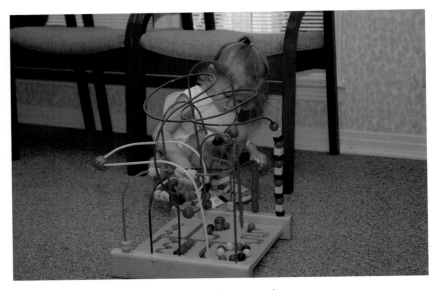

Figure 12.6   Appropriate play materials in consultation room.

MANAGING THE EXPERIENCE

During the first few moments of the initial visit the parents are invited on a tour of the clinic. It is beneficial for parents with babies to have the opportunity to view children of all ages enjoying the rewards of a positive dental

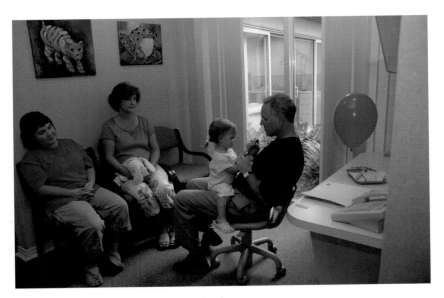

Figure 12.7   Semiprivate consultation bay.

experience, and a tour along the periphery of the clinical area while other children are present is helpful in relieving anxiety. It also provides the parents with a visual cue for what they can expect for their babies in the years to come. After the tour, the family is invited into the consultation room by the staff person (patient representative, clinic coordinator, infant assistant, hygienist, etc.). The family is welcomed to the practice and a dialogue is begun that always begins with the primary concerns of the parents. This question should always be asked: "Is there anything in particular that you wish to discuss with the doctor?" This avoids the embarrassment of covering a plethora of subjects during the course of the visit without ever addressing the issue that got them there in the first place. For practices that wish to delegate the educational aspects of the infant visit, this is the appropriate juncture for those activities. Relevant introductory subjects should include the basics of dental caries, the infectious nature of the disease, and a discussion of the importance of oral health to general health. The first visit is also the suitable moment to cover age-appropriate anticipatory guidance, including the promotion of healthy and safe habits, injury prevention, and general nutrition. *Bright Futures: Guidelines for Health Supervision of Infants, Children, and Adolescents* is a useful publication to use during these discussions. Poor dietary practices that can be related to oral disease should also be emphasized at this juncture. Utilizing the American Academy of Pediatric Dentistry caries-risk assessment tool, the staff person can also assign to the patient the appropriate risk level. It is fitting during this portion of the visit for staff to utilize posters or videos that demonstrates proper brushing techniques for infants and toddlers. The educational portion of the visit is followed by the doctor's examination and oral hygiene technique demonstration. The oral health assessment is then documented with accompanying preventative and treatment recommendations.

CLIMBING THE EXPERIENCE LADDER

Any discussion that explores the various approaches to handling babies and toddlers will invariably rely on the commonly published milestones on human growth and development. However, formulating standardized approaches based on statistical averages is fraught with danger. The assumptions that every 1-year-old will cry when examined and that every child should be comfortable with the dental chair by the third birthday are useless assumptions from a practical standpoint. Just as parents come to the situation with their own points of reference, so do children. That is not to imply that office systems are useless with respect to dealing with babies.

However, as much as operations are standardized, the approach to babies, toddlers, and preschoolers must be individually tailored. The practice that serves a diverse community will have children enrolled who cover the full spectrum of emotional, psychological, physical, and developmental maturity. For example, a 2-year-old child who is the fifth sibling of a farm family, in which all the children are 18 months apart in age, is likely to mirror his older siblings by following them into the clinical area, hopping onto the dental bench, and cooperating fully for an examination. This behavior is a reflection of the child's overall life experience that involves a great deal of sibling mentorship and interdependent behavior modeling. This child is also likely to communicate well verbally and to follow simple instructions with minimal coercion. Children who are reared in a culture in which respect for adult authority, good behavior, and a cooperative spirit are premium values will reflect those values in the dental setting at a very early age. Conversely, the overly indulged and overly protected 4-year-old only child of middle-aged highly educated parents will likely be afraid of most new experiences. Fear of strangers and disrespect for authority are also common observations in children who live in a narcissistic self-absorbed world. Coaxing this child off the mother's legs and accomplishing anything remotely resembling a dental examination can resemble a rodeo and is a far greater challenge than handling an 18-month-old. Admittedly, these two examples represent extreme opposites and most children fall somewhere in-between. In all cases an initial assessment of behavioral readiness must be accomplished before an approach tactic can be formulated. The best opportunity to make such an assessment is during the first few moments after the doctor has entered the consultation room/area. During these first few moments the doctor should avoid the temptation to direct his attention to the child but rather give full attention to only the parent. This skillful maneuver disarms the child and allows a few moments for the child to make his own assessment of the parent's comfort level.

This is obviously a subconscious assessment on the part of the toddler, but it occurs nonetheless, and the balance of the visit hinges on these first few moments. If the doctor barges into the room and immediately focuses his attention on the child (even if only saying hello and calling the child by name), the child is likely to interpret that attention as an act of aggression, and he will adopt a set of defensive maneuvers such as hiding under a chair or clutching the parent's neck. In such an event, the quality of the visit is likely to spiral downward from that point.

It is important to caution parents that during the actual examination some children will be resistant to either the dental team or the parent. Reassuring the parent that this is normal behavior for many children gives her the confidence to use the necessary assertiveness for daily brushing routines at home. Some parents view assertive brushing as an act of violence on the unwilling toddler, and a calm but deliberate demonstration of proper technique is useful in helping parents overcome their own emotions regarding the activity. However, the examination and brushing demonstration should come at the end of the visit. Having a casual conversation with the family and covering all questions and concerns prior to the examination allows for nervous jitters to settle and provides sufficient time for the family to gain a degree of confidence in the doctor. Having parents adequately prepared for the examination/brushing maneuver aids in their receptiveness of the procedure, as well as the likelihood of adopting the doctor's recommendations.

The transition from a knee-to-knee infant examination to the dental chair is never a single step but should occur incrementally over multiple visits. Appropriate modeling is the foundation for building the rungs on the experience ladder and for developing the positive attitudes toward oral care and the dental team/patient relationship. This foundation is equally important for both the child and the parents. Modeling is a much more global subject than the classic explanation of tell/show/do. Tell/show/do is a useful tactic within the context of global modeling but not very effective as a stand-alone method. Global modeling encompasses everything the doctor and staff does, including the manipulation and control of the environment, the use of interpersonal skills, and the manner in which parents and their children are approached. Global modeling is a constellation of efforts that subtly and deftly guides parents and children into accepting oral health and dentistry as important aspects of family health and well-being.

THE MULTIPLE APPROACHES TO THE INFANT/ TODDLER EXAMINATION

Just as tell/show/do is an oversimplification of modeling, so is the knee-to-knee maneuver an oversimplification of the infant/toddler dental experience. The knee-to-knee examination is simply a mechanical maneuver that can be very useful both clinically and at home. However, the technique is only one of several approaches that can be used throughout the continuum of experiences that parallel the various early childhood milestones.

The knee-to-knee position (Figure 12.8) is a very practical technique for examining babies up to about 18 months old. The technique orients the doctor and the parent facing each other in close proximity. The baby's legs are astraddle of the mother's waist while the baby's head rests on the knees of the operator. The operator steadies the baby's head while the mother secures the child's hands. Most mothers are very comfortable with this positioning that allows for uninterrupted contact between the baby and the mother, and yet offers good visualization for both the operator and the parent.

The examination can be accomplished utilizing a gloved finger and a plastic sleeved penlight for both illumination and cheek retraction, eliminating the need for overhead lighting. The position is also useful at home for daily brushing. During the instructional portion of the procedure, the mother is encouraged to follow a pattern of brushing tooth surfaces from top to bottom, right to left, buccal, and lingual to ensure that all surfaces are adequately cleaned. The parents are shown the proper bristle angle along the gingival crevice and are advised of the importance of brushing along the gum line even in the presence of bleeding. Parents will frequently

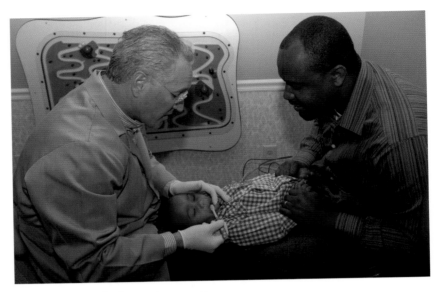

Figure 12.8   The knee-to-knee position.

express difficulty brushing their baby's maxillary anterior teeth, as this area is particularly sensitive, resulting in forceful activation of the orbicularis oris, as well as the baby squirming and crying. It is important to reassure the parents that they are not hurting the child but that the sensation amounts to extreme tickling. For many toddlers it is necessary to use the lip-lift technique in order to adequately access the maxillary incisors for effective brushing (Figure 12.9). It should be noted that in infants and toddlers brushing across a heavy labial frenum may, in fact, be painful. Care should be taken to point out a heavy labial frenum to the parent and to demonstrate proper brushing techniques around this anatomical structure.

For parents wishing to start their babies at the time of or before the emergence of the first teeth, the instructional portion of the visit will often center on the treatment of teething symptoms. During this pre-toothbrush period the use of disposable intraoral wipes is helpful. These prepackaged commercially available wipes are impregnated with xylitol, come in multiple fruit flavors, and are easy to use. Parents are accustomed to carrying disposable prepackaged items in their diaper bags, and the addition of intraoral wipes to their armamentarium is sensible. The parents performing the same with assistance and encouragement follow a demonstration of the use of the intraoral wipe (Figure 12.10). Parents who routinely use the xylitol wipes report positive benefits in alleviating the usual symptoms associated with primary tooth eruption in young infants, and the disposable nature of the wipes makes them a hygienic alternative to the use of a washcloth or finger brush.

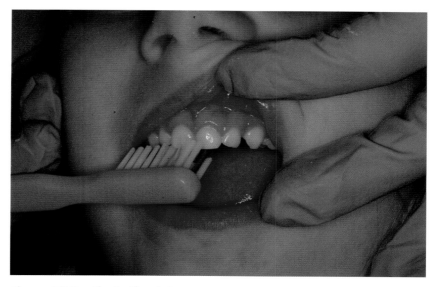

Figure 12.9   The lip-lift technique.

As the child approaches the first birthday, the knee-to-knee position with the baby lying sideways is effective (Figure 12.11).

The 1-year-olds are obviously more aware of their surroundings than they were at 6 months and have become less accustomed to looking at human faces upside down. Many daily activities, however (dressing,

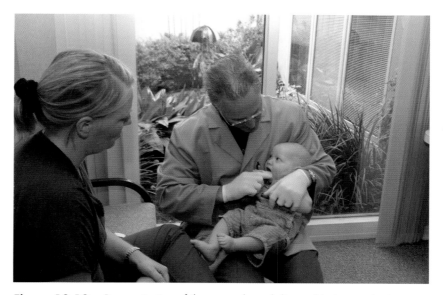

Figure 12.10   Demonstration of the prepackaged disposable intraoral wipe.

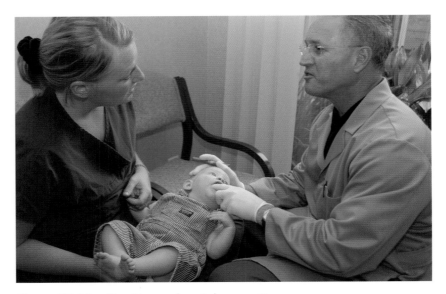

Figure 12.11   The sideways knee-to-knee position.

diaper changes, etc.), occur with the adults approaching from the baby's side or their feet. The sideways position allows the baby to remain on the mother's lap and provides for easy baby/mother eye contact. Most 1-year-old babies are very comfortable and cooperative with the sideways knee-to-knee examination that also offers good clinical visibility and good doctor/parent eye contact.

A curious behavioral milestone occurs with the early toddler at about 18 months. Just as the youngster begins walking, a new era of freedom and mobility begins. During this period babies become resistant to lying on their backs for dressing and diaper changes; babies of this age also resist lying on their backs for toothbrushing. A restrained knee-to-knee examination is interpreted by the resistant toddler as an act of violence and can become very upsetting for both baby and mother. However, most toddlers do not mind sitting in the operator's lap for a few moments, particularly if there is something interesting or curious to capture the child's attention (Figure 12.12). The lap examination is an effective behavior guidance method that bridges the gap from continuous contact with the mother to independent contact with the dentist. The mother is still present, but the doctor/child relationship has stepped up one rung on the experience ladder to one-on-one interaction that is an important milestone.

The first step in the toddler lap examination is to coax the youngster into close proximity to the doctor. This can be accomplished by having something to offer the child that captures his interest such as action figure stickers or an interesting toy or gadget. Once the child is in close proximity to the doctor, it is helpful to allow the toddler to be accustomed to the

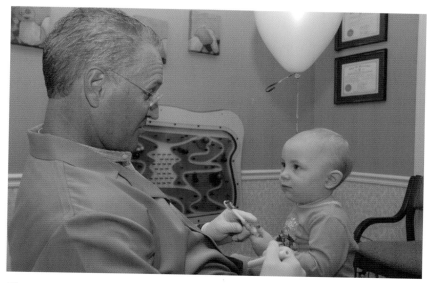

Figure 12.12   The lap examination.

penlight that will be used during the examination (Figure 12.13). Turning on the light and counting the toddler's fingers and then allowing the child to return the favor can accomplish this. At this point the child is placed on the operator's lap and offered a toothbrush (Figure 12.14). The toddler will instinctively begin to brush while the doctor begins the examination. Most

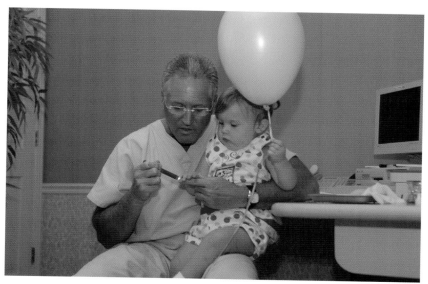

Figure 12.13   Desensitizing the child to the penlight.

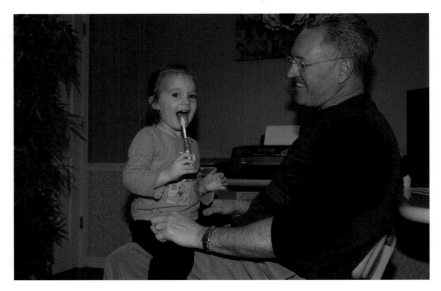

Figure 12.14 The lap examination.

toddlers are remarkably cooperative for a penlight examination while sitting on the operator's lap. The position offers good visibility for the doctor, however less so for the parent.

Another variation of the lap examination is tailored for the toddler who is not quite ready for one-on-one contact with the dentist but cooperates well enough for interaction. In these instances the child is placed on the parent's knee, but facing the dentist (Figure 12.15). In this orientation a similar dialogue is composed with the sharing of stickers, the counting of fingers, etc., and progresses to the oral examination utilizing the sleeved penlight.

The 2-year-old is a delightful, carefree creature who usually approaches new experiences with joyful enthusiasm. The 2-year-olds can also be quite challenging as their developing independence is frustrated by their lack of communication skills. Guiding them through the dental visit is best accomplished by engaging the toddlers in a game-like fashion that appeals to their sense of curiosity. Just as the 18-month-old is coaxed into close proximity to the doctor by capturing the youngster's trust, the same applies to the 2-year-old. However, the terrible 2-year-olds are likely more suspicious of the game and are just as likely to retreat to a corner as they are to eagerly engage the doctor. The operator must avoid the temptation to force the issue but rather continue to negotiate interaction in an easy-going manner. The use of interactive noise making games or toys is a very effective way to lure the 2-year-old into the immediate proximity of the doctor and opens the door for the possibility of one-on-one interaction. Only after the toddler has accepted the premise of personal engagement

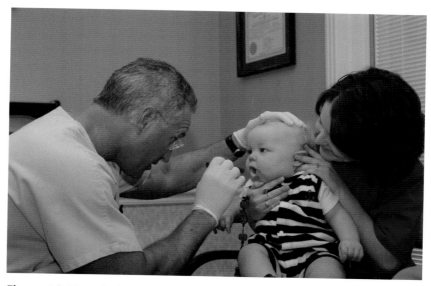

Figure 12.15   The lap examination with the child sitting in parent's lap.

with the operator can an attempt at toothbrushing or an oral examination be accomplished without the use of physical restraint. It should be noted that the 2-year-old is a most unpredictable animal who has mastered the use of the word "no" and is physically resistant to almost anything. Parents will frequently express frustration at toothbrushing efforts. It is not unusual for mother and father to disagree with each other as to whether the activity is worth the effort, and if that occurs, it can add emotional tension to the exercise. There is often concern regarding the psychological effect of restraining the toddler for toothbrushing exercises, and it is common for parents to admit to simply giving up. This is a very important moment for the doctor to offer reassurance that physical resistance by the 2-year-old is normal as noted with a host of other daily activities such dressing, toilet training, eating, and bathing. Impressing upon the parents the importance of effective deliberate brushing by an adult versus simply giving the toddler a toothbrush on which to chew is of paramount importance. At the 2-year-old visit this question should always be asked: "How is toothbrushing going?" If the parent answers, "Oh, he loves to brush his teeth," this is a reliable indicator that the parents are not actively involved in routinely brushing the child's teeth. A majority of well-intentioned parents are simply not inclined to push beyond the resistance of the toddlers to brush the toddlers' teeth against their will. Continual insistence and encouragement from the doctor and staff is essential to help the parents through this difficult period. It is very helpful to demonstrate once again easy and effective positions to accomplish the task. The reverse standing position is a safe and effective maneuver for the 2-year-old and can be

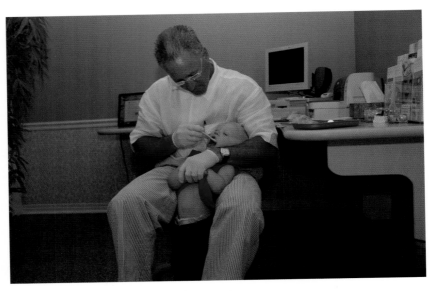

Figure 12.16   The reverse standing position.

accomplished with just one adult if necessary. With the adult comfortably seated, the youngsters stand backward between the parent's legs with their head on the parent's lap. The adult reaches around with one hand in order to secure the toddler's hands and handles the toothbrush with the toothbrush with the alternate hand (Figure 12.16). This position provides exceptional control of the squirming child, provides for good operator visibility, and can be accomplished anywhere in the home. The dentist can also use this positional technique during the visit for the intraoral examination and toothbrushing demonstration (Figure 12.17). With the parent's hand-holding assistance, this is also a very effective position for the application of fluoride varnish because it allows the dentist to use one hand for the lip-lift technique while applying the varnish with the other hand.

As the child approaches 30 months, a much more cooperative attitude begins to emerge. The child's vocabulary has roughly doubled during the last 6 months along with the capability of combining words into simple phrases, questions, and requests. The child is eager to learn and has developed a better sense of social interaction with other children. He is much more likely to imitate older children now, and behavior modeling is beginning to be observed. Even if the child remains precooperative with respect to parental separation or learning about the dental chair, this is the appropriate age for the youngster to observe other children in the clinical environment. Having the children spend time in the clinical

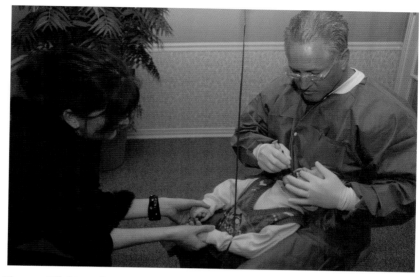

Figure 12.17   The reverse standing position for the clinical examination, with parent holding hands.

area either at the foot of an older sibling (Figure 12.18) or simply playing games or watching movies in the on-deck area is an important transitional exercise in preparing them for the next step. The examination portion of the 30-month-old visit is no different than the previous visit save that the child is now fully cooperative in most instances and relishes the opportunity to

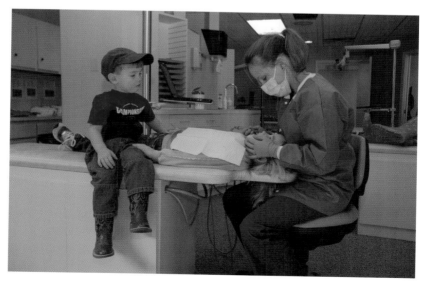

Figure 12.18   Introduction of the preschooler to the clinical setting.

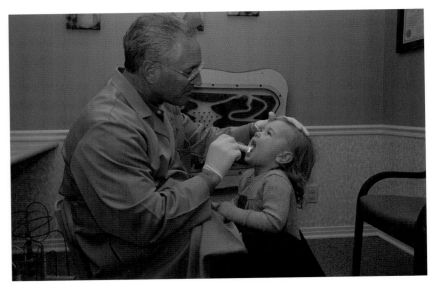

Figure 12.19   Forward facing standing position for the 30-month-old.

demonstrate his or her toothbrushing skills (Figure 12.19). As the examination is accomplished in short order, the remainder of the visit can be used for the initial steps of tell/show/do.

The child is coaxed to the dental bench and invited to take a seat facing the operator (Figure 12.20). If the dental chair is mechanical, it should

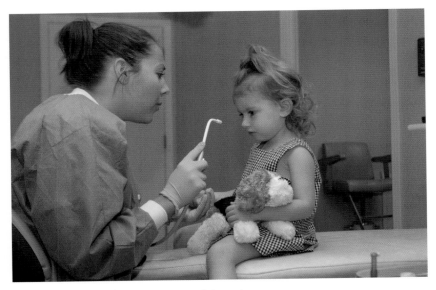

Figure 12.20   Initial steps of the tell-show-do visit.

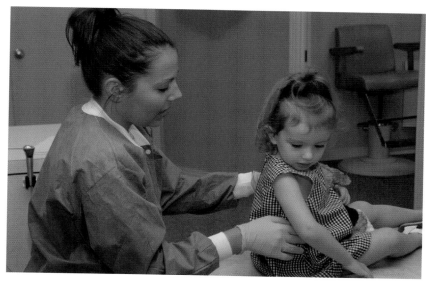

Figure 12.21   Coaxing the child into the recumbent position at the initial tell-show-do visit.

be placed in the horizontal position prior to the exercise. With the child in the upright seated position, the operator introduces the air-water syringe, the saliva ejector, and the rubber cup by using homemade fun names such as squirt gun, sucker straw, and spin brush. The thirty-month-old enjoys hands-on learning and will relish this new experience with great enthusiasm if allowed to participate. Upon completion of these preliminary tell/show/do exercises, the children can be coaxed into turning around and lying down with their head in the operator's lap (Figure 12.21). Having the child willfully roll over is much more acceptable to the child at this age than having the mechanical chair assume a new position once the child is seated. Having the child receive the rubber cup and saliva ejector while in the recumbent position is an important milestone and signifies that the child could be fully cooperative for other procedures if warranted (Figure 12.22).

Although special rooms that are set aside for infant/toddler examinations might be ideal, in an established general practice or in a "first office" made to fit certain physical restraints imposed by an existing office space, this may not be possible. Alternative techniques for the infant/toddler examination in dental chairs can be just as effective. For example, the knee-to-knee examinations for the infant can be performed by positioning two operator stools opposing each with the parent and clinician facing each other, knees touching (Figure 12.23). Infant/toddler examinations can also be performed in the dental chair with the parent holding the child in her lap, with the child's knees bent over the parent's thigh and the child leaning

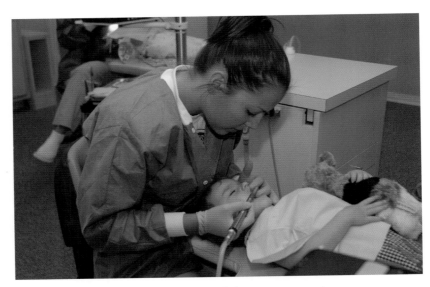

Figure 12.22   The first rubber cup prophylaxis—a major milestone.

back onto the dental chair (Figure 12.24). This allows for the children to remain close to their parent during the examination while reassuring the anxious children that everything is going to be all right. This method is used for both the cooperative and the uncooperative child as the parent can hold the uncooperative child's hands while leaning over and lightly constraining the child's knees (Figure 12.25).

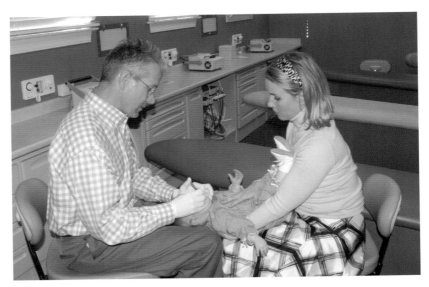

Figure 12.23   The knee-to-knee examination in the clinical area.

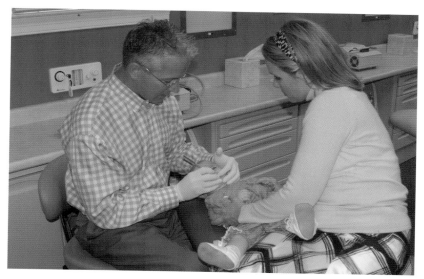

Figure 12.24   The infant examination utilizing the dental bench.

Another method can be helpful for the children who are not comfortable lying down in the dental chair but seem content to sit in their parent's lap or to sit beside their parent on the dental chair. Rather than the child's having an unfavorable dental experience, simply examine the lower dental arch with the child sitting on the parent's lap or beside the parent. To

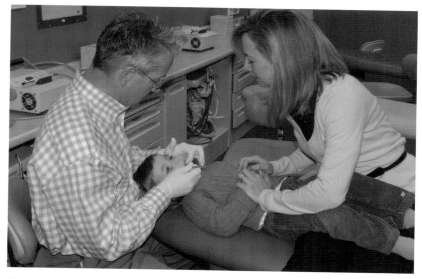

Figure 12.25   Toddler examination with parental assistance utilizing the dental bench.

complete the examination, walk around behind the patient and with one knee on the dental chair, examine the children as they lean back onto the clinician or onto the parent. This method is an easy compromise that allows one to gain all the necessary information needed for an examination while demonstrating to both the parent and child one's flexibility and desire to keep the appointment a happy one.

DOCUMENTATION

During each visit an oral health assessment is documented and a treatment plan is formulated. Utilizing the American Academy of Pediatric Dentistry caries-risk assessment tool, the clinician places the child in the appropriate risk category. With practice, this function becomes quite instinctive and requires very little additional effort on the part of the staff beyond the usual educational activities.

For instance, if a juice cup is visible in the examination room and the toddler has visible plaque on the maxillary incisors with no evidence of effective oral hygiene during the past week, the child is at high risk. If the child has no visible plaque or incipient lesions present, he or she is probably at low risk. This is actually logical. If there ever were a time one would expect a child to be plaque free, it would be on the day of a dental visit. If the dental staff observes dental plaque of long-standing duration, the assumption can be made that the child never receives effective toothbrushing.

Toddlers at low risk are placed on yearly recall intervals. Those at moderate risk are placed on 6-month recall intervals, with fluoride varnish applications scheduled at each visit (Harrison et al., 2007). Educational efforts are continued at each of these visits with a focus on nutritional issues, dietary habits, and, of course, effective plaque removal. High-risk children are placed on 3-month recall intervals. Those visits focus on extensive motivational interviewing with regard to the effectiveness of home care, and the parent's perception of their efforts. Fluoride varnish applications are also accomplished at those visits.

In addition, thorough documentation of other aspects of the dental visit may prove to be helpful as the positive dental experience is a dynamic transformation that usually occurs over several visits. For instance, noting how receptive the patient and the parent are to treatment and which modalities seem to be best received will certainly be of later interest.

Specifically, exactly what type of examination was performed or attempted and whether or not a partial or full rubber cup prophylaxis was completed is worthy of note as each visit should be a step beyond the previous visit. How exactly was the child positioned during the visit? Was the patient afraid of the suction, air-water syringe, prophy angle, or loud noises? Was the parent a "team player" or very timid regarding the dental experience? However, it is important to remember that one should use caution when entering subjective evaluations into the patient's permanent record. Accurate documentation will provide valuable information when planning the specific environment for the patient's next dental visit.

JUST DO IT!

Most dentists' apprehension with the infant/toddler examination may be in part due to their lack of desire to have "fussy kids" in their offices and/or to the fact that these examinations may not be very lucrative for the amount of time that they take. One must realize that as with any new procedure that is introduced into the dental office, it will take some time to become comfortable with seeing very young children. With some experience the clinician will become accustomed to each situation, and these visits will not only become shorter in duration, which is more cost-effective, but also more predictable and relaxed. As with other dental procedures, one simply becomes better with time and practice.

REFERENCES

ADA Council on Scientific Affairs. 2006. Professionally applied topical fluoride: Executive summary of evidence-based clinical recommendations. *J Am Dent Assoc* 8:137 (Special JADA Insert).

Harrison R, Benton T, Everson-Stewart S, and Weinstein P. 2007. Effect of motivational interviewing on rates of early childhood caries: A randomized trial. *Pediatr Dent* 29:16–22.

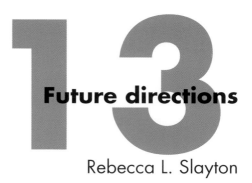

Future directions

Rebecca L. Slayton

INTRODUCTION

Early childhood caries is a serious disease affecting increasing numbers of young children in the United States and the world. It interferes with a child's ability to eat, sleep, and learn. It is expensive to treat because it frequently requires treatment under general anesthesia in a hospital setting, due to the young child's inability to cooperate for care. The disease process puts children at risk for infections that can be life threatening and treatment under general anesthesia puts them at additional risks related to airway complications and general anesthetic medications, among other things.

Because dental caries is a disease, it is not 100% preventable. However, with the proper diet, oral hygiene, fluoride exposure, and management of risk factors, the majority of children can avoid the consequences of dental caries. True prevention begins prior to birth with the oral health and overall health of the mother. Delaying transmission of cariogenic bacteria is a key component in both the timing and the severity of disease for the child.

In the future, in order to prevent and/or manage early childhood caries, it is essential that the dental and medical professions create a shift in the current paradigm surrounding this disease. There has been little change in the understanding of the caries process since first elucidated by Miller in 1881. Our knowledge of the biology of caries has contributed to vast improvements in the prevalence of caries among both adults and children in the United States. Much of this improvement is attributed to fluoride in drinking water and dentifrice but also to improved oral hygiene and dietary habits. In the last decade, we have started losing ground in the fight against caries among young children. In their case, our understanding of the disease process does not seem to be changing diet or behaviors. Many strategies have been proposed and implemented to address this pandemic including screening and risk assessment by physicians and nurses, education by community partners, establishment of a dental home by 1 year of age and media campaigns to inform or motivate families to develop "mouth healthy" habits for their children. Progress in some areas is balanced by failures in others. The possibility of growing-up caries-free seems to only be a reality for a small segment of the population (primarily those with access to care and financial resources).

FUTURE DIRECTIONS

There are a number of questions that remain unanswered that will be a good starting point for future clinical and basic science research efforts. These include the following:

(1) Why do some children in a family get cavities, while others who have the same diet and oral hygiene habits do not?
(2) Why are there disparities in caries prevalence with children from low-income families and minorities being more affected?
(3) Are *mutans streptococci* really the main acidogenic bacteria responsible for caries or are there other bacteria that are not as easily cultivable?
(4) What techniques can we use to detect caries risk prior to the development of disease?
(5) When children at risk for caries are identified early, what can be done to truly prevent the disease from occurring?
(6) Once the disease process has begun, what is the best way to manage the disease and to minimize the consequences of disease?

These questions fall into four basic categories and should guide us toward a better understanding of the management of this disease in the future. First is the identification of the different types and strains of bacteria that contribute to the caries process by producing acid and shifting the pH of the oral environment. Second is a better understanding of the host factors that make a person more susceptible to the caries process. This includes the genetic makeup of the person, the development of enamel, immune factors, behavioral factors, preference for sweet foods, and variations in salivary factors, among others. Third is the ability to accurately predict the risk for caries prior to the manifestations of the disease. This may be through devices that detect changes in enamel mineralization early, through salivary diagnostics or through other measures of host susceptibility. Fourth is the development of materials to arrest or reverse the caries process and to restore teeth to healthy function.

All four of these topics require that we expand our understanding of the caries disease process and set aside the old paradigms that have been with us for the past century. Progress in the fight against early childhood caries depends on us opening our minds to new possibilities and recognizing that even with good oral hygiene and dietary habits, children may still be susceptible to caries.

Identifying new cariogenic microflora

Mutans streptococci and *Lactobacillus* (*L. acidophilus* and *L. casei*) have been recognized for many years as the primary acid-producing bacteria in the oral cavity and, therefore, the most likely candidates for causing caries. These bacteria are easily cultured on appropriate growth medium and have been shown to have higher levels in people with caries and lower levels in healthy mouths. It is normal to find some level of these bacteria in the mouth. In a healthy mouth, there is a balance between the acid-producing bacteria and non-acid-producing bacteria, thus creating a normal "oral ecology" (Marsh, 1994). When something changes to shift this balance, disease is the result. If the caries process were this simple, we would have cured this disease long ago. Millions of dollars have been spent to develop a vaccine against *Streptococcus mutans* with the goal of curing caries. Although this seems like a logical target, the likelihood that caries will be cured by such a vaccine is remote. More than 600 different microbial species inhabit the oral cavity. Less than 50% of these species are accessible to conventional cultivation-based identification and characterization (Kolenbrander, 2000; Aas et al., 2008). The elimination of one acidogenic bacterial species would most likely facilitate the proliferation of others to fill the available niche.

Relatively new technologies are now available both to identify the presence of uncultivable bacterial species and to determine the quantity of these bacteria present in a saliva or plaque sample. These technologies are capable of detecting small quantities of bacteria and allow specific identification of bacterial species. One such technology involves the isolation of bacterial DNA from plaque or saliva followed by polymerase chain reaction (PCR) amplification of 16S RNA genes and then cloning of the PCR products.

Cloned fragments are then sequenced and the bacterial species identified by comparing the sequence to existing databases.

A number of studies using this technology have made interesting discoveries regarding the makeup of the oral microflora in caries-free and caries-active subjects. At least 50% of the bacterial species identified were uncultivable (Aas et al., 2008). In 10% of the subjects with severe caries, *S. mutans* was absent (Aas et al., 2008). There was a significant difference between the bacterial species isolated from cavitated lesions compared to those isolated from intact enamel in caries-free subjects (Becker et al., 2002; Kumar et al., 2006). In one study of microbial diversity in adults, the authors found an abundance of *Lactobacillus*, *Prevotella*, *Fusobacterium*, and *Bifidobacterium*, among others, but rarely detected *S. mutans* (Chhour et al., 2005).

These molecular studies have consistently supported the concept that there are specific bacterial species associated with health and disease and that the oral ecology changes over time as caries progresses. This is in keeping with the ecological plaque hypothesis described by Marsh (1994), which states that a shift in the balance of "normal" microflora, driven by local changes such as decreased pH and acid production, leads to caries and the subsequent demineralization of enamel. Most importantly, there is strong evidence that there are other acid-producing bacteria involved in the etiology of caries that are not cultivable.

Although this technology is extremely powerful and provides amazingly detailed information about the oral microflora, it is currently very expensive and limited to use in research laboratories. The value of this type of research is to gain a better understanding of the dynamics of oral microflora that result in either health or disease. Once more of the disease-associated microbes are identified, there are opportunities to develop diagnostic systems for early detection of changes in the oral ecology, detection of biomarkers for disease, and strategies for managing the disease process.

The identification of correlates between microbial species and caries experience will provide novel insights about previously unidentified cariogenic bacteria and ultimately a better understanding of the caries process.

Host factors and caries susceptibility

There is tremendous variability among people relative to how they look, how they think, and how they behave. Some of these characteristics can be attributed to their basic genetic makeup and some to their environment or upbringing. The question of which factor is stronger—nature or nurture— has long been debated. In reality, it is usually a combination of both.

It is well recognized that caries is a multifactorial disease that requires a host (with teeth), acid-producing microflora, carbohydrates, and time. These factors are moderated by the buffering capacity of the saliva and by the presence of fluoride, calcium, phosphorous, and other salivary components. Some of these factors are genetically determined, while others are more behavioral.

The genetics of caries susceptibility or resistance is an area that is ripe for investigation. Early animal studies and later family studies suggested that there was a significant genetic component to this disease. The most convincing studies compared monozygotic and dizygotic twins reared apart (Boraas et al., 1988; Conry et al., 1993). In these studies, the authors compared the decayed, missing, and filled tooth scores for each of the subjects and found that there was a statistically significant similarity between the monozygotic twin pairs compared to the dizygotic twin pairs. Their data suggest a genetic contribution to caries of 40%. More recent studies of the genetics of caries susceptibility confirm this finding but with varying levels of genetic contribution (Bretz et al., 2005; Slayton et al., 2005).

Because of the complex nature of the caries process, there are many potential candidate genes that could contribute to either susceptibility or resistance to caries. Candidates that have been evaluated to date include genes involved in enamel mineralization (Slayton et al., 2005; Deeley et al., 2008), salivary protein genes (Denny et al., 2006; Zakhary et al., 2007), antimicrobial peptides (Tao et al., 2005), and genes that contribute to host resistance to infection (Lehner et al., 1981).

Caries-risk prediction

Currently, the best predictor of caries is existing caries. Waiting until a disease occurs to be able to accurately predict the risk for the disease is less than ideal. Any efforts at prevention must occur before disease is present. Without knowing who is at risk, preventive efforts are provided more globally, resulting in inefficient use of resources. Our ultimate goal should be to identify risk at an individual level early and then provide targeted, intensive therapies to prevent those individuals from suffering the consequences of this disease.

For at least 30 years, the dental community has struggled to develop a caries-risk assessment tool with both high specificity and high sensitivity. This means that the tool is capable of accurately identifying children at risk for caries and not including those children who are not at risk. When risk is assigned at the group level, for example, saying that children from low-income families are at risk for caries, this does not have a high level of specificity or sensitivity. There are many individuals from low-income families who are caries free, and there are children from high-income families who do have caries. In order to develop effective preventive therapies, it is essential to identify risk on an individual level with both high sensitivity and specificity and to recognize that risk is a dynamic measure that needs to be reassessed on a regular basis. The tools that are currently available and discussed in Chapter 8 are helpful to identify the risk indicators and/or factors that contribute to an individual's risk. None have the ideal level of sensitivity or specificity to reliably identify individuals at high risk prior to disease manifestation.

What would the ideal caries-risk assessment tool look like? It would have to measure characteristics of the individual that are objective and repeatable and that do not rely on self-report. It would need to provide an assessment of the oral environment and a profile of the host genetics from which a probability of disease manifestation could be calculated. The oral environmental factors include the oral microflora, salivary pH, salivary flow and buffering capacity, composition of saliva, and anatomy of tooth surfaces. Host genetic factors include genes involved in the development and mineralization of enamel, genes that code for immune factors and for salivary components, among others.

Research is ongoing to identify the diverse components of the oral microflora. Since many of these microbes are not cultivable, they must be identified using molecular biology techniques. The presence of a particular microbe in high numbers does not necessarily imply causation of disease. Therefore, it will require comparisons of large numbers of subjects with and without caries, conducted over time in order to identify those bacteria that cause disease and those that are protective or that contribute to the normal oral ecology. Once the key microbes are identified, assays can be developed to detect them as part of routine well-child examinations.

For this type of assay to be practical in a clinical setting, it should be relatively inexpensive, available as a chair side test and ideally, be something practitioners can be reimbursed for. To get a glimpse of what a test like this might look like, we can turn to the field of bioengineering. By combining current advances in microelectronics with the need for inexpensive, portable diagnostic devices, researchers have developed a variety of tools that have been used in both developed and developing countries to diagnose and treat disease. The "lab on a chip" (LOC) is a miniaturized device with rapid analysis times and reduced reagent and sample volume requirements. It has been shown to be cost-effective and useful for point of care testing. Devices like this are capable of measuring pH, biomarkers, and other analytes. Christodoulides et al. (2007) used an LOC assay system to measure levels of C-reactive protein, interleukin-1β, and matrix metalloproteinase-8 in patients with periodontal disease and healthy controls. They compared the results to the gold standard ELISA and found that the LOC assay was comparable to the ELISA for two of the markers and superior in the detection of C-reactive protein. Devices such as this have potential for diagnosing disease or risk for disease once the relevant biomarkers are identified for a specific disease.

Saliva is increasingly becoming the diagnostic fluid of choice for a number of diseases. The benefits of this are that collection of saliva is noninvasive and straightforward; it does not require specialized training to collect and the detection devices are sensitive enough to detect very low levels of analytes. Since saliva is such an important component of oral health and disease, it is also advantageous to use this fluid for diagnostic purposes. In a recent keynote address, Dr David Wong predicted that "the use of saliva for disease diagnostics and normal health surveillance is about 5 years away." He was referring to the diagnosis of medical as well as oral diseases. Before this type of diagnostics is a reality for dental caries, it is necessary that we identify the relevant biomarkers for this disease (Segal and Wong, 2008).

One such biomarker has been identified by Dr Paul Denny at the University of Southern California. His laboratory is developing a test that measures salivary glycoprotein oligosaccharides and can be used to predict caries in children and adults (Denny et al., 2006). These are genetically determined salivary components that have been shown to have a strong association with caries experience. The predictive ability of this test in subjects who do not yet have the disease is yet to be determined.

Markers for caries risk or for caries activity may be used in the future to both predict the risk for caries and facilitate early preventive approaches or to monitor and manage the caries process once disease is present. A marker such as salivary glucotransferase B (GtfB) from *S. mutans* is one example of a marker that could be used to monitor the effectiveness of therapies intended to manage the disease process by reducing acidogenic microflora (Vacca Smith et al., 2007). In this study, the authors showed that levels of GtfB were strongly correlated with both the presence of caries in children and the number of caries lesions. Other biomarkers, whether related to host genetics or microbial genetics, are still to be identified.

Dental materials and disease management

Realistically, no matter how well we understand a disease and no matter how aggressive we are with our preventive protocols, there will always be individuals who get the disease anyway. This is especially true in a disease like dental caries, where there are dietary risk factors, environmental risk factors, and other behavioral factors that are out of our control. There will continue to be a need to manage this disease and to restore teeth that have been damaged by the acid produced by cariogenic bacteria.

Fluoride-releasing materials

Dental materials have traditionally been used to restore the function and/or esthetics of the dentition. They generally consist of alloys such as amalgam or gold or resins such as composites, compomers, resin-modified glass ionomers, and glass ionomers. Materials that contain and release fluoride may be viewed as both a restorative and a therapeutic restoration. In some studies, it has been shown that resin-modified glass ionomer materials used to restore interproximal lesions can provide a protective effect to the adjacent tooth (Donly et al., 1999). A therapeutic effect can also be seen by performing an indirect pulp cap when deep caries is present in vital teeth.

The key factor in this procedure is the sealing of the infected dentin from the oral environment to stop the progression of caries. This has been done effectively either with resin-modified glass ionomers or with calcium hydroxide (Marchii et al., 2006).

The atraumatic restorative technique, as described in Chapter 3, was initially developed for use in underdeveloped countries but has become more widely used in the United States in the past decade. In this country, it is frequently used to delay the progression of caries lesions until the child is old enough to cooperate in the traditional dental setting or while the child is waiting for treatment in the operating room under general anesthesia. In both of these cases, the goal is to arrest or delay the progression of caries and to "buy time" until the tooth can be restored definitively or it exfoliates naturally. In a time of scarce resources and more demands for services than can be met in a timely way, materials and techniques that will slow or arrest the progression of caries are essential.

Caries-arresting agents

Silver diamine fluoride (SDF) is a caries-arresting agent that has been shown to be effective without the removal of carious dentin and with annual application (Chu et al., 2002). It has been used for this purpose in China, Japan, and Cuba and in research studies in the United States (Moritani et al., 1970; Klein et al., 1999; Chu et al., 2002). In the clinical studies reported, SDF treatment resulted in a significant reduction in caries-active lesions when compared to controls. It was also found that annual applications of SDF was more effective than an every 3-month application of 5% sodium fluoride (Chu et al., 2002). In the in vitro study by Klein et al. (1999), SDF was similar in effectiveness to chlorhexidine (CHX) but less effective than silver nitrate ($AgNO_3$) and silver fluoride/stannous fluoride (AgF/SnF_2). Currently, SDF is not available commercially in the United States but can be used off-label as a desensitizing agent. Efforts are underway to make this product available for use in the United States (Peter Milgrom, personal communication).

Fluoride varnish (5% sodium fluoride) is approved for use in the United States as a desensitizing agent. It is used off-label to remineralize white spot lesions in enamel and to delay progression of cavities in enamel and dentin. A number of studies have also found it to be effective in arresting or preventing caries lesions (Chu et al., 2002; Marinho et al., 2003; Weintraub et al., 2006). Current protocols recommend application of fluoride varnish every 6 months. There are alternative protocols being tested in clinical trials that are currently underway. Some states permit medical professionals to apply fluoride varnish and to bill for this service at the time of a well-child examination. In children considered to be at high risk for caries and who have limited access to dental care, this is a valuable service and one that should be encouraged and expanded to other states.

Materials to inhibit bacterial adhesion

Management of biofilm formation is a serious problem in both medicine, dentistry, and industrial settings. The first step in biofilm formation is adhesion of bacteria to a surface, followed by colonization of multiple bacterial species, and establishment of a complex organization. Biofilms tend to be resistant to removal and disruption and can lead to infection. Antibiotics have had limited success in the elimination of biofilms once established. One approach that has shown promise is the use of antifouling agents to prevent or minimize bacterial adhesion. In a recent study, Vejborg and Klemm (2008) used an antiadhesive coating made from fish muscle α-tropomyosin to reduce biofilm formation on Foley catheters exposed to a range of urinary tract bacterial strains. They found that there was a dramatic and significant reduction in biofilm formation on treated catheters compared to untreated catheters. In some cases there was a 100-fold reduction in the biofilm (Vejborg and Klemm, 2008).

Hannig et al. (2007) investigated the ability of a nanocomposite coating material, applied to enamel or titanium surfaces, to inhibit biofilm formation when compared to uncoated control specimens. The specimens were attached to intraoral splints and worn by study subjects for a 24 h period prior to evaluation. They found both a significant reduction in biofilm formation and an enhanced ability to clean the surfaces that were coated versus those that were uncoated (Hannig et al., 2007).

Whether coatings such as these are applied professionally or at home via a paste or rinse, there is good evidence to suggest that this type of strategy will contribute to our ability to prevent and/or manage the caries disease process.

SUMMARY

Our goal, as oral health care professionals, is to provide our patients and their families with the education and tools to increase the probability that they will have the best oral health possible. This translates into identifying the risk for disease early so that we can prevent the manifestations of disease. When we do not succeed in this, we need to have effective tools to treat and manage the disease process. Research in medicine, biotechnology, and materials science has both direct and indirect applications in dentistry that are yet to be investigated.

Prevention and management of this devastating disease in children will be best accomplished by coordinating efforts with the many individuals and groups who are dedicated to the well-being of children. Many of these groups were discussed in this book and include nondental health care providers, community partners, families, teachers, public health workers, and researchers. With the dedication of all of these individuals, we can make a difference in the lives of our youngest citizens.

REFERENCES

Aas JA, Griffen AL, Dardis SR, Lee AM, Olsen I, Dewhirst FE, Leys EJ, and Paster BJ. 2008. Bacteria of dental caries in primary and permanent teeth in children and young adults. *J Clin Microbiol* 46(4):1407–17.

Becker MR, Paster BJ, Leys EJ, Moeschberger ML, Kenyon SG, Galvin JL, Boches SK, Dewhirst FE, and Griffen AL. 2002. Molecular analysis of bacterial species associated with childhood caries. *J Clin Microbiol* 40: 1001–9.

Boraas JC, Messer LB, and Till MJ. 1988. A genetic contribution to dental caries, occlusion and morphology as demonstrated by twins reared apart. *J Dent Res* 67:1150–55.

Bretz WA, Corby PM, Schork NJ, Robinson MT, Coelho M, Costa S, Melo Filho MR, Weyant RJ, and Hart TC. 2005. Longitudinal analysis of heritability for dental caries traits. *J Dent Res* 84(11):1047–51.

Chhour KL, Nadkarni MA, Byun R, Martin FE, Jacques NA, and Hunter N. 2005. Molecular analysis of microbial diversity in advanced caries. *J Clin Microbiol* 43:843–9.

Christodoulides N, Floriano PN, Miller CS, Ebersole JL, Mohanty S, Dharshan P, Griffin M, Lennart A, Ballard KL, King CP, Jr, Langub MC, Kryscio RJ, Thomas MV, and McDevitt JT. 2007. Lab-on-a-chip methods for point-of-care measurements of salivary biomarkers of periodontitis. *Ann N Y Acad Sci* 1098:411–28.

Chu CH, Lo EC, and Lin HC. 2002. Effectiveness of silver diamine fluoride and sodium fluoride varnish in arresting dentin caries in Chinese pre-school children. *J Dent Res* 81:767–70.

Conry JP, Messer LB, Boraas JC, Aeppli DP, and Bouchard TJ, Jr. 1993. Dental caries and treatment characteristics in human twins reared apart. *Arch Oral Biol* 38:937–43.

Deeley K, Letra A, Rose EK, Brandon CA, Resick JM, Marazita ML, and Vieira AR. 2008. Possible association of amelogenin to high caries experience in a Guatemalan-Mayan population. *Caries Res* 42(1):8–13.

Denny PC, Denny PA, Takashima J, Si Y, Navazesh M, and Galligan JM. 2006. A novel saliva test for caries risk assessment. *J Calif Dent Assoc* 34(4):287–90, 292–4.

Donly KJ, Segura A, Wefel JS, and Hogan MM. 1999. Evaluating the effects of fluoride-releasing dental materials on adjacent interproximal caries. *J Am Dent Assoc* 130:817–25.

Hannig M, Kriener L, Hoth-Hannig W, Becker-Willinger C, and Schmidt H. 2007. Influence of nanocomposite surface coating on biofilm formation in situ. *J Nanosci Nanotechnol* 7(12):4642–8.

Klein U, Kanellis MJ, and Drake D. 1999. Effects of four anticaries agents on lesion depth progression in an in vitro caries model. *Pediatr Dent* 21(3):176–80.

Kolenbrander PE. 2000. Oral microbial communities: Biofilms, interactions, and genetic systems. *Annu Rev Microbiol* 54:413–37.

Kumar PS, Leys EJ, Bryk JM, Martinez FJ, Moeschberger ML, and Griffen AL. 2006. Changes in periodontal health status are associated with bacterial community shifts as assessed by quantitative 16 S cloning and sequencing. *J Clin Microbiol* 44:3665–73.

Lehner T, Lamb JR, Welsh KL, and Batchelor RJ. 1981. Association between HLA-DR antigens and helper cell activity in the control of dental caries. *Nature* 292:770–72.

Marchii JJ, de Araujo FB, Froner AM, Straffon LH, and Nor JE. 2006. Indirect pulp capping in the primary dentition: A 4 year follow-up study. *J Clin Pediatr Dent* 31(2):68–71.

Marinho VC, Higgins JP, Logan S, and Sheiham A. 2003. Topical fluoride (toothpastes, mouthrinses, gels, or varnishes) for preventing dental caries in children and adolescents. Cochrane Database Systemic Review 4, CD002782.

Marsh PD. 1994. Microbial ecology of dental plaque and its significance in health and disease. *Adv Dent Res* 8:263–71.

Moritani Y, Doi M, Yao K, Yoshihara M, Miyazaki K, Ito M. 1970. Clinical evaluation of diamine silver fluoride (Saforide) in controlling caries of deciduous teeth [in Japanese]. *Rinsho Shika* 266:48–53.

Segal A and Wong DT. 2008. Salivary diagnostics: Enhancing disease detection and making medicine better. *Eur J Dent Educ* 12(Suppl 1):22–9.

Slayton RL, Cooper ME, and Marazita ML. 2005. Tuftelin, mutans streptococci, and dental caries susceptibility. *J Dent Res.* 84(8):711–4.

Tao R, Jurevic RJ, Coulton KK, Tsutsui MT, Roberts MC, Kimball JR, Wells N, Berndt J, and Dale BA. 2005. Salivary antimicrobial peptide expression and dental caries experience in children. *Antimicrob Agents Chemother* 49(9): 3883–8.

Vacca Smith AM, Scott-Anne KM, Whelehan MT, Berkowitz RJ, Feng C, and Bowen WH. 2007. Salivary glucosyltransferase B as a possible marker for caries activity. *Caries Res* 41(6):445–50.

Vejborg VM and Klemm P. 2008. Blocking of bacterial biofilm formation by a fish protein coating. *Appl Environ Microbiol* 74(11): 3551–8.

Weintraub JA, Ramos-Gomez F, and Jue B, Shain S, Hoover CI, Featherstone JD, and Gansky SA. 2006. Fluoride varnish efficacy in preventing early childhood caries. *J Dent Res* 85(2):172–6.

Zakhary GM, Clark RM, Bidichandani SI, Owen WL, Slayton RL, and Levine M. 2007. Acidic proline-rich protein Db and caries in young children. *J Dent Res* 86(12):1176–80.

Index